The Quality of Medical Care in the United States:

A Report on the Medicare Program

The Dartmouth Atlas of Health Care 1999

The Center for the Evaluative Clinical Sciences
Dartmouth Medical School

The views expressed in this publication are strictly those of the authors and do not necessarily represent official positions of the American Hospital Association.

Library of Congress Cataloging-in-Publication Data

Dartmouth Medical School. Center for the Evaluative Clinical Sciences.
     The Dartmouth Atlas of Health Care 1999 / The Center for the Evaluative Clinical
     Sciences, Dartmouth Medical School.

     ISBN 1-55648-257- 4
     1. Medical care—United States—Marketing—Maps. 2. Health facilities—United States—
Statistics. I. Title.

Catalog no. 044401

Printed in the USA

press™

The Dartmouth Atlas of Health Care in the United States

John E. Wennberg, M.D., M.P.H., *Principal Investigator and Series Editor*

Megan McAndrew Cooper, M.B.A., M.S., *Editor*

and other members of the Dartmouth Atlas of Health Care Working Group

John D. Birkmeyer, M.D.
Kristen K. Bronner, M.A.
Thomas A. Bubolz, Ph.D.
Diane E. Campbell, Ph.D.
Elliott S. Fisher, M.D., M.P.H.
Gerald T. O'Connor, Ph.D., D. Sc.
James F. Poage, Ph.D.
Sandra M. Sharp, S.M.
Jonathan S. Skinner, Ph.D.
Thérèse A. Stukel, Ph.D.
David E. Wennberg, M.D., M.P.H.

Atlas design and print production by

Jonathan Sa'adah and Elizabeth Adams
Intermedia Communications

*The research on which the Dartmouth Atlas of Health Care
is based was made possible by a grant from*

The Robert Wood Johnson Foundation

The Center for the Evaluative Clinical Sciences
Dartmouth Medical School
Hanover, New Hampshire 03756
(603) 650-1820
http://www.dartmouth.edu/~atlas/

Published by AHA Press, a division of Health Forum, Inc.

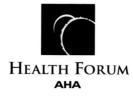

HEALTH FORUM
AHA

Chicago, Illinois

Table of Contents

Maps

Figures

Tables

Introduction and Overview

The Quality of Medical Care in the United States

The United States leads the world, by a substantial measure, in its monetary commitment to medical care. If, as we have long believed, *more* care is *better* care, then American medicine must surely be the best in the world. *But where is the "best" of American medicine?*

Previous editions of the Atlas have demonstrated conclusively that in American health care, geography is destiny. Both the amounts and kinds of care provided to residents of the United States are highly dependent on two factors: the capacity of the local health care system (which influences *how much* care is provided) and the practice style of local physicians (which determines *what kind* of care is provided). Variations in the intensity of use of hospitals, the striking differences in care at the end of life, and the nearly random patterns of elective surgery all raise questions about the outcomes and value of care — about quality. Is more in fact better? What is the value received for the money spent? What, as Joseph Juran asked, is the cost of poor quality?

These questions are receiving increasing public attention. The National Academy of Sciences convened the National Roundtable on Health Care Quality to assess the problem of quality of care. Reporting its findings in the American Journal of Medicine, the Roundtable concluded:

> "Serious and widespread quality problems exist throughout American medicine. These problems, which may be classified as underuse, overuse and misuse, occur in small and large communities alike, in all parts of the country and with approximately equal frequency in managed care and fee-for-service systems of care."

The Roundtable estimated that "very large numbers of Americans are harmed as a direct result" of poor quality care:

"Millions of Americans are not reached by proven effective interventions that can save lives and prevent disability. Perhaps an equal number suffer needlessly because they are exposed to the harms of unnecessary health services. Large numbers are injured because preventable complications are not averted."

The concern about quality is not restricted to experts or to those who speak on the part of patients or the American public. Ordinary citizens are concerned. The American Hospital Association's "Reality✓" investigation revealed that patients have significant problems with "The way the 'system' works (or fails to work), and the way decisions are made about their care." Patients interviewed for this study reported that they "see a confusing, expensive, unreliable and often impersonal dis-assembly of medical professionals and institutions." Moreover, patients expressed a strong concern over their own roles in making health care decisions.

Asked who should control decisions about health care in an "ideal world," AHA focus group participants answered that they, themselves, should call the shots, along with their doctors. Patients are more aware than they have been in the past about the variations and alternatives in treatments for many disorders, and they are more likely to question doctors about decisions regarding their treatment ... [a] senior citizen who had recently drawn up a living will with the help of her seniors' group commented, "I didn't know before that I could *refuse!* Now I know!"

These findings call into question the underlying assumption that more care is better care, and that access and cost are the most fundamental problems of the American health care system. Patients as well as health services researchers have begun to ask whether more really is better, and whether the "system" really is a system. Until we can answer those questions with any certainty, we will not be able to achieve real quality in American medical care.

Overview of the 1999 Atlas

In reaching its conclusions about the extent of the quality problem in American medicine, the Roundtable did not consider geographic variations. This edition of the Atlas considers what these variations imply about the quality of medical care in the United States.

■ Chapter One examines geographic variations in spending by the Medicare program for enrollees receiving fee-for-service care. There are substantial differences in the amount of money spent on Medicare enrollees, depending on where they live — and spending is independent of the price of care and overall population health.

■ Chapter Two examines the peculiar distribution and utilization of acute care hospital resources and the physician workforce. As in previous editions of the Atlas, there is overwhelming evidence that the "system" of care in the United States is not a system at all, but a largely unplanned and irrational sprawl of resources, undisciplined by the laws of supply and demand.

■ Chapter Three considers the relationship between the supply of resources in medical care markets and the ways in which those resources are used to treat medical conditions. The supply of acute care hospital beds has a substantial influence on rates of hospitalization for medical (non-surgical) conditions.

■ Chapter Four provides an assessment of the quality of ambulatory care provided to Medicare enrollees in fee-for-service medicine. The chapter demonstrates large scale underuse of preventive services that are known to reduce morbidity and mortality. Strangely, the use of these services is *not* related to the supply of resources, to measures of access to and continuity of care, or to overall spending levels. By contrast, higher hospitalization rates for "ambulatory care sensitive conditions" — conditions that many believe are useful indicators of the quality of ambulatory care — are related to greater hospital capacity, rather than to poor access to care or suboptimal use of primary care.

■ Chapter Five provides an interpretation of the significance of geographic variations with regard to the quality of surgical care. The variations are traced to three factors: the poor quality of clinical decision making (which results in patients getting treatments they don't want); the poor quality of the scientific basis for clinical practice (which results in unnecessary uncertainty about what the outcomes of care really are); and the poor quality of the skill with which surgical care is delivered (which results in unnecessary morbidity, mortality and costs).

■ Chapter Six examines whether Americans at the ends of their lives are receiving the care that they have said that they want. The dispiriting answer is that, all too often, they are not. The supply of resources and the practice patterns of physicians seem to play a more important role than patient preferences in determining the amount and type of care received at the end of life.

■ Chapter Seven provides a summary assessment of the quality of care in fee-for-service Medicare. It provides evidence of extensive underuse of services that are known to work and that patients want. The chapter also finds evidence of widespread overuse of certain surgical procedures, of acute care hospitalizations for medical conditions, and of intensive care and physicians' services during the last six months of life.

Will improving quality increase the cost of care? When value is considered in terms of the benefit gained per dollar spent, it is hard to find evidence that more resources are required to improve the quality of care in fee-for-service Medicare. There is, instead, evidence of large-scale waste and inefficiency in the delivery system; scarcity, where it exists, is the result of misallocation, not under-allocation. To improve overall quality, it will be necessary to improve the quality of clinical science, the quality of clinical decision making, and the quality of medical resource allocation.

The Geography of Health Care in the United States

Most of the tools used to measure and explore variation in this edition of the Atlas will be familiar to most readers. We have again based our measurements on the experience of populations — how health care is used by defined populations, rather than the physical location of health care resources. This methodology, which is generally known as small area analysis, is at the core of our work. Readers who are unfamiliar with the strategies of studying population-based rates of resource distribution and utilization are urged to read the Appendix on Methods. The endnote provides references for further reading.

The first task of the Atlas project, undertaken in 1993, was to establish the geographic boundaries of naturally occurring health care markets in the United States. Based on a study of where Medicare patients were hospitalized, 3,436 geographic hospital service areas were defined. The hospital service areas were then grouped into 306 hospital referral regions on the basis of where Medicare patients were hospitalized for major cardiovascular surgical procedures and neurosurgery, markers for regionalization. The Appendix on the Geography of Medical Care in the United States, which is reprinted in part from the first edition of the Atlas, describes how this was done, and contains a series of maps that detail each hospital referral region in the United States. One important finding was that most hospital service areas and hospital referral regions, as defined by where patients actually receive their care, correspond poorly to political configurations, such as counties, which have traditionally been used to measure health care resources and utilization.

About Rates in the Atlas

In order to make comparisons easier, all rates in the Atlas are expressed in terms that result in at least one digit to the left of the decimal point (e.g., 1.6 cardiologists per hundred thousand residents, 3.9 hospital beds per thousand residents). In order to achieve this result, different denominators were used in calculating rates.

The levels of supply of hospital beds and hospital full time equivalent employees are expressed as beds and employees per thousand residents of the hospital referral region, based on American Hospital Association and Medicare data.

Reimbursements are expressed as dollars per capita, or per resident of the hospital referral region, based on Medicare claims data and census calculations.

The numbers of physicians providing services to residents of hospital referral regions are expressed as physicians per hundred thousand residents, based on American Medical Association and American Osteopathic Association data and census calculations.

The numbers of surgical and diagnostic procedures performed are expressed as procedures per thousand Medicare enrollees in the hospital referral region, or as procedures per thousand male or female Medicare enrollees in the region (for procedures like prostatectomy or mastectomy that apply only to one sex) based on Medicare claims data.

Patient day rates are expressed as total inpatient days per thousand Medicare enrollees.

Making Fair Comparisons between Regions

Some areas of the country have greater needs for health care services and resources than others; for example, in some communities in Florida, as many as 60% of residents are over 65. Other parts of the country — including some with large college populations, or ski resorts — have much larger proportions of younger people. To ensure fair comparisons between areas, all rates in the Atlas have been adjusted to remove the differences that might be due to the different age and sex composition of local populations. This adjustment avoids identifying some areas as having high rates of utilization simply because of their larger proportions of elderly residents. When data were available, rates have also been adjusted for differences in race. (See the Appendix on Methods.)

This edition of the Atlas provides an important new method for adjusting for differences in illness based on a community health index. The index is used to adjust for differences in mortality and for the incidence of certain diseases, such as coronary artery disease and stroke.

Some areas, such as major urban centers, have higher costs of living than others. Such areas are likely to have high health care expenditures because the costs of personnel, real estate, and supplies are higher, and not necessarily because they are providing more services. Adjusting for such variation provides a more comparable measure of differences in real health care spending that is not simply due to differences in costs of living among areas. Medicare reimbursement rates were adjusted to take into account the differences between hospital service areas in costs of living.

The methods used to adjust for age, sex, race, illness and price of medical care are detailed in the Appendix on Methods.

About the Dartmouth Atlas on CD-ROM

A sophisticated CD-ROM data viewer has been developed which makes it possible to query, manipulate, and display the Dartmouth Atlas data base using point-and-click techniques. The viewer contains both the hospital referral region and hospital service area levels of data used to create the Dartmouth Atlas. For more information about the CD-ROM, contact AHA Order Services at 1-800-242-2626.

Communicating With Us About the Atlas

Our Atlas Home Page on the World Wide Web contains Atlas information, including a summary of Dartmouth-related research and electronic copies of some hard-to-find references. Please send us your comments on the Atlas, particularly suggestions on how to improve it in the future.

We are at http://www.dartmouth.edu/~atlas.

Variations in Medicare Spending

Variations In Medicare Spending

In 1996, most Americans over the age of 65 were enrolled in the Medicare program. Most received their care from "traditional" Medicare — that is, from providers who charged on a fee-for-service basis, either as independent practitioners or as members of health maintenance organizations that were not capitated. In 1996, according to Health Care Financing Administration records, $138.3 billion — over 87.8% of Medicare outlays for people over age 65 who were enrolled in both Part A and Part B of the Medicare program — was reimbursed on a fee-for-service basis.

This chapter examines the large differences in Medicare reimbursements among hospital referral regions, in total and by program component (reimbursements for inpatient care, professional and laboratory services, and other components). In each sector, and in total, there were substantial variations in Medicare payments for enrollees' care.

■ Reimbursements per capita varied by a factor of 2.9.
■ Reimbursements per capita for acute hospital care varied by a factor of 2.4.
■ Reimbursements per capita for professional and laboratory services varied by a factor of 4.2.
■ Reimbursements per capita for home health services by a factor of 38.1.

The differences in Medicare spending were not explained by local differences in population age, sex, race, illness or prices. In fact, adjustment for these factors has almost no effect on the range of variation in Medicare spending.

Another hypothesis is that some areas use fewer acute care hospital services because they have substituted other services, such as outpatient care, hospice care, or home health services, for costly inpatient care. There is very little evidence of such substitution, and in fact the opposite is often the case: regions with higher reimbursements for acute care hospital services in 1996 tended also to have higher reimbursements for hospital-based outpatient care, as well as higher reimbursements for physicians' services and for home health services.

Medicare Reimbursements for Noncapitated Medicare

In 1996, Medicare payments for services reimbursed on a fee-for-service basis (including non-risk bearing health maintenance organizations) averaged $4,993 per enrollee. This represented an increase of slightly more than 4% over the average reimbursement in 1995 ($4,790 per enrollee). Per enrollee reimbursements varied remarkably among hospital referral regions, even after adjustment for differences in population age, sex, race, and illness factors, and for differences in regional prices. Reimbursements were almost three times higher among residents of the McAllen, Texas hospital referral region ($9,033) than among residents of the Lynchburg, Virginia hospital referral region ($3,074).

Among the hospital referral regions with the highest per capita Medicare reimbursements for all services, five were in Louisiana and four were in Texas. Reimbursements were also high among residents of the Miami hospital referral region ($7,783).

Among the large hospital referral regions with lower than average price adjusted Medicare reimbursements per capita were Appleton, Wisconsin ($3,404); Lafayette, Indiana ($3,467); Eugene, Oregon ($3,506); Honolulu ($3,526); and San Luis Obispo, California ($3,553).

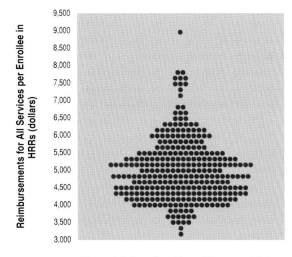

Figure 1.1. Age, Sex, Race, Illness and Price Adjusted Reimbursements for Noncapitated Medicare Among Hospital Referral Regions (1996)

Per enrollee Medicare reimbursements for all services varied by a factor of three, from about $3,000 to more than $9,000. Each point represents one of the 306 hospital referral regions in the United States.

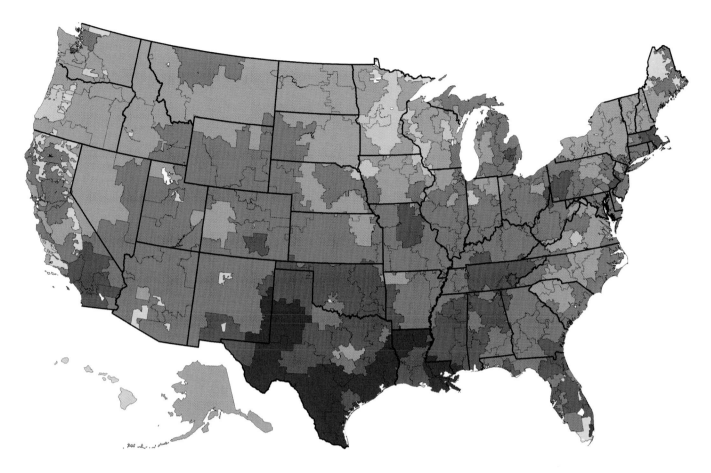

Map 1.1. Age, Sex, Race, Illness and Price Adjusted Reimbursements for Noncapitated Medicare (1996)

Payments by the Medicare program were generally higher in the South and Midwest than in the North and West. Total reimbursements for all services were substantially higher than the national average in several Northern cities and in parts of Texas and Louisiana.

Ratio of Rates of Price Adjusted Reimbursements for Noncapitated Medicare to the U.S. Average

by Hospital Referral Region (1996)

■ 1.30 to   1.81   (17)
■ 1.10 to < 1.30   (54)
■ 0.90 to < 1.10   (142)
■ 0.75 to < 0.90   (81)
□ 0.61 to < 0.75   (12)
□ Not Populated

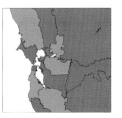

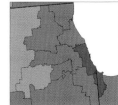

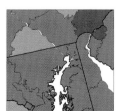

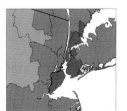

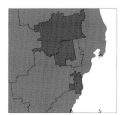

San Francisco   **Chicago**   **New York**   **Washington-Baltimore**   **Detroit**

Medicare Reimbursements for Inpatient Hospital Services

In 1996, Medicare reimbursements to hospitals for acute, short-stay care paid for on a fee-for-service basis totaled $67.8 billion. The average per enrollee reimbursement for inpatient services was $2,450, an increase of about 7.5% from 1995. These payments represented about 50% of the Medicare program's total outlays for traditional Medicare. Price adjusted reimbursements to hospitals per Medicare enrollee were almost two and one-half times higher in the highest rate hospital referral region than in the region with the lowest rate.

Among the hospital referral regions with the highest rates of per enrollee reimbursements for inpatient hospital care were the Bronx, New York ($3,780); McAllen, Texas ($3,727); Houma, Louisiana ($3,648); Manhattan ($3,612); Monroe, Louisiana ($3,516); and Shreveport, Louisiana ($3,429).

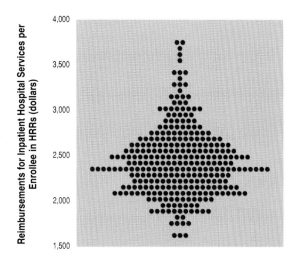

Hospital referral regions with lower than average per enrollee payments for inpatient hospital care included Lafayette, Indiana ($1,583); San Luis Obispo, California ($1,612); Lynchburg, Virginia ($1,625); Appleton, Wisconsin ($1,719); and Olympia, Washington ($1,743).

Figure 1.2. Age, Sex, Race, Price and Illness Adjusted Medicare Reimbursements for Inpatient Hospital Services Among Hospital Referral Regions (1996)

Per enrollee Medicare reimbursements for acute care hospital services varied by a factor of more than 2.3, from less than $1,600 to almost $3,800. Each point represents one of the 306 hospital referral regions in the United States.

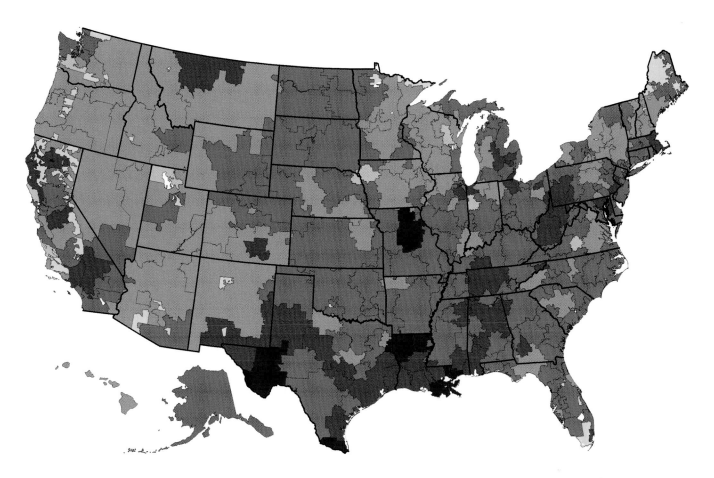

Map 1.2. Age, Sex, Race, Price and Illness Adjusted Medicare Reimbursements for Inpatient Hospital Services (1996)

Rates of reimbursements for inpatient hospital care were generally lower in the Western and Mountain states than elsewhere, with the exception of California, and generally higher in the South and East, with the exception of parts of Texas and the Mid-South. Contiguous regions in many cases had widely different levels of spending on inpatient care.

Ratio of Rates of Price Adjusted Reimbursements for Inpatient Hospital Services to the U.S. Average

by Hospital Referral Region (1996)

- 1.30 to   1.55   (13)
- 1.10 to < 1.30   (45)
- 0.90 to < 1.10   (159)
- 0.75 to < 0.90   (81)
- 0.64 to < 0.75   (8)
- Not Populated

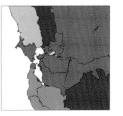

San Francisco

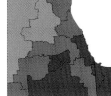

Chicago

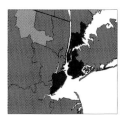

New York

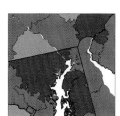

Washington-Baltimore

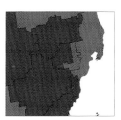

Detroit

Medicare Reimbursements for Professional and Laboratory Services

Reimbursements for professional services include payments to surgeons and medical doctors for activities such as office consultations, vaccinations, and open heart surgery; among the most common laboratory services are biopsy evaluations and blood tests. In 1996, reimbursements for professional and laboratory services paid for on a fee-for-service basis totaled $28.1 billion. The average per enrollee reimbursement was $1,015, an increase of about 1.3% over 1995. These payments represented 20.3% of Medicare outlays for traditional (noncapitated) Medicare.

Among the seven hospital referral regions with the highest price adjusted reimbursements for professional and laboratory services, four were in Florida, and three were in California. They were Miami ($1,990); Fort Lauderdale, Florida ($1,696); Los Angeles ($1,534); Palm Springs-Rancho Mirage, California ($1,503); Hudson, Florida ($1,463); Orange County, California ($1,450); and Clearwater, Florida ($1,421).

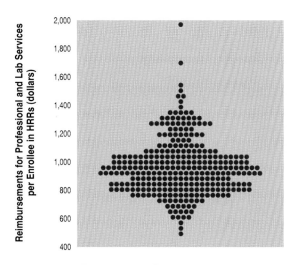

Hospital referral regions with lower than average per enrollee reimbursements included Grand Junction, Colorado ($474); Dubuque, Iowa ($547); Duluth, Minnesota ($580); Ogden, Utah ($599); Lafayette, Indiana ($606); and Lebanon, New Hampshire ($619).

Figure 1.3. Age, Sex, Race, Price and Illness Adjusted Part B Medicare Reimbursements for Professional and Laboratory Services Among Hospital Referral Regions (1996)
Reimbursements for professional and laboratory services varied by a factor of more than four, from less than $500 per Medicare enrollee to almost $2,000. Each point represents one of the 306 hospital referral regions in the United States.

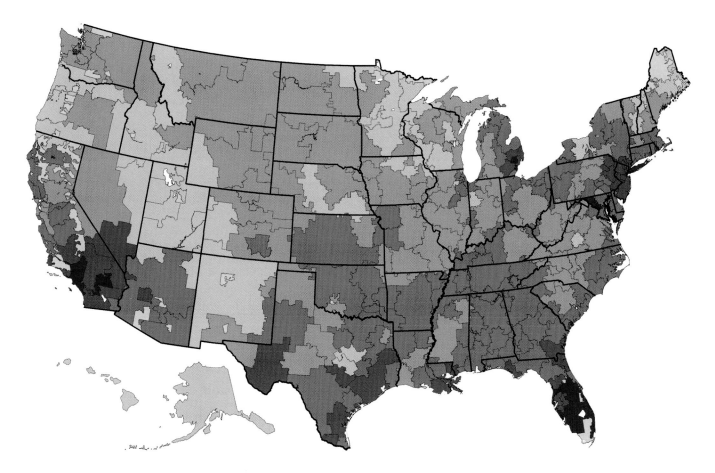

Map 1.3. Age, Sex, Race, Price and Illness Adjusted Part B Reimbursements for Professional and Laboratory Services (1996)

Reimbursements for professional and laboratory services followed essentially the same pattern as reimbursements for inpatient hospital care; rates were generally higher in the East and South than in the West and Northwest. Regions in California, Florida, and the New York metropolitan area had some of the highest rates.

Ratio of Rates of Price Adjusted Reimbursements for Professional and Laboratory Services to the U.S. Average

by Hospital Referral Region (1996)

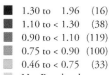

- 1.30 to   1.96   (16)
- 1.10 to < 1.30   (38)
- 0.90 to < 1.10   (119)
- 0.75 to < 0.90   (100)
- 0.46 to < 0.75   (33)
- Not Populated

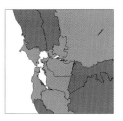

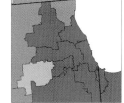

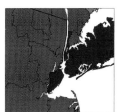

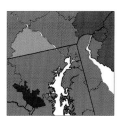

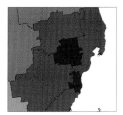

San Francisco   **Chicago**   **New York**   **Washington-Baltimore**   **Detroit**

Medicare Reimbursements for Outpatient Services

In 1996, Medicare reimbursements for the use of outpatient services paid for on a fee-for-service basis totaled $12.3 billion. The average per enrollee reimbursement was $444, an increase of about 12% over 1995 ($396). These reimbursements represented 8.9% of total outlays for traditional (noncapitated) Medicare. Price adjusted reimbursements for residents of the Miami hospital referral region ($795) were 3.4 times higher than for residents of the Las Vegas hospital referral region ($237).

Among the hospital referral regions with the highest price adjusted Medicare reimbursements for outpatient services per enrollee were Minot, North Dakota ($785); San Angelo, Texas ($739); Iowa City, Iowa ($726); Columbia, Missouri ($712); and Houma, Louisiana ($707).

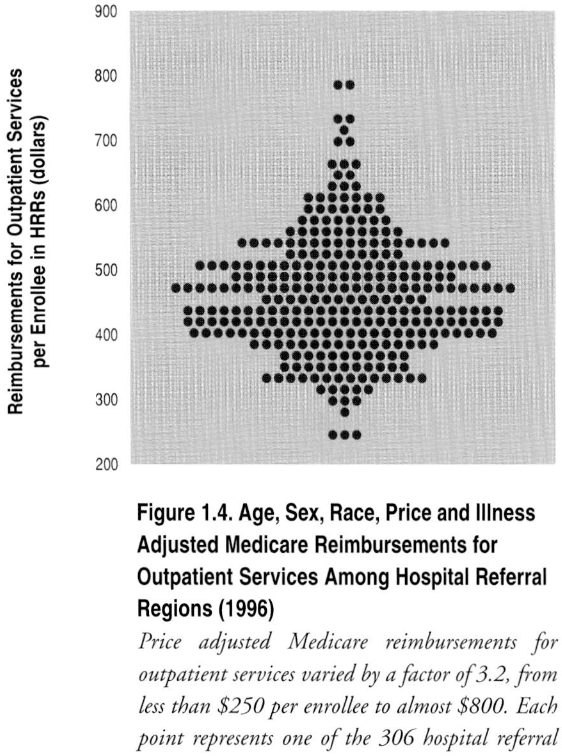

Among the hospital referral regions with lower than average per enrollee reimbursements for outpatient services were Sun City, Arizona ($240); Mesa, Arizona ($249); Montgomery, Alabama ($282); San Luis Obispo, California ($298); New Brunswick, New Jersey ($299); and Winchester, Virginia ($304).

Figure 1.4. Age, Sex, Race, Price and Illness Adjusted Medicare Reimbursements for Outpatient Services Among Hospital Referral Regions (1996)

Price adjusted Medicare reimbursements for outpatient services varied by a factor of 3.2, from less than $250 per enrollee to almost $800. Each point represents one of the 306 hospital referral regions in the United States.

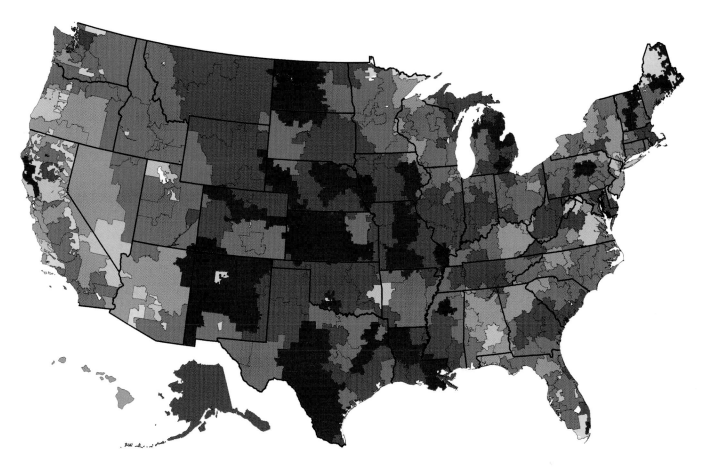

Map 1.4. Age, Sex, Race, Price and Illness Adjusted Medicare Reimbursements for Outpatient Services (1996)

In general, reimbursements for outpatient services were higher in the Midwest and West than on either coast. Hospital referral regions in the lowest quintile of outpatient reimbursements were widely scattered and often contiguous with areas in the highest quintile of spending.

Ratio of Rates of Price Adjusted Reimbursements for Outpatient Services to the U.S. Average

by Hospital Referral Region (1996)

- 1.30 to 1.80 (34)
- 1.10 to < 1.30 (77)
- 0.90 to < 1.10 (124)
- 0.75 to < 0.90 (52)
- 0.53 to < 0.75 (19)
- Not Populated

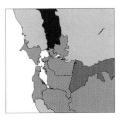

San Francisco

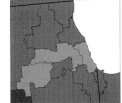

Chicago

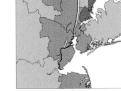

New York

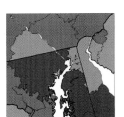

Washington-Baltimore

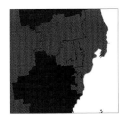

Detroit

Medicare Reimbursements for Home Health Services

In 1996, Medicare reimbursements for home health care services paid for on a fee-for-service basis totaled $14.7 billion. The average per enrollee reimbursement was $532, a 7.5% increase over the 1995 average of $495. These reimbursements represented 10.7% of noncapitated Medicare program outlays. Variations in the levels of Medicare reimbursements for home health care services were extreme; the average age, sex, race, illness and price adjusted reimbursement in McAllen, Texas ($3,090) was 38 times higher than the average reimbursement in Appleton, Wisconsin ($81).

Among the hospital referral regions with the highest Medicare reimbursements for home health services per enrollee were Baton Rouge, Louisiana ($2,404); Harlingen, Texas ($2,212); Beaumont, Texas ($1,973); Corpus Christi, Texas ($1,967); and Monroe, Louisiana ($1,794).

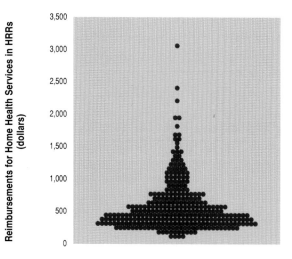

Among the hospital referral regions with lower than average per enrollee rates of reimbursement for home health services were Rochester, Minnesota ($115); Cedar Rapids, Iowa ($126); Lynchburg, Virginia ($143); Minot, North Dakota ($156); and Sioux Falls, South Dakota ($174).

Figure 1.5. Age, Sex, Race, Price and Illness Adjusted Medicare Reimbursements for Home Health Services Among Hospital Referral Regions (1996)

Price adjusted Medicare reimbursements for home health care varied by a factor of 38, from $81 per enrollee to more than $3,000. Each point represents one of the 306 hospital referral regions in the United States.

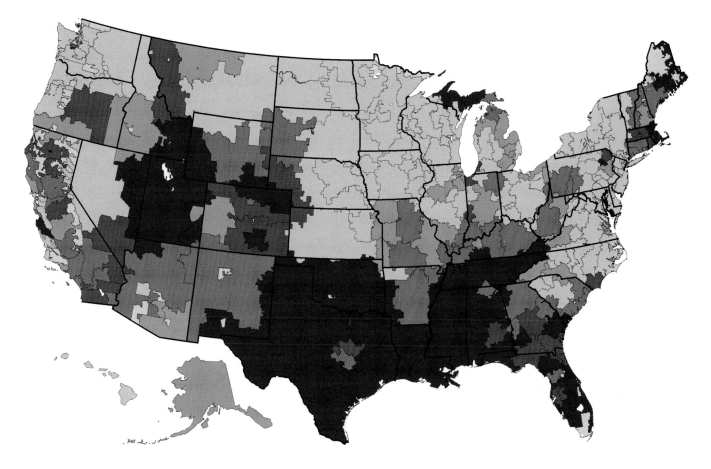

Map 1.5. Age, Sex, Race, Price and Illness Adjusted Medicare Reimbursements for Home Health Services (1996)

Home health services reimbursements were generally higher in Texas, Louisiana, Mississippi, Alabama, Utah and Tennessee than elsewhere. Some states had hospital referral regions in both the highest and lowest quintiles of spending; only a few, including North Dakota, Minnesota, Wisconsin and New York, were uniformly low in reimbursements.

Ratio of Rates of Price Adjusted Reimbursements for Home Health Care Services to the U.S. Average
by Hospital Referral Region (1996)

- 1.30 to 5.81   (78)
- 1.10 to < 1.30   (26)
- 0.90 to < 1.10   (43)
- 0.75 to < 0.90   (39)
- 0.15 to < 0.75   (120)
- Not Populated

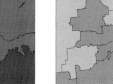
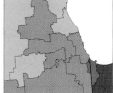
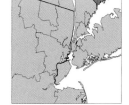
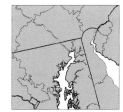
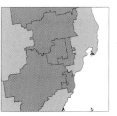

San Francisco   **Chicago**   **New York**   **Washington-Baltimore**   **Detroit**

Differences in Population Health and Regional Differences in Prices Do Not Explain Variations in Medicare Spending

Little of the variation in spending is explained by regional differences in population health; crude rates of spending do not differ substantially from rates adjusted for differences in population illness rates. Spending is simply higher in some areas than in others, for reasons that have little to do with need, or "demand," for care.

Similarly, little of the variation is explained by regional differences in prices. Adjustment for regional differences in the costs of delivering care have only a modest effect on the patterns of variation.

Figure 1.6 demonstrates the effect of adjustment for differences in illness and price on variations in Medicare spending. The left-hand column shows the distribution of unadjusted spending per enrollee (obtained by dividing total Medicare spending in each region by the number of enrollees living in the region). Average per enrollee reimbursements ranged from less than $3,000 to more than $8,500. The second

Figure 1.6. Unadjusted, Adjusted, and Illness Predicted Medicare Spending Among Hospital Referral Regions (1996)

The distribution on the left shows the range of Medicare spending without any statistical adjustments for population or price differences. Proceeding from left to right, the next distribution shows the range of variation after adjustment for population characteristics — differences in population age, sex, race, and illness factors. The third distribution shows the effect of adding adjustments for differences in regional prices — it is the age, sex, race, illness and price adjusted distribution in Figure 1.1. The rightmost distribution is the expected range of variation, if spending in fact reflected a demand for care based on population needs.

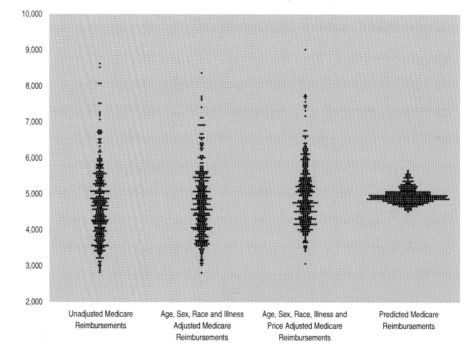

Unadjusted Medicare Reimbursements	Age, Sex, Race and Illness Adjusted Medicare Reimbursements

	Unadjusted Medicare Reimbursements	Age, Sex, Race and Illness Adjusted Medicare Reimbursements	Age, Sex, Race, Illness and Price Adjusted Medicare Reimbursements	Predicted Medicare Reimbursements
Index of Variation				
Coefficient of variation	0.218	0.199	0.178	0.042
Range of Variation				
Extremal ratio (highest to lowest rate)	3.04	2.99	2.94	1.26
Interquartile ratio (75th to 25th percentile rate)	1.34	1.31	1.26	1.05
Number of Regions with High and Low Rates				
Rates more than 25% below the national average	56	46	12	0
Rates 30% or more above the national average	19	17	17	0

Table 1.1. Measures of Variations in Medicare Spending (Part A and Part B) by Strategies for Adjustment (1996)

column shows the distribution of reimbursements after adjustment for differences in population age, sex, race and health status (including mortality rates and the incidence of acute myocardial infarction, stroke, certain cancers, and hip fractures). Adjustment for these factors reduces the coefficient of varation about 9%, from .218 to .119. The extremal range of variation remains about three-fold (Table 1.1). The third column shows the range of per capita Medicare spending after adjustment for age, sex, race, illness and price. Adding the adjustment for regional variations in price reduces the coefficient of variation to .178 (which is about an 18% reduction in variation compared to the unadjusted spending rate). The extremal ratio decreases slightly, to 2.9, and the number of regions with rates 25% less than the national average decreases from 56 to 12. Age, sex, race, illness and price adjustment has little effect on the number of regions with Medicare spending rates 30% or more above the national average.

Another way to look at the problem of variation in Medicare spending is to ask what we might expect the distribution of spending to look like, if variations in population health and prices drove regional spending for health care services. The rightmost column in Figure 1.6 shows the predicted range of variation, if spending were based on patient need differences among regions. The total expected variation in Medicare spending is much smaller than the actual variation. The extremal range is 1.26; the coeffecient of variation is .042, only about 20% that of actual (unadjusted) spending. If spending were determined by illness, only nine regions would have spending rates more than 10% above or below the national average. No regions would have spending less than 25% below or 30% above the national average.

Map 1.6a shows the unadjusted pattern of per capita Medicare spending for all services in 1996. In 56 of the 306 hospital referral regions in the United States, Medicare spending was at least 25% below the national average. In 19 regions, spending was more than 30% above the national average. In the highest-rate region, spending was 1.3 times higher than spending in the lowest-rate region. Map 1.6b shows the predicted distribution of spending rates based on differences in demographic characteristics (population age, sex, race, and illness) which would drive demand for care. Predicted rates vary much less than the actual rates; in the predicted distribution, no areas are more than 25% below the national average, and no areas are more than 30% above it.

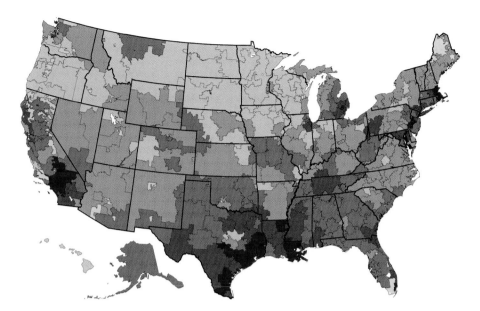
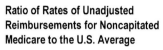
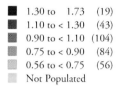

Ratio of Rates of Unadjusted Reimbursements for Noncapitated Medicare to the U.S. Average

by Hospital Referral Region (1996)

- 1.30 to   1.73   (19)
- 1.10 to < 1.30   (43)
- 0.90 to < 1.10 (104)
- 0.75 to < 0.90   (84)
- 0.56 to < 0.75   (56)
- Not Populated

Map 1.6a. Unadjusted Medicare Spending (1996)

There are clear regional patterns of unadjusted Medicare spending; the South, parts of the East Coast, Texas, and Southern California had substantially higher spending levels than the Upper Midwest, Montana, and Oregon.

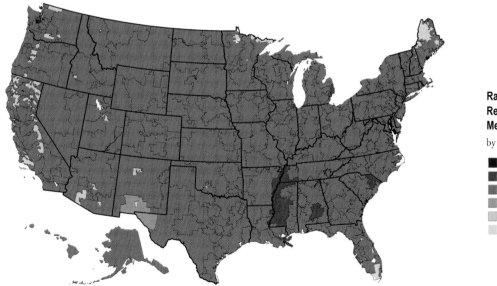
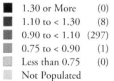

Ratio of Rates of Predicted Reimbursements for Noncapitated Medicare to the U.S. Average

by Hospital Referral Region (1996)

- 1.30 or More   (0)
- 1.10 to < 1.30   (8)
- 0.90 to < 1.10 (297)
- 0.75 to < 0.90   (1)
- Less than 0.75   (0)
- Not Populated

Map 1.6b. Age, Sex, Race, and Illness Predicted Spending (1996)

Predicted rates of spending predicted by actual population demand for care based on health needs related to age, sex, race and illness rates are far less variable than actual spending. Only nine hospital referral regions would be predicted to have spending more than 10% above or below the national average; no regions would be predicted to have spending less than 25% below or 30% above the national average.

Are There Tradeoffs Between Sectors of Care?

It has often been proposed that overall expenditures for health care could be reduced by substituting less costly care, such as outpatient services and home health care, for more costly inpatient hospital care. It has also been suggested that reimbursements for physicians' services might be lower in regions with greater use of home health services. It has also been theorized that regions with relatively low per capita investment in physicians' services have higher costs for hospital care. The documented patterns of variation in reimbursements for Medicare services provide no evidence that such substitutions are occurring.

Greater levels of expenditures for outpatient services were not associated with lower levels of expenditures for inpatient services. In fact, the opposite is the case: there was a slight positive correlation (R^2 = .12) between higher levels of reimbursement for outpatient and higher reimbursements for acute hospital care (Figure 1.7).

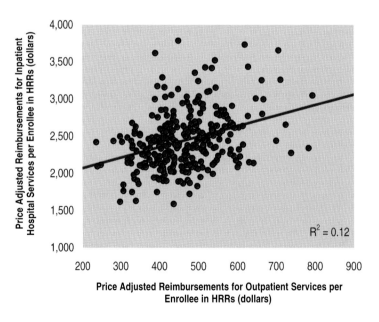

Figure 1.7. The Association Between Price Adjusted Medicare Reimbursements for Outpatient and Inpatient Hospital Services (1996)
There was a slight correlation between inpatient and outpatient reimbursements. Regions with higher reimbursements for outpatient care tended also to have higher inpatient reimbursements (R^2 = .12).

A number of regions that were in the top 20% of spending for outpatient services were also in the top quintile for spending on inpatient care; examples include Columbia, Missouri; McAllen, Texas; Shreveport, Louisiana; and Miami.

Similarly, several regions in the lowest 20% of reimbursements for inpatient care were also in the lowest 20% for outpatient care. These included Honolulu; Eugene, Oregon; Ogden, Utah; Lynchburg, Virginia; and San Luis Obispo, California.

There was no evidence of tradeoffs between other alternatives to acute hospital care and inpatient care. Inverse correlations would indicate that out-of-hospital services were providing a substitute for inpatient care, but in fact there was a positive correlation between the level of reimbursement for acute hospital care and payments for home health care ($R^2 = .24$), and there was no correlation between acute care expenditures and payments for hospice care ($R^2 = .00$), or long-stay care ($R^2 = .01$).

Greater reimbursements for home health agency services were not associated with lower physician reimbursements. There was a very weak positive correlation ($R^2 = .05$), indicating that the use of home health services did not result in less use of physicians' services.

Regions with higher reimbursements for physicians' services tended also to have higher reimbursements for acute hospital care. Figure 1.8 illustrates that there is a modest positive correlation between price adjusted Medicare reimbursements for inpatient hospital services and price adjusted reimbursements for professional and laboratory services (R^2 = .19).

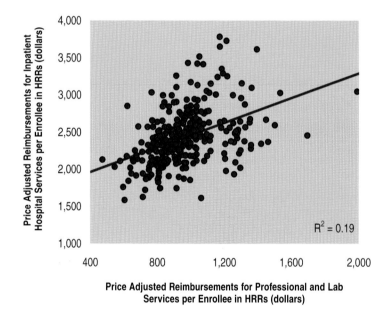

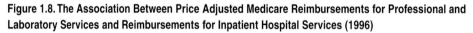

Figure 1.8. The Association Between Price Adjusted Medicare Reimbursements for Professional and Laboratory Services and Reimbursements for Inpatient Hospital Services (1996)

Communities with greater per enrollee outlays for short-term hospital care tended also to have higher reimbursements for professional and laboratory services (R^2 = .19).

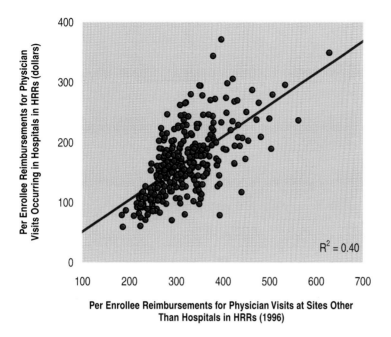

Figure 1.9. The Association Between Price Adjusted Medicare Part B Reimbursements for Physician Visits Provided in the Inpatient Setting and Elsewhere (1996)

There was a relationship between Part B outpatient visits and Part B reimbursements for inpatient physician visits ($R^2 = .40$).

Regions with higher Medicare Part B reimbursements for inpatient physician visits tended also to have higher reimbursements for physician visits provided elsewhere (Figure 1.9). Part B reimbursements per Medicare enrollee for visits occurring in the hospital varied more than five-fold among the 306 hospital referral regions; reimbursements for care provided at other sites also varied more than three-fold. There was a fairly strong correlation between Medicare Part B reimbursements for inpatient visits and care provided elsewhere in 1996 ($R^2 = .40$), indicating that outpatient visits were not effectively being used as a substitute for inpatient visits or as a way of keeping enrollees out of the hospital.

Medicare Enrollment in Capitated Managed Care Plans

Since the early 1970s, Medicare beneficiaries have been offered the option of joining risk bearing, or capitated, health maintenance organizations. Under the capitation plan, the federal government pays health maintenance organizations a fixed annual amount per enrollee. In exchange, the health maintenance organization must provide all required services. If the total costs of care exceed the amount the government pays, then the health maintenance organization must absorb the loss; if they are less, then the health maintenance organization may retain the difference.

In 1996, about 3.4 million, or 10.7%, of all Medicare enrollees were covered by risk bearing health maintenance organizations, an approximate doubling since 1993, when 1.6 million enrollees, or about 5.2%, had such coverage. The distribution of enrollment in managed care remained geographically uneven. In general, enrollment in health maintenance organizations was higher on the West Coast, the Midwest, and Florida than elsewhere.

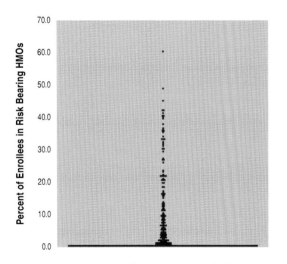

Figure 1.10. Medicare Enrollment in Managed Care Plans (1996)

Enrollment in managed care ranged from less than 1% to 60%. Each point represents one of the 306 hospital referral regions in the United States.

Medicare residents of the San Bernardino, California hospital referral region, where 60.5% of enrollees were in risk bearing health maintenance organizations, had the highest rate of such coverage. Other hospital referral regions where enrollment in health maintenance organizations was higher than the national average included San Diego, California (48.7%); Orange County, California (45.0%); Mesa, Arizona (42.2%); and Tucson, Arizona (42.1%).

In 1993, more than 60% of Medicare enrollees lived in hospital referral regions where fewer than 1% of beneficiaries were enrolled in risk bearing health maintenance organizations. In 1996, the proportion was only 32.6%.

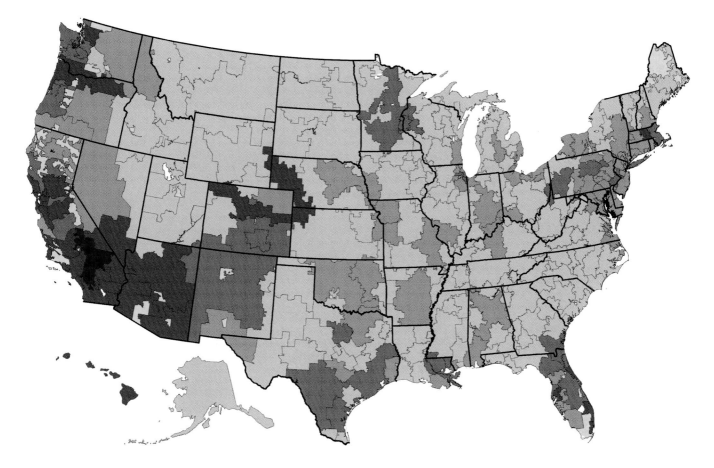

Map 1.7. Medicare Enrollment in Managed Care Plans (1996)

In some hospital referral regions, more than 45% of the Medicare population were members of risk bearing health maintenance organizations (dark green). Enrollment in managed care was more common in California, Arizona, New Mexico, Colorado, Florida, the Northeast, Minneapolis, and the Northwest than elsewhere.

Percent of Medicare Beneficiaries Enrolled in Risk Bearing Health Maintenance Organizations

by Hospital Referral Region (1996)

- ■ 50 or More   (1)
- ■ 25 to < 50   (30)
- ■ 10 to < 25   (40)
- ■ 1 to < 10   (78)
- ☐ Less than 1 (157)
- ☐ Not Populated

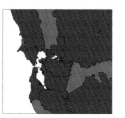

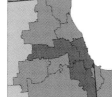

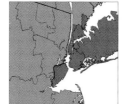

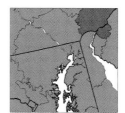

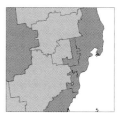

San Francisco   **Chicago**   **New York**   **Washington-Baltimore**   **Detroit**

Chapter One Table   Reimbursements are expressed in rates per person, and are adjusted for regional differences in age, sex, race, and prices. Medicare data exclude enrollees who were members of risk bearing health maintenance organizations.

Specific codes used to define the numerator for rates, and methods of age, sex, race and price adjustment are included in the Appendix on Methods.

CHAPTER ONE TABLE

Medicare Reimbursements by Hospital Referral Regions (1996)

Hospital Referral Region	Medicare Enrollees (1996)	Price Adj; Reimb. for Noncapitated Medicare per Enrollee (1996)	Price Adj; Medicare Reimb. for Inpatient Hospital Services per Enrollee (1996)	Price Adj; Medicare Reimb. for Professional and Lab. Services per Enrollee (1996)	Price Adj; Medicare Reimb. for Outpatient Services per Enrollee (1996)	Price Adj; Medicare Reimb. for Home Health Care Services per Enrollee (1996)	Price Adj; Medicare Reimb. for Physician Visits in the Inpatient Setting per Enrollee (1996)	Price Adj; Medicare Reimb. for Physician Visits at Sites Other than Hospitals per Enrollee (1996)	Percent of Medicare Population Enrolled in Health Maintenance Organizations (1996)
Alabama									
Birmingham	260,180	5,597	2,749	1,079	397	785	189	314	3.6
Dothan	44,540	5,075	2,255	921	389	888	160	312	0.1
Huntsville	53,840	4,967	2,500	1,010	431	525	178	286	0.1
Mobile	78,380	6,308	3,050	1,095	432	1,087	231	317	5.7
Montgomery	46,840	5,074	2,429	1,111	282	642	155	337	0.1
Tuscaloosa	28,380	5,186	2,525	1,033	351	796	200	296	0.1
Alaska									
Anchorage	27,460	4,309	2,356	707	513	411	116	227	0.4
Arizona									
Mesa	50,180	4,653	2,108	1,080	249	440	137	343	42.2
Phoenix	176,180	4,871	2,197	1,036	395	498	144	337	26.2
Sun City	44,680	4,350	2,090	1,267	240	286	137	380	30.2
Tucson	68,400	5,254	2,398	1,031	451	464	153	333	42.1
Arkansas									
Fort Smith	44,320	6,187	2,477	973	318	1,626	218	272	0.2
Jonesboro	29,000	5,168	2,504	920	539	506	203	265	0.1
Little Rock	188,440	5,112	2,557	986	432	483	177	288	1.0
Springdale	46,660	4,173	1,895	809	411	388	134	270	0.2
Texarkana	34,600	6,146	2,693	957	502	906	177	283	0.1
California									
Orange Co.	125,760	6,017	2,665	1,450	430	532	245	497	45.0
Bakersfield	56,960	5,380	2,512	1,213	412	523	188	409	27.4
Chico	33,740	5,172	2,333	912	507	596	148	329	16.1
Contra Costa Co.	50,040	4,330	2,233	796	365	397	113	321	36.2
Fresno	68,900	4,238	1,871	958	478	410	100	348	19.6
Los Angeles	437,640	6,200	3,024	1,534	416	535	301	530	40.4
Modesto	52,780	5,461	2,775	1,062	382	683	172	386	27.0
Napa	33,300	5,467	2,767	975	628	489	131	355	13.0
Alameda Co.	83,740	4,685	2,566	843	338	344	147	344	33.9
Palm Spr/Rancho Mir	28,880	5,993	2,592	1,503	468	558	197	500	40.1
Redding	41,900	5,301	2,747	985	478	604	128	318	2.0
Sacramento	150,700	4,791	2,431	910	329	494	132	343	29.5
Salinas	29,720	4,779	2,302	950	342	736	111	349	9.6
San Bernardino	79,060	6,116	2,994	1,252	390	557	206	447	60.5
San Diego	151,400	5,678	2,649	1,199	427	601	178	446	48.7
San Francisco	94,340	4,557	2,478	848	382	395	146	357	33.3
San Jose	77,140	4,233	2,084	858	361	313	123	339	36.4
San Luis Obispo	20,160	3,553	1,612	1,063	298	243	81	392	33.4
San Mateo Co.	47,780	3,873	1,921	766	336	399	120	346	41.1
Santa Barbara	29,220	4,471	1,975	1,211	335	333	125	432	35.9

Hospital Referral Region	Medicare Enrollees (1996)	Price Adj. Reimb. for Noncapitated Medicare per Enrollee (1996)	Price Adj. Medicare Reimb. for Inpatient Hospital Services per Enrollee (1996)	Price Adj. Medicare Reimb. for Professional and Lab. Services per Enrollee (1996)	Price Adj. Medicare Reimb. for Outpatient Services per Enrollee (1996)	Price Adj. Medicare Reimb. for Home Health Care Services per Enrollee (1996)	Price Adj. Medicare Reimb. for Physician Visits in the Inpatient Setting per Enrollee (1996)	Price Adj. Medicare Reimb. for Physician Visits at Sites Other than Hospitals per Enrollee (1996)	Percent of Medicare Population Enrolled in Health Maintenance Organizations (1996)
Santa Cruz	20,480	4,638	2,178	997	319	566	135	389	15.5
Santa Rosa	33,020	4,023	1,744	915	330	410	115	351	35.8
Stockton	33,480	5,324	2,590	1,003	430	509	163	383	20.4
Ventura	41,220	4,715	2,016	1,297	437	436	216	479	40.2
Colorado									
Boulder	13,980	4,849	2,073	835	495	570	154	305	20.8
Colorado Springs	53,820	4,891	2,203	830	485	613	138	269	11.1
Denver	132,160	5,339	2,317	913	583	606	145	314	31.3
Fort Collins	25,080	5,225	2,232	887	551	759	121	275	0.7
Grand Junction	30,180	4,053	2,126	474	493	422	63	184	0.6
Greeley	28,620	5,218	2,380	877	531	725	144	295	1.5
Pueblo	16,560	5,833	2,766	931	480	795	174	301	21.6
Connecticut									
Bridgeport	81,860	4,497	2,114	1,035	357	580	170	351	1.9
Hartford	185,420	4,663	2,216	935	439	531	146	354	1.6
New Haven	170,080	4,766	2,293	1,026	425	544	152	362	1.9
Delaware									
Wilmington	73,780	4,511	2,371	1,083	359	300	191	333	4.5
District of Columbia									
Washington	197,040	4,548	2,382	1,114	423	202	206	379	3.9
Florida									
Bradenton	46,520	4,922	1,930	1,260	405	671	151	386	5.5
Clearwater	82,080	5,904	2,339	1,421	376	710	206	451	20.7
Fort Lauderdale	299,720	6,109	2,453	1,696	554	715	244	555	30.5
Fort Myers	171,760	5,385	2,275	1,360	419	713	170	418	1.1
Gainesville	47,120	5,639	2,437	1,078	392	948	178	367	11.6
Hudson	77,300	5,843	2,365	1,463	418	787	207	429	21.8
Jacksonville	109,640	5,848	2,618	1,253	480	682	231	422	18.3
Lakeland	42,020	5,268	2,338	1,207	331	615	156	366	4.6
Miami	201,940	7,783	3,045	1,990	795	946	349	627	37.7
Ocala	82,580	5,208	2,211	1,290	418	491	166	361	6.5
Orlando	350,800	5,491	2,251	1,298	422	756	190	399	11.4
Ormond Beach	45,380	5,328	2,176	1,098	547	740	163	384	33.3
Panama City	22,960	6,358	2,557	1,232	488	1,146	201	385	0.2
Pensacola	73,160	5,464	2,458	1,095	399	876	177	359	0.2
Sarasota	95,960	5,602	2,322	1,361	469	745	174	418	2.1
St Petersburg	61,160	5,910	2,373	1,321	473	685	196	435	22.0
Tallahassee	70,800	4,958	2,187	969	457	623	150	314	0.3
Tampa	81,860	5,658	2,484	1,264	416	613	220	417	26.9
Georgia									
Albany	21,560	5,304	2,731	943	576	694	188	268	0.1
Atlanta	359,520	4,890	2,423	1,024	388	583	166	314	0.5
Augusta	63,320	4,981	2,438	943	524	520	147	284	0.1
Columbus	33,900	4,770	2,364	981	401	546	164	311	0.1
Macon	69,920	5,119	2,433	991	513	656	140	322	0.1
Rome	30,580	5,515	2,852	999	416	766	146	315	0.1

Hospital Referral Region	Medicare Enrollees (1996)	Price Adj. Reimb. for Noncapitated Medicare per Enrollee (1996)	Price Adj. Medicare Reimb. for Inpatient Hospital Services per Enrollee (1996)	Price Adj. Medicare Reimb. for Professional and Lab. Services per Enrollee (1996)	Price Adj. Medicare Reimb. for Outpatient Services per Enrollee (1996)	Price Adj. Medicare Reimb. for Home Health Care Services per Enrollee (1996)	Price Adj. Medicare Reimb. for Physician Visits in the Inpatient Setting per Enrollee (1996)	Price Adj. Medicare Reimb. for Physician Visits at Sites Other than Hospitals per Enrollee (1996)	Percent of Medicare Population Enrolled in Health Maintenance Organizations (1996)
Savannah	70,920	5,409	2,627	1,108	568	705	165	329	0.2
Hawaii									
Honolulu	87,180	3,526	1,897	742	344	190	127	342	32.5
Idaho									
Boise	70,940	4,305	1,886	752	449	458	99	246	0.4
Idaho Falls	17,840	5,129	2,427	790	442	927	97	219	0.3
Illinois									
Aurora	17,660	4,182	2,322	746	366	333	156	247	1.2
Bloomington	19,220	4,158	2,011	951	475	356	109	297	0.1
Blue Island	88,240	5,042	2,665	1,021	423	425	256	322	13.2
Chicago	208,560	5,549	3,169	999	396	456	274	355	13.1
Elgin	41,500	4,552	2,147	924	415	437	187	307	6.6
Evanston	110,380	4,699	2,451	1,023	410	320	214	374	9.6
Hinsdale	31,880	5,211	2,773	1,033	420	416	238	345	7.3
Joliet	47,620	5,245	2,939	1,021	460	436	254	320	1.8
Melrose Park	126,160	4,788	2,478	938	399	402	231	320	10.2
Peoria	94,920	4,612	2,285	847	562	420	130	268	0.1
Rockford	82,980	4,082	2,057	833	428	310	141	279	0.2
Springfield	123,420	4,662	2,510	881	514	369	151	263	0.1
Urbana	55,080	4,547	2,344	901	496	307	146	283	0.1
Indiana									
Evansville	96,420	4,670	2,154	767	507	563	128	261	0.1
Fort Wayne	98,620	4,256	1,860	804	461	489	120	287	0.1
Gary	54,560	5,289	2,721	994	435	660	225	308	1.8
Indianapolis	284,300	4,796	2,319	882	510	434	144	301	1.1
Lafayette	22,700	3,467	1,583	606	437	363	80	239	0.1
Muncie	21,780	4,534	2,454	828	435	342	141	280	0.1
Munster	38,400	5,817	3,129	1,040	449	585	244	315	3.3
South Bend	80,540	4,148	1,975	810	414	388	117	266	0.1
Terre Haute	25,020	5,231	2,366	975	494	596	188	297	0.1
Iowa									
Cedar Rapids	33,640	4,031	2,124	820	604	126	107	242	0.1
Davenport	70,040	4,170	2,135	800	488	321	140	258	0.1
Des Moines	136,800	4,206	2,139	831	542	273	149	263	0.1
Dubuque	21,620	3,583	2,030	547	460	222	76	184	0.1
Iowa City	40,340	4,760	2,649	830	726	258	137	262	0.1
Mason City	26,740	4,135	2,114	712	537	330	93	234	0.1
Sioux City	39,480	3,692	1,824	807	498	188	111	247	0.1
Waterloo	31,840	4,136	2,135	682	642	225	101	246	0.1
Kansas									
Topeka	54,780	4,143	2,110	788	470	321	120	251	0.1
Wichita	174,540	5,070	2,612	954	604	388	146	266	0.1
Kentucky									
Covington	34,940	4,831	2,518	923	467	232	215	308	0.5
Lexington	153,280	4,793	2,487	812	394	507	161	281	0.1
Louisville	182,100	5,378	2,600	1,028	420	545	206	324	3.2

Hospital Referral Region	Medicare Enrollees (1996)	Price Adj. Reimb for Noncapitated Medicare per Enrollee (1996)	Price Adj. Medicare Reimb. for Inpatient Hospital Services per Enrollees (1996)	Price Adj. Medicare Reimb. for Professional and Lab. Services per Enrollee (1996)	Price Adj. Medicare Reimb. for Outpatient Services per Enrollee (1996)	Price Adj. Medicare Reimb. for Home Health Care Services per Enrollee (1996)	Price Adj. Medicare Reimb for Physician Visits in the Inpatient Setting per Enrollee (1996)	Price Adj. Medicare Reimb for Physician Visits at Sites Other than Hospitals per Enrollee (1996)	Percent of Medicare Population Enrolled in Health Maintenance Organizations (1996)
Owensboro	17,680	4,759	2,461	976	420	415	157	276	0.1
Paducah	55,600	5,100	2,477	1,002	474	568	171	302	0.1
Louisiana									
Alexandria	33,360	6,423	2,992	885	668	1,219	157	288	0.1
Baton Rouge	59,160	7,700	2,795	1,031	665	2,404	184	338	18.5
Houma	23,360	7,568	3,648	1,174	707	1,628	208	316	3.5
Lafayette	58,440	6,227	2,935	975	508	1,082	171	302	0.1
Lake Charles	24,740	5,784	3,103	913	529	751	205	272	0.1
Metairie	38,120	7,454	3,248	1,217	664	1,651	264	385	16.0
Monroe	32,820	7,723	3,516	1,051	543	1,794	232	284	0.1
New Orleans	72,940	7,317	3,239	1,159	501	1,565	239	379	16.6
Shreveport	82,240	6,602	3,429	982	629	992	206	273	0.1
Slidell	15,300	6,597	3,349	1,184	492	1,013	229	372	6.6
Maine									
Bangor	55,100	4,813	2,233	750	591	798	124	262	0.1
Portland	129,060	4,377	2,131	845	438	539	131	293	0.2
Maryland									
Baltimore	260,740	5,119	2,777	1,096	555	261	198	369	4.7
Salisbury	53,020	4,560	2,297	989	516	284	189	350	3.5
Takoma Park	59,800	4,962	2,563	1,326	409	207	231	430	4.9
Massachusetts									
Boston	499,540	5,949	2,766	1,008	566	816	185	404	11.9
Springfield	90,000	4,769	2,221	862	417	607	148	363	7.2
Worcester	62,100	5,576	2,638	951	548	600	165	393	32.0
Michigan									
Ann Arbor	131,080	5,267	2,632	1,175	614	433	193	376	0.9
Dearborn	72,420	5,553	2,870	1,324	513	423	261	407	1.9
Detroit	222,380	5,246	2,642	1,296	496	391	216	378	1.4
Flint	57,860	5,627	2,955	1,301	494	428	226	344	0.1
Grand Rapids	113,640	4,156	2,078	832	483	289	112	267	0.1
Kalamazoo	75,020	4,819	2,532	889	554	364	135	295	0.1
Lansing	62,800	5,196	2,847	1,034	567	377	171	334	5.7
Marquette	32,420	5,033	2,432	792	498	1,042	116	271	0.1
Muskegon	35,840	4,103	2,073	852	460	351	126	299	0.1
Petoskey	25,220	5,031	2,435	956	577	542	135	292	0.1
Pontiac	36,440	5,975	3,094	1,364	524	411	245	408	0.8
Royal Oak	80,800	5,422	2,628	1,352	540	440	194	422	1.0
Saginaw	93,480	5,136	2,650	1,009	581	468	179	291	0.1
St Joseph	19,760	5,062	2,672	961	432	625	160	280	0.1
Traverse City	32,240	4,851	2,620	934	590	404	133	294	0.1
Minnesota									
Duluth	53,900	3,760	2,108	580	387	319	87	191	0.2
Minneapolis	276,580	3,700	2,016	641	411	212	100	215	11.5
Rochester	54,920	4,148	2,416	775	406	115	91	256	0.3
St Cloud	24,320	3,659	1,887	750	454	220	121	241	0.4
St Paul	73,240	3,954	2,250	669	389	239	109	220	20.5

Hospital Referral Region	Medicare Enrollees (1996)	Price Adj. Reimb. for Noncapitated Medicare per Enrollee (1996)	Price Adj. Medicare Reimb. for Inpatient Hospital Services per Enrollee (1996)	Price Adj. Medicare Reimb. for Professional and Lab. Services per Enrollee (1996)	Price Adj. Medicare Reimb. for Outpatient Services per Enrollee (1996)	Price Adj. Medicare Reimb. for Home Health Care Services per Enrollee (1996)	Price Adj. Medicare Reimb. for Physician Visits in the Inpatient Setting per Enrollee (1996)	Price Adj. Medicare Reimb. for Physician Visits at Sites Other than Hospitals per Enrollee (1996)	Percent of Medicare Population Enrolled in Health Maintenance Organizations (1996)
Mississippi									
Gulfport	19,060	6,746	3,412	1,074	536	997	254	310	0.3
Hattiesburg	31,280	5,937	2,782	1,107	571	828	214	299	0.1
Jackson	117,720	6,015	2,592	913	535	1,195	185	267	0.1
Meridian	26,160	5,913	2,661	1,049	427	1,060	210	281	0.1
Oxford	17,840	6,252	2,677	1,034	585	1,350	199	293	0.1
Tupelo	45,800	5,716	2,842	869	481	951	173	266	0.0
Missouri									
Cape Girardeau	37,040	4,642	2,260	780	582	558	123	251	0.1
Columbia	86,060	5,974	3,255	912	712	565	175	272	0.1
Joplin	49,360	5,085	2,528	864	508	469	140	278	0.2
Kansas City	226,660	5,128	2,488	995	504	466	191	308	8.3
Springfield	108,060	4,807	2,383	804	615	484	126	245	0.2
St Louis	380,240	4,943	2,571	867	500	466	165	289	7.3
Montana									
Billings	61,560	4,336	2,116	779	537	383	120	244	0.2
Great Falls	19,880	5,399	3,031	767	502	434	168	244	0.2
Missoula	41,360	4,307	2,030	754	434	616	93	247	0.3
Nebraska									
Lincoln	75,960	3,930	1,989	751	537	244	97	225	0.1
Omaha	150,320	4,730	2,520	813	582	297	148	256	2.4
Nevada									
Las Vegas	79,300	5,349	2,414	1,277	237	675	229	376	35.3
Reno	57,600	4,363	2,135	848	394	343	122	291	8.4
New Hampshire									
Lebanon	53,000	4,243	2,172	619	596	531	98	229	0.2
Manchester	82,180	4,167	2,049	798	410	410	126	311	1.1
New Jersey									
Camden	328,380	4,808	2,459	1,274	373	300	263	423	8.8
Hackensack	147,620	4,541	2,362	1,260	357	251	273	425	5.3
Morristown	103,940	4,341	2,210	1,200	329	276	237	394	2.2
New Brunswick	93,760	4,693	2,493	1,280	299	261	340	376	6.2
Newark	160,160	4,656	2,530	1,283	337	267	369	394	2.7
Paterson	39,180	4,216	2,139	1,205	319	189	298	408	4.1
Ridgewood	41,980	4,777	2,509	1,271	351	226	315	415	5.8
New Mexico									
Albuquerque	107,220	4,591	2,081	760	601	566	116	262	21.7
New York									
Albany	230,100	4,026	2,014	972	343	278	187	353	1.0
Binghamton	55,040	3,949	2,039	802	525	220	164	297	0.2
Bronx	89,060	6,093	3,780	1,172	450	297	238	471	12.6
Buffalo	198,880	4,199	2,188	946	399	258	178	305	4.7
Elmira	52,900	3,826	1,893	929	419	250	191	323	0.1
East Long Island	432,520	4,997	2,673	1,354	331	293	269	473	14.9
New York	399,320	6,055	3,612	1,396	391	373	288	501	11.3
Rochester	140,620	4,046	2,230	712	433	373	126	258	9.4

Hospital Referral Region	Medicare Enrollees (1996)	Price Adj. Reimb. for Noncapitated Medicare per Enrollee (1996)	Price Adj. Medicare Reimb. for Inpatient Hospital Services per Enrollee (1996)	Price Adj. Medicare Reimb. for Professional and Lab. Services per Enrollee (1996)	Price Adj. Medicare Reimb. for Outpatient Services per Enrollee (1996)	Price Adj. Medicare Reimb. for Home Health Care Services per Enrollee (1996)	Price Adj. Medicare Reimb. for Physician Visits in the Inpatient Setting per Enrollee (1996)	Price Adj. Medicare Reimb. for Physician Visits at Sites Other than Hospitals per Enrollee (1996)	Percent of Medicare Population Enrolled in Health Maintenance Organizations (1996)
Syracuse	129,400	4,125	2,083	972	359	297	168	336	0.1
White Plains	112,780	4,601	2,374	1,241	332	251	252	446	9.7
North Carolina									
Asheville	92,260	4,533	2,090	927	457	466	143	307	0.2
Charlotte	194,940	4,432	2,260	896	416	418	160	304	0.1
Durham	144,840	4,325	2,377	839	441	316	132	298	0.1
Greensboro	63,260	4,181	2,136	856	364	346	135	286	0.1
Greenville	83,060	4,761	2,617	996	446	374	148	334	0.1
Hickory	31,480	4,414	2,393	850	351	315	138	313	0.1
Raleigh	134,380	4,491	2,363	917	450	379	151	320	0.1
Wilmington	41,820	5,231	2,636	1,053	416	616	157	366	0.1
Winston-Salem	119,640	4,510	2,405	904	380	383	157	310	0.7
North Dakota									
Bismarck	30,960	4,333	2,223	834	607	325	110	248	0.1
Fargo Moorhead -Mn	69,840	4,314	2,342	791	484	321	110	237	0.1
Grand Forks	24,500	4,372	2,571	688	539	347	111	231	0.1
Minot	19,540	4,445	2,336	883	785	156	107	249	0.1
Ohio									
Akron	86,440	5,102	2,832	975	437	345	207	334	2.8
Canton	85,760	4,261	2,180	968	376	300	175	347	0.2
Cincinnati	179,500	4,521	2,290	865	513	324	136	339	2.7
Cleveland	264,060	5,068	2,522	1,016	464	433	184	366	9.8
Columbus	295,360	4,667	2,461	886	434	294	151	321	0.1
Dayton	136,900	4,597	2,335	935	445	322	158	333	0.1
Elyria	29,020	4,967	2,471	1,095	410	351	182	340	1.2
Kettering	47,640	4,617	2,314	952	470	331	171	334	0.4
Toledo	122,900	5,224	2,804	991	505	302	193	342	3.1
Youngstown	117,340	5,064	2,579	1,050	536	423	205	373	0.5
Oklahoma									
Lawton	23,440	5,247	2,318	823	605	1,105	125	278	0.1
Oklahoma City	197,080	6,254	2,692	966	492	1,448	164	288	3.5
Tulsa	138,680	5,748	2,540	929	511	1,182	162	291	8.3
Oregon									
Bend	20,980	4,231	2,094	780	366	672	91	252	1.4
Eugene	78,600	3,506	1,840	629	307	329	77	224	13.4
Medford	56,060	3,910	1,938	716	394	469	84	264	9.0
Portland	143,800	3,923	2,120	656	404	246	87	250	39.5
Salem	25,100	3,647	1,940	648	387	244	81	208	23.4
Pennsylvania									
Allentown	143,420	5,163	2,558	1,181	418	416	266	373	7.0
Altoona	45,220	4,673	2,300	766	466	548	178	302	2.0
Danville	64,520	4,478	2,146	905	631	348	178	329	16.0
Erie	112,720	4,969	2,544	974	475	387	211	332	0.1
Harrisburg	120,660	4,501	2,239	939	472	268	179	324	4.2
Johnstown	42,300	5,184	2,898	841	545	517	197	274	0.2
Lancaster	67,380	4,527	2,377	985	447	267	187	356	5.4

Hospital Referral Region	Medicare Enrollees (1996)	Price Adj. Reimb. for Noncapitated Medicare per Enrollee (1996)	Price Adj. Medicare Reimb. for Inpatient Hospital Services per Enrollee (1996)	Price Adj. Medicare Reimb. for Professional and Lab. Services per Enrollee (1996)	Price Adj. Medicare Reimb. for Outpatient Services per Enrollee (1996)	Price Adj. Medicare Reimb. for Home Health Care Services per Enrollee (1996)	Price Adj. Medicare Reimb. for Physician Visits in the Inpatient Setting per Enrollee (1996)	Price Adj. Medicare Reimb. for Physician Visits at Sites Other than Hospitals per Enrollee (1996)	Percent of Medicare Population Enrolled in Health Maintenance Organizations (1996)
Philadelphia	394,520	5,792	3,154	1,304	414	352	280	465	22.9
Pittsburgh	451,520	5,720	2,954	1,081	472	566	264	333	12.6
Reading	75,860	4,405	2,086	961	435	306	191	341	8.6
Sayre	27,100	4,060	2,119	771	382	358	161	281	1.3
Scranton	53,200	5,257	2,445	1,118	387	593	282	352	6.6
Wilkes-Barre	42,100	5,471	2,242	1,119	465	750	280	350	10.1
York	48,520	4,107	2,078	821	366	269	130	311	2.8
Rhode Island									
Providence	140,380	5,056	2,472	1,055	417	644	176	367	9.1
South Carolina									
Charleston	83,260	5,024	2,476	982	514	485	158	347	0.5
Columbia	112,280	4,302	2,072	912	410	364	151	296	0.7
Florence	39,860	5,191	2,689	1,028	443	514	190	321	0.1
Greenville	86,800	4,468	2,261	932	372	368	158	298	0.1
Spartanburg	42,840	4,151	2,251	845	357	395	145	278	0.1
South Dakota									
Rapid City	22,080	4,724	2,634	800	462	484	134	232	0.2
Sioux Falls	113,260	4,177	2,264	789	520	174	120	227	0.1
Tennessee									
Chattanooga	75,280	5,775	2,340	979	540	1,355	171	313	0.1
Jackson	45,100	5,227	2,378	960	488	980	177	337	0.1
Johnson City	30,720	5,421	2,772	870	437	756	186	294	0.1
Kingsport	66,840	5,443	2,567	775	561	953	152	271	0.1
Knoxville	150,620	5,558	2,497	960	467	1,174	190	313	0.1
Memphis	177,920	5,361	2,594	1,027	403	806	223	315	0.1
Nashville	242,400	6,258	2,795	980	548	1,229	179	339	0.2
Texas									
Abilene	43,700	6,329	2,903	913	587	1,274	158	261	0.1
Amarillo	51,340	5,540	2,378	904	513	1,086	146	266	0.1
Austin	77,940	5,146	2,076	1,016	510	801	168	311	5.3
Beaumont	56,520	7,394	3,028	1,110	471	1,973	235	327	3.3
Bryan	17,780	6,097	2,656	958	589	862	145	299	0.7
Corpus Christi	46,440	7,648	3,004	1,150	648	1,967	229	382	13.7
Dallas	276,980	6,037	2,549	1,063	474	1,064	176	331	6.4
El Paso	81,000	5,940	2,898	898	478	998	182	292	1.1
Fort Worth	118,300	6,093	2,350	999	545	1,192	152	333	17.2
Harlingen	43,480	7,472	3,421	1,039	519	2,212	184	341	0.2
Houston	309,280	6,617	3,149	1,118	545	1,054	223	346	16.2
Longview	23,720	5,018	1,905	868	473	1,139	123	286	0.2
Lubbock	76,380	6,537	2,928	1,041	512	1,279	213	277	0.1
McAllen	34,140	9,033	3,727	1,213	620	3,090	257	353	0.2
Odessa	31,480	7,149	3,287	1,191	409	1,403	249	310	0.2
San Angelo	21,500	5,875	2,271	876	739	1,455	150	291	0.1
San Antonio	158,540	6,736	2,610	1,077	594	1,673	196	337	21.6
Temple	30,780	4,750	2,849	622	406	510	94	217	0.2
Tyler	71,060	6,432	2,435	1,055	701	1,279	152	318	0.2

Hospital Referral Region	Medicare Enrollees (1996)	Price Adj. Reimb. for Noncapitated Medicare per Enrollee (1996)	Price Adj. Medicare Reimb. for Inpatient Hospital Services per Enrollee (1996)	Price Adj. Medicare Reimb. for Professional and Lab. Services per Enrollee (1996)	Price Adj. Medicare Reimb. for Outpatient Services per Enrollee (1996)	Price Adj. Medicare Reimb. for Home Health Care Services per Enrollee (1996)	Price Adj. Medicare Reimb. for Physician Visits in the Inpatient Setting per Enrollee (1996)	Price Adj. Medicare Reimb. for Physician Visits at Sites Other than Hospitals per Enrollee (1996)	Percent of Medicare Population Enrolled in Health Maintenance Organizations (1996)
Victoria	18,300	6,171	2,665	916	483	1,401	159	267	0.3
Waco	41,220	4,259	1,867	734	478	658	98	229	0.2
Wichita Falls	28,260	5,437	2,168	903	468	1,088	158	288	0.1
Utah									
Ogden	27,980	3,948	1,759	599	308	846	66	221	0.6
Provo	26,600	5,444	2,569	743	434	1,194	98	220	0.4
Salt Lake City	136,420	4,499	1,913	676	400	880	75	232	0.9
Vermont									
Burlington	69,100	4,308	2,350	778	476	383	146	302	0.2
Virginia									
Arlington	100,140	3,844	1,853	997	347	280	171	356	3.9
Charlottesville	59,560	4,771	2,509	806	529	335	144	311	0.1
Lynchburg	30,460	3,074	1,625	716	340	143	114	254	0.1
Newport News	51,240	4,347	2,174	1,014	421	426	180	353	2.6
Norfolk	106,580	4,514	2,277	1,033	431	375	193	·359	3.7
Richmond	153,480	4,032	2,130	906	328	330	175	304	1.0
Roanoke	94,420	4,469	2,328	799	405	444	158	275	0.1
Winchester	38,340	4,283	2,419	798	304	366	170	274	0.2
Washington									
Everett	37,500	4,768	2,446	815	516	360	110	307	31.4
Olympia	33,200	3,886	1,743	817	394	324	82	318	19.5
Seattle	191,420	4,340	2,227	824	402	305	102	306	22.0
Spokane	138,960	4,276	2,099	841	408	257	99	277	7.8
Tacoma	52,840	4,335	2,115	866	479	330	102	338	16.4
Yakima	27,600	4,029	2,043	829	402	249	71	290	0.6
West Virginia									
Charleston	124,840	5,408	2,993	834	499	507	170	280	0.0
Huntington	50,100	4,765	2,624	953	340	293	208	310	0.0
Morgantown	57,000	5,379	2,844	831	558	450	172	285	0.2
Wisconsin									
Appleton	36,800	3,404	1,719	730	478	81	84	218	0.1
Green Bay	66,940	3,960	2,058	766	500	216	94	222	0.1
La Crosse	47,540	3,679	2,103	659	351	208	110	225	0.1
Madison	110,780	3,983	2,185	677	439	256	98	222	0.1
Marshfield	53,460	4,000	2,024	834	429	267	103	269	0.1
Milwaukee	277,600	4,525	2,339	908	486	192	156	273	1.5
Neenah	29,160	4,034	1,946	810	506	259	110	231	0.1
Wausau	27,160	4,006	2,013	823	467	195	106	257	0.1
Wyoming									
Casper	21,260	5,053	2,655	771	533	546	111	245	0.2
United States									
	27,691,820	4,993	2,450	1,015	444	532	183	340	10.7

Variations in Acute Care Hospital Resources and the Physician Workforce

Acute Care Hospital Resources

The dramatic differences in levels of acute care hospital resources that were documented in the 1996 and 1998 editions of the Dartmouth Atlas of Health Care (which used data from 1992 through 1995) are demonstrated in this section to have persisted through 1996, although the health care industry has undergone a period of profound change. The numbers of acute care hospital beds, hospital employees, and registered nurses employed by acute care hospitals varied substantially among regions, and in many cases within states. Generally the supply of hospital resources was higher in the East, South, and Midwest than in the West and on the West Coast; but the idiosyncratic nature of the distribution of resources remained a constant attribute of the American health care system.

Data from the American Hospital Association and the Medicare program were used to estimate the number of staffed acute care hospital beds, full time equivalent hospital employees, and registered nurses employed in acute care hospitals allocated to care for the population of each region.

Acute Care Hospital Beds

There were 759,292 acute care hospital beds in the United States in 1996, an average of 2.8 beds per 1,000 residents. This represented a 9% decline since 1993, when there were more than 827,000 acute care hospital beds, an average of 3.3 per 1,000 residents. Reduction in hospital bed capacity over this period was observed in hospital referral regions with both high and low rates of allocated beds. The supply of beds in the Bronx, New York, for example, was reduced from 4.8 per thousand to 4.3; but the supply in Arlington, Virginia fell from 1.9 in 1995 to 1.7 in 1996, the same rate of decrease. The numbers of hospital beds per 1,000 persons in 1996, after adjusting for differences in age and sex, varied by a factor of 3.4, from 1.5 beds per 1,000 residents to 5.1.

The supply of hospital beds exceeded 4.5 per 1,000 residents in nine hospital referral regions, including Minot, North Dakota (5.1); Monroe, Louisiana (5.0); Newark, New Jersey (4.6); Hattiesburg, Mississippi (4.6); and New Orleans (4.6).

Eleven hospital referral regions had 1.7 or fewer beds per 1,000 residents, including Everett, Washington (1.4); Contra Costa County, California (1.5); Mesa, Arizona (1.5); Boulder, Colorado (1.6); and Sacramento, California (1.6).

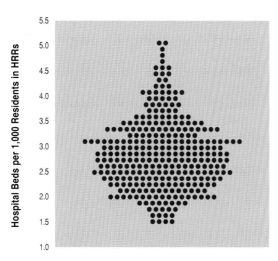

Figure 2.1. Acute Care Hospital Beds Allocated to Hospital Referral Regions (1996)

The number of hospital beds per thousand residents, after adjusting for differences in the age and sex of the local population, ranged from 1.5 to 5.1. Each point represents one of the 306 hospital referral regions in the United States.

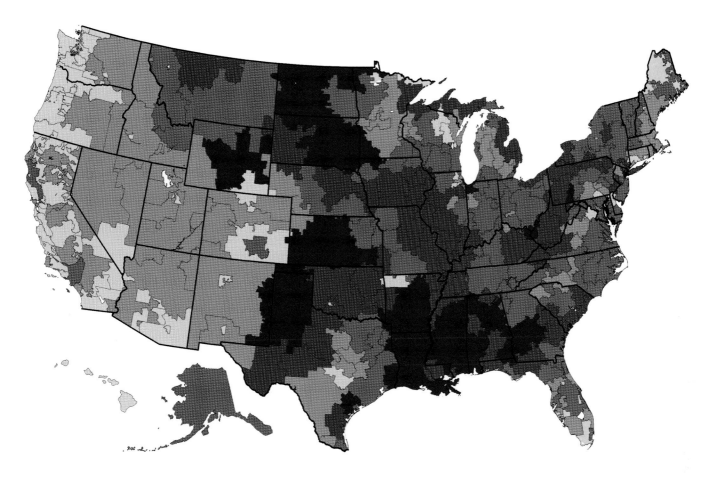

Map 2.1. Acute Care Hospital Beds (1996)

Thirty-nine hospital referral regions had supplies of hospital beds at least 30% higher than the national average. Most of these areas were in the South and rural Midwest, although a number of urban areas also had higher than average supplies of beds. Lower than average rates prevailed in the Western states and on the West Coast.

Ratio of Rates of Acute Care Hospital Beds per 1,000 Residents to the U.S. Average

by Hospital Referral Region (1996)

- 1.30 to 1.82 (39)
- 1.10 to < 1.30 (67)
- 0.90 to < 1.10 (90)
- 0.75 to < 0.90 (69)
- 0.51 to < 0.75 (41)
- Not Populated

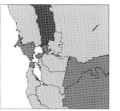
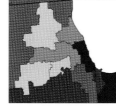
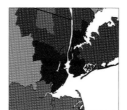
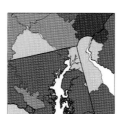
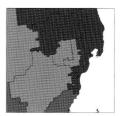

San Francisco   **Chicago**   **New York**   **Washington-Baltimore**   **Detroit**

Hospital Employees

There were more than 3.56 million full time equivalent acute care hospital employees in 1996, the same number employed in acute care hospitals in 1993, in spite of the fact that the number of acute care beds declined about 9% during the same period. There was substantial variation in how this workforce was deployed; the numbers of full time equivalent hospital employees per 1,000 residents, after adjusting for differences in population age and sex, varied by a factor of four, from fewer than 6.5 to more than 25.0.

Five hospital referral regions had more than 20.0 hospital employees per 1,000 residents, including the Bronx, New York (25.7); Chicago (21.9); New Orleans (21.4); Manhattan (20.8); and Meridian, Mississippi (20.6).

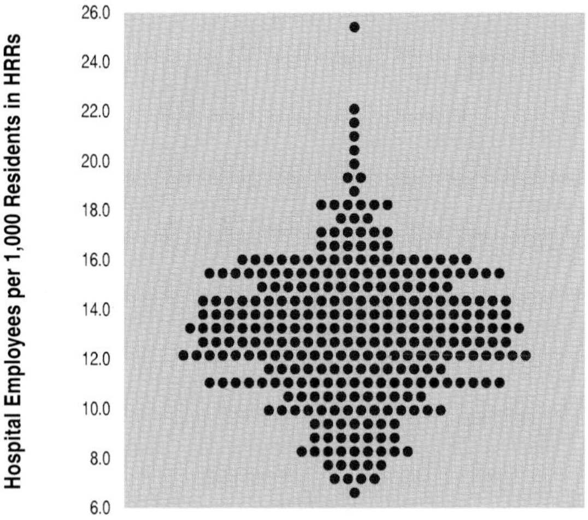

Ten hospital referral regions had fewer than 8.0 full-time equivalent employees per 1,000 residents, including seven in California, as well as Mesa, Arizona (6.3); Las Vegas (7.4); and Arlington, Virginia (7.5).

Figure 2.2. Hospital Employees Allocated to Hospital Referral Regions (1996)
The number of full time equivalent hospital employees per 1,000 residents, after adjusting for differences in the age and sex of the local population, ranged from fewer than 6.5 to more than 25.0. Each point represents one of the 306 hospital referral regions in the United States.

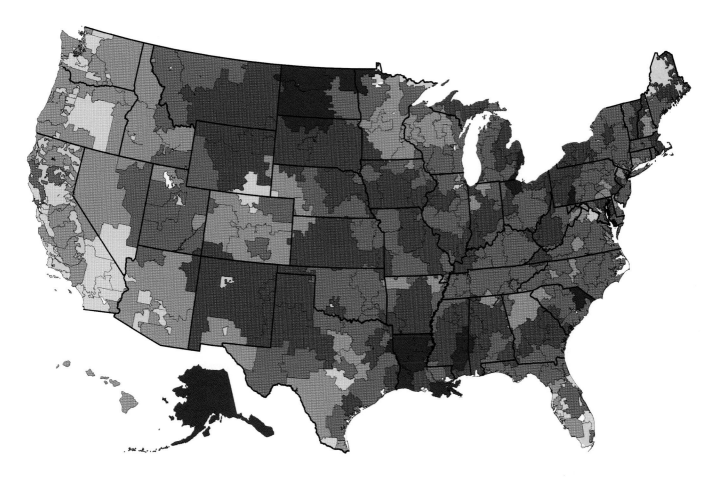

Map 2.2. Acute Care Hospital Employees (1996)

Twenty hospital referral regions had rates at least 30% higher than the national average; many of these areas were in Louisiana, North Dakota, and urban centers of the Eastern United States. Rates of employment in acute care hospitals were generally lower than the national average in the West.

Ratio of Rates of Acute Care Hospital Employees per 1,000 Residents to the U.S. Average

by Hospital Referral Region (1996)

- 1.30 to 1.95 (20)
- 1.10 to < 1.30 (70)
- 0.90 to < 1.10 (117)
- 0.75 to < 0.90 (62)
- 0.47 to < 0.75 (37)
- Not Populated

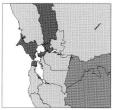

San Francisco

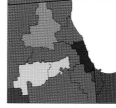

Chicago

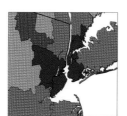

New York

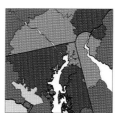

Washington-Baltimore

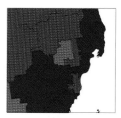

Detroit

Registered Nurses Employed in Acute Care Hospitals

There were more than 877,900 full time equivalent registered nurses employed in acute care hospitals in 1996, an average of 3.3 per 1,000 residents. This represented a slight decrease from the 882,000 employed in 1995. The numbers of hospital-based registered nurses per 1,000 residents, after adjusting for differences in age and sex of the local populations, varied by a factor of more than three, from 1.7 per 1,000 residents to 5.4.

Twelve hospital referral regions had more than 4.5 registered nurses per 1,000 residents, including Meridian, Mississippi (5.4); Chicago (5.0); Toledo, Ohio (4.8); Bangor, Maine (4.7); New Orleans (4.7); Newark, New Jersey (4.7); and the Bronx, New York (4.6).

Eight hospital referral regions had fewer than 2.1 hospital-employed registered nurses per 1,000 residents, including five in California as well as Mesa, Arizona (1.9); and Austin, Texas (2.0).

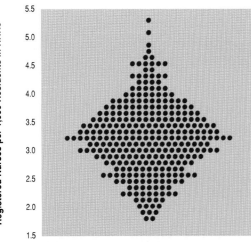

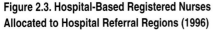

Figure 2.3. Hospital-Based Registered Nurses Allocated to Hospital Referral Regions (1996)

The acute care hospital-employed registered nurse workforce varied from fewer than 1.8 per 1,000 residents to almost 5.5. Each point represents one of the 306 hospital referral regions in the United States.

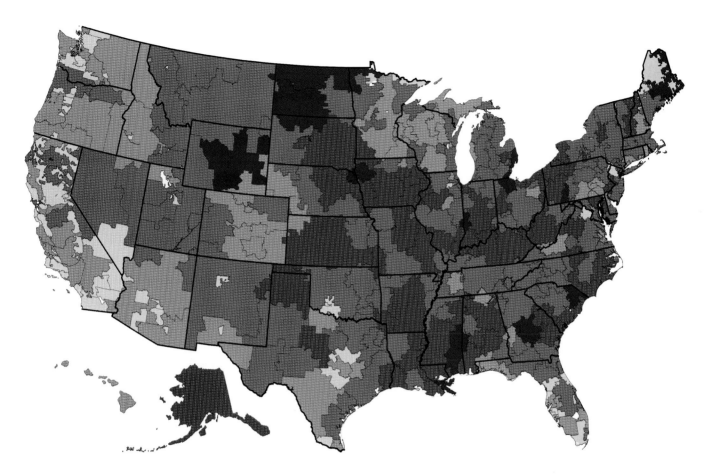

Map 2.3. Registered Nurses Employed in Acute Care Hospitals (1996)

The distribution of the registered nurse workforce closely resembled the distribution of hospital beds and employees. Twenty-one hospital referral regions had supplies of hospital-based registered nurses at least 30% higher than the national average; 31 regions were at least 25% lower than the average.

Ratio of Rates of Registered Nurses per 1,000 Residents to the U.S. Average

by Hospital Referral Region (1996)

- 1.30 to 1.65 (21)
- 1.10 to < 1.30 (60)
- 0.90 to < 1.10 (129)
- 0.75 to < 0.90 (65)
- 0.53 to < 0.75 (31)
- Not Populated

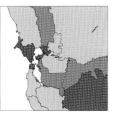

San Francisco

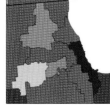

Chicago

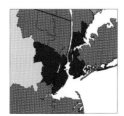

New York

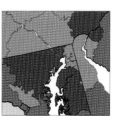

Washington-Baltimore

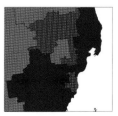

Detroit

The Physician Workforce

In 1970, there were 235,241 physicians active in patient care in the United States. By 1993, the number had increased to 469,603, an increase that was largely attributable to growth in medical schools, an increase in class sizes, and policies that encouraged international medical graduates to enter the professional workforce in the United States. In 1996, there were 495,507 physicians in active practice in the United States. Although the per capita number of physicians was 188.9 per 100,000 residents of the United States, the workforce was not uniformly deployed. Some areas had very high numbers of physicians per capita, and some areas had many fewer; the workforce-to-population ratio varied by a factor of 3.8 among hospital referral regions.

The uneven distribution of the physician workforce raises the question of whether the deployment patterns of physicians might be explained by differences in population need — that some areas might have many more physicians because residents of those areas are much sicker, on average, than residents of areas with fewer physicians per 100,000 residents. Research conducted in conjunction with the Atlas indicates that, in fact, very little of the variation in the physician workforce deployment can be explained by differences in population illness.

This section examines the physician workforce in the nation's 306 hospital referral regions. The data come from the American Medical Association, the American Osteopathic Association, and the Medicare program, and are for 1996. A clinically active physician is defined as one who reported that he or she spent at least 20 hours a week in patient care. The population count is the Claritas® estimate for 1995.

The estimates of the number of physicians allocated to populations per 100,000 persons take into account patient migration across the boundaries of the regions, using a method similar to that used for hospital beds. For example, medical specialists and primary care physicians were allocated on the basis of medical admissions.

The estimates have been adjusted for differences in the age and sex of the populations of hospital referral regions (see the Appendix on Methods).

The Physician Workforce Active in Patient Care

In 1996, there were 495,507 physicians in active practice, an increase of 5.5% since 1993. The distribution of the physician workforce did not change in any dramatic way between 1993 and 1996; there was some growth in the number of physicians per 100,000 residents of parts of the Western and Mountain states, but for the most part the workforce remained concentrated in urban areas.

Among the hospital referral regions with the highest total numbers of active physicians per 100,000 residents in 1996 were White Plains, New York (333.5); Hackensack, New Jersey (299.6); Royal Oak, Michigan (288.5); San Francisco (282.2); and Takoma Park, Maryland (277.8).

Some regions of the United States had fewer than half as many physicians per 100,000 residents. The McAllen, Texas hospital referral region had the lowest supply (88.2). Other regions with fewer than average physicians per 100,000 residents included Provo, Utah (131.5); San Bernardino, California (144.7); Wichita, Kansas (147.5); and Dayton, Ohio (147.7).

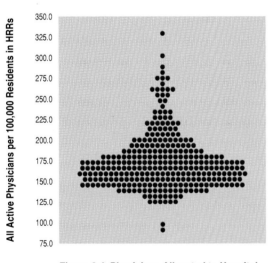

Figure 2.4. Physicians Allocated to Hospital Referral Regions (1996)

The number of physicians in active practice per 100,000 residents, after adjusting for differences in age and sex of the local population, ranged from fewer than 90 to more than 330. Each point represents one of the 306 hospital referral regions in the United States.

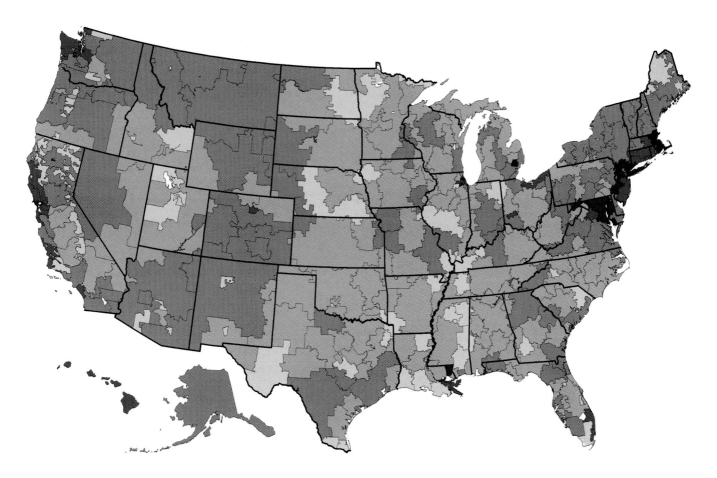

Map 2.4. The Physician Workforce (1996)

In 1996, there were higher than average numbers of physicians per 100,000 residents of the East and West Coasts, parts of the Mountain and Southwestern states, and in the Pacific Northwest. Some regions with high supplies of physicians were contiguous with areas that had much lower supplies, as in Nebraska, New Mexico, and Idaho.

Ratio of Rates of Physicians per 100,000 Residents to the U.S. Average

by Hospital Referral Region (1996)

- ■ 1.30 to 1.77 (18)
- ■ 1.10 to < 1.30 (27)
- ■ 0.90 to < 1.10 (98)
- ■ 0.75 to < 0.90 (132)
- ■ 0.46 to < 0.75 (31)
- ■ Not Populated

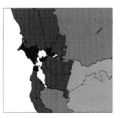

San Francisco

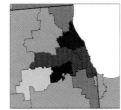

Chicago

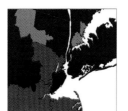

New York

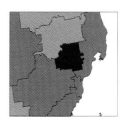

Washington-Baltimore

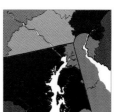

Detroit

Primary Care Physicians

The number of active primary care physicians increased by 62% between 1970 and 1993, and by 3.9% between 1993 and 1996. The proportion of physicians who were in primary care, 35% of the workforce, did not change between 1993 and 1996. Among hospital referral regions, the supply of physicians clinically active in primary care in 1996 varied from 33.8 per 100,000 residents in McAllen, Texas, to 105.1 in White Plains, New York; the national average among hospital referral regions was 65.0 per 100,000 residents.

Among hospital referral regions with the highest number of primary care physicians per 100,000 residents were Royal Oak, Michigan (102.9); San Francisco (102.1); Hackensack, New Jersey (99.9); Evanston, Illinois (98.1); Philadelphia (89.4); and Napa, California (89.0).

Few hospital referral regions with large populations had lower than average supplies of physicians in primary care; the exceptions included El Paso, Texas (41.6); Las Vegas, Nevada (47.4); Shreveport, Louisiana (47.9); Fort Wayne, Indiana (48.2); and Salt Lake City (48.3).

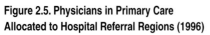

Figure 2.5. Physicians in Primary Care Allocated to Hospital Referral Regions (1996)
The number of primary care physicians in active practice per 100,000 residents, after adjusting for differences in age and sex of the local population, ranged from fewer than 34 to more than 105. Each point represents one of the 306 hospital referral regions in the United States.

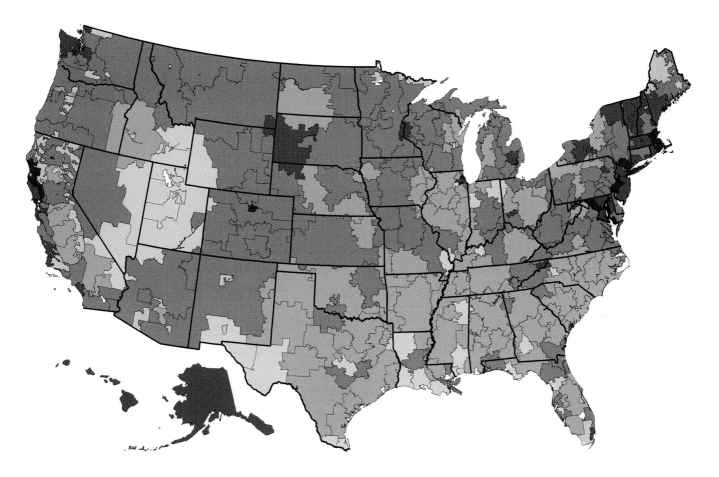

Map 2.5. Physicians in Primary Care (1996)

In 1996, the numbers of primary care physicians per 100,000 residents were greatest in the Northeast, the Mountain States, the Pacific Northwest, northern California, Alaska and Hawaii. There were relatively few primary care physicians in the Southeastern United States, Texas, southern Idaho, western Wyoming, Utah, and Eastern Nevada.

Ratio of Rates of Primary Care Physicians per 100,000 Residents to the U.S. Average

by Hospital Referral Region (1996)

- ■ 1.30 to 1.62 (14)
- ■ 1.10 to < 1.30 (35)
- ■ 0.90 to < 1.10 (123)
- ■ 0.75 to < 0.90 (106)
- □ 0.51 to < 0.75 (28)
- □ Not Populated

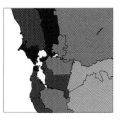

San Francisco

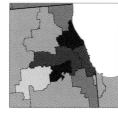

Chicago

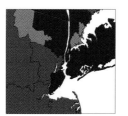

New York

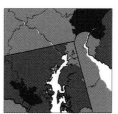

Washington-Baltimore

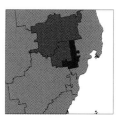

Detroit

Specialist Physicians

In 1970, there were 130,784 clinically active physicians who were identified as specialists; by 1993 the number had increased to 302,511, representing about 65% of the physician workforce. Between 1993 and 1996, the number of specialists (medical and surgical) increased 6.6%, in spite of efforts to encourage medical graduates to enter primary care. The population ratio increased by about 1%, from 121.7 specialists per hundred thousand in 1993 to 122.9 in 1996.

Among the areas with the highest numbers of specialists per 100,000 residents were White Plains, New York (227.0); Hackensack, New Jersey (198.3); Royal Oak, Michigan (185.2); Takoma Park, Maryland (184.7); Washington, D.C. (182.7); and Metairie, Louisiana (181.8). The per capita number of specialists serving the population of White Plains was about 84% higher than the national average of 122.9.

The number of specialists allocated to the McAllen, Texas hospital referral region (53.3) actually declined slightly between 1993 and 1996. Other areas with lower than average numbers of specialists included Fort Wayne, Indiana (82.4); Wichita, Kansas (84.9); Springfield, Illinois (87.3); and Springfield, Missouri (87.6).

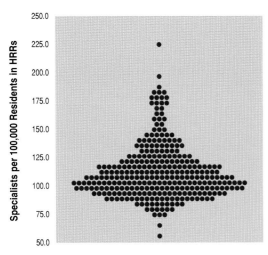

Figure 2.6. Specialist Physicians Allocated to Hospital Referral Regions (1996)

The number of specialist physicians per 100,000 residents, after adjusting for differences in age and sex of the local population, ranged from about 50 to more than 225. Each point represents one of the 306 hospital referral regions in the United States.

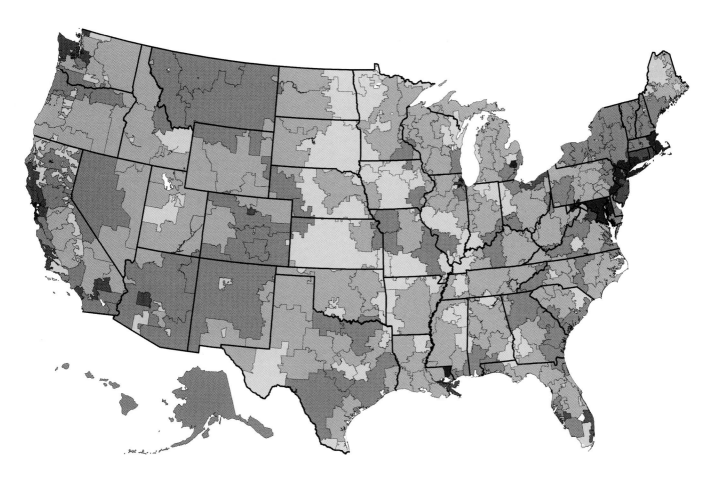

Map 2.6. Specialist Physicians (1996)

In 1996, the supply of specialists per 100,000 residents was highest on the East and West Coasts and lowest in the Midwest, the East South Central states, and the Upper Midwest. The Northeast and California also had very high supplies of specialists.

Ratio of Rates of Specialist Physicians per 100,000 Residents to the U.S. Average

by Hospital Referral Region (1996)

- 1.30 to 1.85 (20)
- 1.10 to < 1.30 (25)
- 0.90 to < 1.10 (85)
- 0.75 to < 0.90 (126)
- 0.43 to < 0.75 (50)
- Not Populated

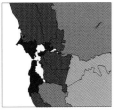
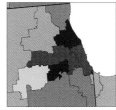
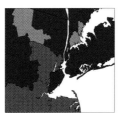
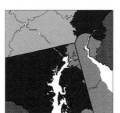
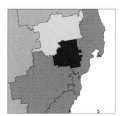

San Francisco   **Chicago**   **New York**   **Washington-Baltimore**   **Detroit**

Chapter Two Table   All measures of allocated hospital resources are expressed in rates per 1,000 residents. The physician supply is expressed in rates per 100,000 residents. All rates are adjusted for differences in the age and sex of the population. Estimates of allocated hospital employees and registered nurses are expressed as full time equivalents (FTEs).

See the Appendix on Methods for details on the methods used for allocating resources, estimating populations and adjusting rates, and for other details concerning the rates in these tables.

CHAPTER TWO TABLE

Acute Care Hospital Resources and the Physician Workforce by Hospital Referral Regions (1996)

Hospital Referral Region	Resident Population (1996)	Acute Care Hospital Beds per 1,000 Residents (1996)	Acute Care Hospital Employees per 1,000 Residents (1996)	Registered Nurses Employed in Acute Care Hospitals per 1,000 Residents (1996)	Physicians per 100,000 Residents (1996)	Primary Care Physicians per 100,000 Residents (1996)	Specialist Physicians per 100,000 Residents (1996)
Alabama							
Birmingham	2,113,094	4.0	15.8	4.1	157.5	54.9	101.8
Dothan	342,388	3.9	14.6	3.5	145.6	53.0	91.6
Huntsville	536,579	3.1	11.3	2.9	145.2	54.3	90.0
Mobile	751,227	3.7	15.7	4.1	164.1	51.3	111.8
Montgomery	426,307	3.6	13.5	3.9	142.7	49.6	92.3
Tuscaloosa	235,761	3.5	15.0	3.0	156.4	56.6	98.7
Alaska							
Anchorage	612,273	2.7	18.1	3.6	186.9	73.0	112.2
Arizona							
Mesa	946,270	1.5	6.3	1.9	151.2	53.0	97.2
Phoenix	2,429,986	2.2	10.6	2.7	177.9	59.5	117.5
Sun City	184,945	2.0	8.5	2.3	201.0	64.3	135.7
Tucson	1,010,007	1.9	10.1	2.5	179.9	63.3	115.7
Arkansas							
Fort Smith	328,687	3.3	12.8	3.0	145.9	57.7	86.9
Jonesboro	213,837	3.3	11.6	3.0	133.3	53.9	78.7
Little Rock	1,407,504	3.7	15.4	3.9	163.9	57.7	105.2
Springdale	375,514	2.1	11.7	3.1	146.0	58.4	86.5
Texarkana	252,628	4.4	15.3	3.8	137.7	53.4	83.3
California							
Orange Co.	2,908,769	2.2	8.5	2.3	211.8	73.1	137.9
Bakersfield	874,305	2.2	10.9	2.6	145.9	49.5	95.5
Chico	266,611	2.2	13.3	3.4	171.9	55.3	115.6
Contra Costa Co.	892,780	1.5	7.1	1.8	214.9	69.2	144.6
Fresno	1,027,730	2.0	10.7	2.4	152.4	54.6	96.7
Los Angeles	9,288,694	2.7	11.0	2.9	197.6	64.9	131.9
Modesto	728,080	2.3	10.7	3.0	148.9	54.3	93.5
Napa	255,209	2.6	12.5	2.5	243.9	89.0	154.2
Alameda Co.	1,376,059	2.0	8.9	2.5	223.9	82.2	141.1
Palm Spr/Rancho Mir	270,662	2.0	8.7	2.2	197.5	55.5	141.0
Redding	319,558	2.4	11.8	3.4	185.8	68.4	116.4
Sacramento	2,073,264	1.6	8.5	2.1	184.2	64.9	118.3
Salinas	320,662	2.1	11.7	2.6	192.5	60.4	131.4
San Bernardino	2,402,938	2.1	8.8	2.5	144.7	49.8	93.9
San Diego	3,086,657	1.8	7.8	2.3	194.1	61.1	132.1
San Francisco	1,315,188	2.2	12.1	3.0	282.2	102.1	180.0
San Jose	1,619,112	2.0	8.2	2.4	196.2	69.2	126.1
San Luis Obispo	218,934	1.9	7.4	2.5	227.7	77.6	149.3
San Mateo Co.	775,025	1.7	8.9	2.0	234.7	72.3	161.2
Santa Barbara	405,511	2.4	7.7	1.7	215.2	73.3	140.9

Hospital Referral Region	Resident Population (1996)	Acute Care Hospital Beds per 1,000 Residents (1996)	Acute Care Hospital Employees per 1,000 Residents (1996)	Registered Nurses Employed in Acute Care Hospitals per 1,000 Residents (1996)	Physicians per 100,000 Residents (1996)	Primary Care Physicians per 100,000 Residents (1996)	Specialist Physicians per 100,000 Residents (1996)
Santa Cruz	249,750	1.9	7.5	1.9	223.6	73.9	149.0
Santa Rosa	437,664	1.8	6.9	1.9	228.2	84.1	143.0
Stockton	475,253	2.2	11.2	2.7	149.8	50.3	98.8
Ventura	751,104	2.0	7.9	2.4	203.5	68.4	134.2
Colorado							
Boulder	253,571	1.6	9.4	2.7	231.8	85.0	145.7
Colorado Springs	694,232	2.0	11.2	2.6	174.9	59.0	115.0
Denver	2,231,794	2.2	11.2	2.8	203.2	69.1	133.1
Fort Collins	273,695	1.8	9.6	2.5	169.4	61.8	106.5
Grand Junction	256,524	2.1	11.1	3.0	182.1	71.3	109.7
Greeley	266,422	2.4	12.5	3.2	169.4	62.6	105.7
Pueblo	145,620	2.6	13.2	2.8	193.4	70.9	121.5
Connecticut							
Bridgeport	630,305	2.1	11.0	2.6	258.8	83.2	174.4
Hartford	1,378,608	2.2	13.1	3.0	217.8	68.3	148.2
New Haven	1,352,675	2.0	11.4	2.5	236.8	74.6	161.0
Delaware							
Wilmington	688,879	2.0	11.7	2.8	186.9	65.5	120.4
District of Columbia							
Washington	2,261,708	2.7	13.5	3.4	268.6	84.5	182.7
Florida							
Bradenton	217,801	2.5	8.4	2.0	163.4	48.3	114.1
Clearwater	479,607	2.4	8.5	2.2	190.7	63.9	125.7
Fort Lauderdale	2,278,268	2.5	9.6	2.8	215.4	68.4	145.8
Fort Myers	759,101	2.5	10.7	2.6	171.4	54.5	115.9
Gainesville	470,775	2.6	12.2	3.2	170.1	61.8	107.3
Hudson	325,174	2.4	9.2	2.3	166.2	55.0	110.1
Jacksonville	1,304,471	2.8	13.5	3.3	181.0	59.9	120.2
Lakeland	315,828	2.5	9.5	2.5	146.7	48.8	97.2
Miami	2,654,961	3.0	12.1	3.3	229.7	83.0	146.3
Ocala	364,574	2.1	10.2	2.3	147.1	45.6	100.5
Orlando	2,640,954	2.5	12.3	3.2	162.8	54.0	107.9
Ormond Beach	309,939	2.5	9.6	2.3	160.2	54.9	104.4
Panama City	192,583	3.0	12.6	2.8	148.2	45.2	102.5
Pensacola	680,836	3.5	12.6	2.9	174.3	58.5	114.8
Sarasota	350,693	2.1	8.6	2.1	205.4	61.4	142.4
St Petersburg	396,332	2.8	11.9	3.2	202.9	69.0	132.9
Tallahassee	699,165	3.4	14.2	3.0	155.8	57.7	97.1
Tampa	979,089	2.7	11.3	2.8	181.4	60.0	120.4
Georgia							
Albany	209,269	3.9	15.5	3.3	124.1	40.6	83.1
Atlanta	4,568,206	2.7	11.9	3.2	173.0	56.6	115.5
Augusta	600,232	3.5	16.8	4.0	179.0	56.6	121.6
Columbus	318,114	4.1	12.1	2.9	144.7	52.0	91.8
Macon	649,109	3.7	15.9	4.5	167.5	58.3	108.2
Rome	238,137	2.9	12.7	3.0	159.9	63.2	95.7

Hospital Referral Region	Resident Population (1996)	Acute Care Hospital Beds per 1,000 Residents (1996)	Acute Care Hospital Employees per 1,000 Residents (1996)	Registered Nurses Employed in Acute Care Hospitals per 1,000 Residents (1996)	Physicians per 100,000 Residents (1996)	Primary Care Physicians per 100,000 Residents (1996)	Specialist Physicians per 100,000 Residents (1996)
Savannah	686,526	3.4	15.0	3.9	169.9	54.2	115.1
Hawaii							
Honolulu	1,190,945	2.0	11.5	2.9	208.7	75.8	132.0
Idaho							
Boise	654,939	2.1	10.5	2.8	156.8	51.0	105.0
Idaho Falls	180,953	2.7	11.1	3.2	127.6	37.9	89.6
Illinois							
Aurora	215,728	2.0	8.7	2.1	136.9	45.1	91.3
Bloomington	178,289	2.2	13.2	2.8	143.7	50.2	92.7
Blue Island	864,630	2.8	13.5	3.1	184.7	67.0	116.7
Chicago	2,571,452	4.4	21.9	5.0	225.4	84.5	140.2
Elgin	646,287	2.0	10.2	2.7	150.7	51.8	98.1
Evanston	878,796	2.4	13.2	3.1	276.1	98.1	177.4
Hinsdale	418,065	1.7	9.7	2.7	253.5	89.0	163.8
Joliet	494,800	3.2	13.5	3.0	166.6	54.7	111.0
Melrose Park	1,254,647	2.4	13.3	3.3	223.2	81.2	141.2
Peoria	608,273	3.1	15.7	3.9	148.0	53.3	93.7
Rockford	666,923	2.9	13.4	3.3	154.9	52.8	101.3
Springfield	839,901	3.1	14.3	3.5	140.3	52.0	87.3
Urbana	426,114	2.9	12.5	3.4	159.5	56.5	102.1
Indiana							
Evansville	661,028	3.5	15.0	3.7	143.4	53.8	88.5
Fort Wayne	804,774	2.6	12.0	3.0	131.5	48.2	82.4
Gary	497,400	3.9	15.0	4.0	146.0	50.6	94.5
Indianapolis	2,499,556	2.9	15.1	3.7	170.4	58.9	110.6
Lafayette	213,605	2.2	11.3	3.1	141.8	46.4	94.6
Muncie	168,681	2.9	13.3	3.4	160.8	59.0	101.0
Munster	300,199	3.6	15.4	4.3	159.6	58.4	100.3
South Bend	663,559	2.7	11.9	3.2	147.0	55.9	90.1
Terre Haute	179,339	3.0	15.4	4.6	153.2	55.2	96.8
Iowa							
Cedar Rapids	270,235	3.1	13.1	3.9	143.3	51.3	91.1
Davenport	493,041	3.3	15.7	3.6	155.0	52.9	101.3
Des Moines	971,099	3.3	16.0	3.7	155.9	63.3	91.6
Dubuque	150,147	3.3	13.3	3.9	152.4	48.9	102.7
Iowa City	320,338	3.1	14.9	4.0	174.0	58.5	114.5
Mason City	140,670	2.9	13.3	2.9	147.0	64.1	81.8
Sioux City	261,773	3.0	14.3	4.3	127.7	52.4	74.0
Waterloo	204,638	3.3	15.4	3.8	149.5	60.2	88.4
Kansas							
Topeka	423,555	3.0	14.0	3.5	154.0	52.1	101.1
Wichita	1,218,945	3.8	14.7	3.7	147.5	61.2	84.9
Kentucky							
Covington	352,122	2.5	13.0	3.6	159.1	58.7	99.4
Lexington	1,387,517	3.5	14.1	3.7	153.0	57.4	94.5
Louisville	1,560,881	3.1	14.1	3.7	176.0	59.6	115.5

Hospital Referral Region	Resident Population (1996)	Acute Care Hospital Beds per 1,000 Residents (1996)	Acute Care Hospital Employees per 1,000 Residents (1996)	Registered Nurses Employed in Acute Care Hospitals per 1,000 Residents (1996)	Physicians per 100,000 Residents (1996)	Primary Care Physicians per 100,000 Residents (1996)	Specialist Physicians per 100,000 Residents (1996)
Owensboro	139,868	2.9	12.9	3.9	134.8	40.9	93.2
Paducah	358,858	3.6	14.8	3.4	141.5	50.2	90.3
Louisiana							
Alexandria	275,946	4.4	17.6	3.9	164.1	59.5	103.5
Baton Rouge	788,489	3.2	14.4	3.7	152.5	52.7	99.0
Houma	252,997	3.8	17.8	3.8	132.2	37.0	95.3
Lafayette	570,302	4.0	15.2	3.1	141.3	48.2	92.3
Lake Charles	262,933	4.2	17.4	3.9	138.7	43.9	94.0
Metairie	428,303	3.9	16.2	3.7	251.8	68.5	181.8
Monroe	271,201	5.0	18.2	3.8	137.4	49.9	86.5
New Orleans	819,298	4.6	21.4	4.7	220.4	59.4	159.6
Shreveport	654,500	3.8	17.6	3.3	157.4	47.9	108.6
Slidell	168,087	3.4	14.6	3.7	164.9	46.7	117.5
Maine							
Bangor	391,225	2.9	16.0	4.7	170.3	65.4	103.9
Portland	981,998	2.5	13.3	3.1	200.8	73.0	126.9
Maryland							
Baltimore	2,315,565	2.9	16.0	4.1	250.3	82.6	166.7
Salisbury	344,316	2.7	13.8	3.1	189.1	62.6	125.5
Takoma Park	833,532	2.1	9.7	2.5	277.8	92.2	184.7
Massachusetts							
Boston	4,536,227	2.4	16.2	3.5	260.4	84.7	174.7
Springfield	714,878	2.6	12.5	3.0	202.0	71.9	129.2
Worcester	734,010	2.2	12.4	3.0	215.6	81.2	133.5
Michigan							
Ann Arbor	1,328,193	2.4	14.2	3.1	189.7	66.3	122.4
Dearborn	558,108	3.1	15.6	3.6	174.0	60.9	112.2
Detroit	1,902,947	3.4	18.6	4.4	175.8	61.2	113.6
Flint	578,915	3.3	16.3	3.7	163.8	71.6	90.7
Grand Rapids	1,069,910	2.1	12.2	3.1	154.1	57.4	95.6
Kalamazoo	649,268	2.7	12.7	3.4	166.8	60.2	105.6
Lansing	676,246	2.5	16.0	3.2	174.9	68.0	105.9
Marquette	196,487	3.4	17.0	2.9	153.0	59.5	92.5
Muskegon	258,550	2.8	12.9	2.7	155.0	63.7	89.9
Petoskey	168,676	2.7	12.2	3.1	168.0	65.3	101.6
Pontiac	453,016	2.4	13.8	3.3	252.5	84.2	167.1
Royal Oak	678,431	2.3	15.9	3.8	288.5	102.9	185.2
Saginaw	656,599	3.1	15.9	3.5	155.7	59.9	94.8
St Joseph	148,901	2.9	15.3	3.5	164.1	58.1	105.0
Traverse City	203,676	2.4	14.0	3.3	180.1	70.1	109.1
Minnesota							
Duluth	329,499	3.1	12.6	3.1	167.0	69.4	96.5
Minneapolis	2,842,544	2.4	11.4	2.6	169.7	68.0	100.5
Rochester	372,335	2.8	10.1	2.9	205.0	70.4	133.6
St Cloud	225,721	2.3	11.3	3.0	150.3	64.6	83.9
St Paul	930,373	2.3	11.5	2.5	188.4	80.4	106.6

Hospital Referral Region	Resident Population (1996)	Acute Care Hospital Beds per 1,000 Residents (1996)	Acute Care Hospital Employees per 1,000 Residents (1996)	Registered Nurses Employed in Acute Care Hospitals per 1,000 Residents (1996)	Physicians per 100,000 Residents (1996)	Primary Care Physicians per 100,000 Residents (1996)	Specialist Physicians per 100,000 Residents (1996)
Mississippi							
Gulfport	192,214	3.9	16.2	4.5	173.7	46.1	126.7
Hattiesburg	278,033	4.6	19.3	4.3	137.7	42.6	94.5
Jackson	1,018,753	4.6	16.9	3.7	149.0	52.3	95.8
Meridian	197,604	4.9	20.6	5.4	140.1	54.3	84.5
Oxford	133,965	4.5	16.2	3.3	139.7	50.2	88.6
Tupelo	377,136	4.1	15.5	3.8	123.3	46.1	76.3
Missouri							
Cape Girardeau	260,875	3.3	14.5	3.5	136.8	48.4	87.4
Columbia	632,078	3.1	16.4	3.9	157.3	59.4	96.9
Joplin	332,080	3.5	17.1	3.8	150.2	58.4	90.6
Kansas City	2,182,185	2.8	14.0	3.5	180.1	65.1	114.1
Springfield	722,224	2.8	14.3	3.2	144.3	55.7	87.6
St Louis	3,230,235	3.5	15.2	3.6	182.3	63.5	117.9
Montana							
Billings	507,831	2.9	14.9	3.2	177.7	65.0	111.7
Great Falls	151,459	3.2	14.5	3.1	175.4	61.8	112.5
Missoula	332,310	2.6	12.5	3.2	191.7	64.3	126.5
Nebraska							
Lincoln	535,346	3.1	12.3	3.3	134.4	56.3	76.8
Omaha	1,178,908	3.3	15.6	3.9	160.2	58.6	100.6
Nevada							
Las Vegas	1,221,192	1.9	7.4	2.2	148.8	47.4	100.6
Reno	593,823	2.4	11.3	3.0	179.9	59.6	119.3
New Hampshire							
Lebanon	372,811	3.0	14.9	3.6	200.8	74.2	125.6
Manchester	780,685	2.3	11.3	2.8	186.3	64.4	120.9
New Jersey							
Camden	2,628,556	2.8	14.0	3.5	218.8	73.5	144.2
Hackensack	1,163,380	3.3	14.2	3.6	299.6	99.9	198.3
Morristown	952,294	2.5	11.0	2.4	249.2	83.7	164.3
New Brunswick	911,993	2.8	12.2	2.9	236.4	82.8	152.7
Newark	1,436,059	4.6	19.6	4.7	216.6	74.7	141.0
Paterson	383,268	3.2	14.6	3.3	189.2	69.0	119.2
Ridgewood	400,623	2.7	11.6	3.3	263.2	84.6	177.5
New Mexico							
Albuquerque	1,447,898	2.3	15.6	3.2	194.6	71.0	122.5
New York							
Albany	1,740,557	3.0	13.3	3.4	201.4	66.2	134.1
Binghamton	365,205	2.8	14.0	3.0	172.7	58.5	113.3
Bronx	1,203,020	4.3	25.7	4.6	201.1	66.7	133.5
Buffalo	1,419,836	3.5	16.2	3.9	189.9	67.1	121.9
Elmira	330,134	3.4	15.5	3.8	185.7	59.1	125.7
East Long Island	4,310,790	3.1	14.2	3.4	273.7	96.4	176.6
New York	4,613,362	3.9	20.8	4.5	260.5	84.6	175.0
Rochester	1,265,140	2.8	15.3	3.4	195.6	72.6	122.1

Hospital Referral Region	Resident Population (1996)	Acute Care Hospital Beds per 1,000 Residents (1996)	Acute Care Hospital Employees per 1,000 Residents (1996)	Registered Nurses Employed in Acute Care Hospitals per 1,000 Residents (1996)	Physicians per 100,000 Residents (1996)	Primary Care Physicians per 100,000 Residents (1996)	Specialist Physicians per 100,000 Residents (1996)
Syracuse	1,064,721	2.9	14.0	3.3	173.2	57.7	114.5
White Plains	1,062,330	3.2	13.7	3.4	333.5	105.1	227.0
North Carolina							
Asheville	546,031	2.6	13.5	3.5	181.8	67.6	113.5
Charlotte	1,794,228	2.5	12.0	3.3	158.0	53.2	103.9
Durham	1,151,381	2.8	14.5	3.6	167.0	53.6	112.2
Greensboro	525,241	2.5	11.3	3.4	160.6	55.2	104.4
Greenville	732,499	3.1	14.2	3.8	155.7	52.0	102.9
Hickory	265,426	2.8	11.2	3.6	137.1	47.7	88.6
Raleigh	1,507,574	2.6	12.3	3.0	157.5	53.9	102.7
Wilmington	339,434	2.9	14.4	3.9	164.7	54.0	109.9
Winston-Salem	963,941	2.8	13.4	3.5	147.3	49.1	97.3
North Dakota							
Bismarck	202,507	4.8	19.3	4.3	154.5	54.4	98.9
Fargo Moorhead -Mn	487,416	2.9	12.7	3.3	138.7	60.4	76.5
Grand Forks	178,305	4.0	17.4	4.5	147.2	65.8	79.0
Minot	126,329	5.1	18.2	4.4	170.8	69.1	100.7
Ohio							
Akron	684,104	2.8	16.0	3.5	182.0	65.3	115.8
Canton	630,650	3.0	12.1	2.9	148.6	54.2	93.5
Cincinnati	1,589,519	2.8	14.1	3.1	192.8	64.8	127.1
Cleveland	2,128,355	3.3	16.4	3.9	210.2	71.0	138.1
Columbus	2,710,309	2.9	13.3	3.5	158.2	57.9	99.3
Dayton	1,107,868	3.0	15.3	4.2	147.7	55.3	91.4
Elyria	243,919	3.0	14.3	3.6	162.1	56.6	104.7
Kettering	392,795	2.4	12.6	3.2	210.5	76.7	133.0
Toledo	990,622	3.0	18.2	4.8	179.6	63.6	115.1
Youngstown	685,030	3.0	15.6	4.2	175.6	66.1	108.6
Oklahoma							
Lawton	190,085	3.4	15.6	2.3	154.1	62.6	90.0
Oklahoma City	1,658,264	3.3	14.3	3.2	160.9	58.0	101.8
Tulsa	1,221,114	3.1	13.9	3.0	161.9	62.8	98.0
Oregon							
Bend	158,393	2.3	9.8	2.9	171.1	60.2	110.0
Eugene	662,909	1.9	10.0	2.9	179.1	70.1	107.9
Medford	390,923	2.1	10.9	2.8	166.7	62.5	103.0
Portland	2,245,921	1.9	10.2	3.0	190.4	68.0	121.4
Salem	270,313	1.7	8.6	2.4	169.3	57.4	111.0
Pennsylvania							
Allentown	1,057,227	2.7	13.2	3.3	180.7	64.0	115.8
Altoona	299,897	2.9	13.1	3.4	148.4	53.2	94.3
Danville	550,736	2.8	13.7	3.2	170.3	60.9	108.6
Erie	733,910	3.5	14.6	3.8	159.8	54.2	104.7
Harrisburg	925,611	2.5	12.0	2.8	172.5	65.6	106.1
Johnstown	236,716	3.7	18.0	4.5	178.2	66.1	111.3
Lancaster	576,884	2.1	10.5	2.5	157.8	59.3	97.5

Hospital Referral Region	Resident Population (1996)	Acute Care Hospital Beds per 1,000 Residents (1996)	Acute Care Hospital Employees per 1,000 Residents (1996)	Registered Nurses Employed in Acute Care Hospitals per 1,000 Residents (1996)	Physicians per 100,000 Residents (1996)	Primary Care Physicians per 100,000 Residents (1996)	Specialist Physicians per 100,000 Residents (1996)
Philadelphia	3,873,168	3.2	16.2	4.2	263.5	89.4	173.1
Pittsburgh	2,998,859	3.5	16.2	4.1	191.9	64.5	126.4
Reading	532,259	2.6	11.8	2.7	166.0	62.4	102.8
Sayre	194,643	3.2	12.3	3.4	158.3	58.1	99.1
Scranton	297,688	3.2	13.4	3.5	190.2	69.6	119.7
Wilkes-Barre	248,402	3.5	13.0	3.1	200.1	78.6	120.9
York	376,089	2.0	10.6	2.6	161.7	64.3	96.4
Rhode Island							
Providence	1,144,116	2.4	13.1	2.8	209.6	72.4	136.3
South Carolina							
Charleston	756,108	3.3	14.1	3.9	180.0	57.9	121.2
Columbia	1,069,366	2.9	13.6	3.3	163.4	55.1	107.4
Florence	359,522	3.6	18.4	4.4	132.7	50.9	80.4
Greenville	760,317	2.3	11.2	3.1	164.9	58.8	105.2
Spartanburg	334,961	3.0	13.8	3.6	146.2	51.4	93.9
South Dakota							
Rapid City	197,999	3.5	14.6	3.4	172.0	71.6	98.9
Sioux Falls	724,678	3.8	14.9	4.1	149.6	63.6	84.5
Tennessee							
Chattanooga	603,002	3.1	13.7	3.2	161.2	55.8	104.6
Jackson	304,310	3.3	12.9	2.9	135.0	55.0	79.0
Johnson City	237,376	3.3	12.5	3.5	189.9	72.0	117.3
Kingsport	476,614	3.6	14.8	3.5	160.8	62.5	97.5
Knoxville	1,188,258	3.1	13.9	3.0	164.7	60.1	103.7
Memphis	1,689,602	3.6	14.5	3.4	149.9	49.5	99.6
Nashville	2,260,204	3.1	12.8	3.4	168.4	57.7	109.8
Texas							
Abilene	285,708	3.2	15.3	3.6	154.0	55.8	97.2
Amarillo	414,423	4.0	15.8	3.7	152.0	54.0	97.0
Austin	1,134,631	1.7	8.1	2.0	179.3	62.6	115.7
Beaumont	451,778	4.2	14.9	3.6	162.8	55.7	106.2
Bryan	203,261	2.3	10.7	2.6	145.3	58.7	85.7
Corpus Christi	546,890	3.1	13.9	3.3	156.8	55.1	100.8
Dallas	3,590,270	2.6	12.4	3.3	168.3	54.0	113.4
El Paso	969,472	2.4	10.1	2.5	141.7	41.6	99.8
Fort Worth	1,633,143	2.2	11.5	3.0	152.8	53.0	99.0
Harlingen	474,701	2.6	10.2	2.5	100.4	34.0	65.8
Houston	4,890,132	2.9	13.8	3.3	171.3	53.4	117.1
Longview	184,802	2.7	13.2	3.6	138.0	48.9	88.1
Lubbock	658,346	4.2	15.9	3.3	153.0	54.5	97.3
McAllen	458,251	2.3	8.0	2.2	88.2	33.8	53.3
Odessa	322,637	3.4	13.8	3.2	124.3	36.4	87.6
San Angelo	156,797	3.6	13.9	3.2	156.5	50.7	104.9
San Antonio	2,131,335	2.4	10.9	2.7	182.7	55.9	126.0
Temple	384,620	2.2	12.0	2.6	124.1	44.9	78.1
Tyler	467,199	3.0	16.4	3.3	164.1	57.9	105.1

Hospital Referral Region	Resident Population (1996)	Acute Care Hospital Beds per 1,000 Residents (1996)	Acute Care Hospital Employees per 1,000 Residents (1996)	Registered Nurses Employed in Acute Care Hospitals per 1,000 Residents (1996)	Physicians per 100,000 Residents (1996)	Primary Care Physicians per 100,000 Residents (1996)	Specialist Physicians per 100,000 Residents (1996)
Victoria	143,410	4.1	16.3	3.4	156.7	54.9	101.0
Waco	315,426	2.5	11.9	2.2	151.4	54.9	95.7
Wichita Falls	200,911	3.4	12.9	2.5	172.2	60.1	111.1
Utah							
Ogden	359,938	2.4	10.9	2.9	137.1	41.7	95.3
Provo	397,951	2.2	12.1	3.5	131.5	43.5	87.6
Salt Lake City	1,658,407	2.4	12.3	3.4	155.6	48.3	107.1
Vermont							
Burlington	615,795	2.7	13.7	3.3	192.7	74.0	117.7
Virginia							
Arlington	1,739,167	1.7	7.5	2.1	208.3	70.2	137.1
Charlottesville	476,957	2.5	13.9	3.7	188.2	63.1	124.0
Lynchburg	223,604	2.5	10.8	3.6	145.6	53.6	91.1
Newport News	515,588	2.6	10.1	2.8	181.0	62.3	117.7
Norfolk	1,206,838	2.7	12.1	3.3	192.7	63.1	128.8
Richmond	1,409,630	3.1	12.6	3.6	174.7	63.7	110.1
Roanoke	667,289	3.2	13.4	2.8	177.1	63.0	113.2
Winchester	332,681	2.8	11.8	3.4	159.1	51.2	107.0
Washington							
Everett	538,759	1.4	8.5	2.1	173.3	65.1	106.9
Olympia	333,084	1.9	9.7	2.2	170.7	63.0	106.6
Seattle	2,400,372	1.7	10.4	2.5	219.3	80.9	137.6
Spokane	1,289,475	2.4	10.3	2.7	172.2	65.8	105.2
Tacoma	680,235	1.8	9.7	2.2	179.7	59.8	119.0
Yakima	266,554	2.1	10.2	2.6	161.4	63.7	96.0
West Virginia							
Charleston	861,102	3.6	16.3	4.1	167.0	65.5	100.5
Huntington	355,189	3.9	15.2	4.0	167.3	61.5	104.9
Morgantown	384,194	3.1	14.3	3.4	174.1	64.9	108.5
Wisconsin							
Appleton	289,435	2.0	10.0	2.5	142.4	58.4	82.7
Green Bay	483,369	2.5	12.1	3.1	143.0	51.9	90.2
La Crosse	333,001	2.8	12.7	3.1	159.2	60.8	97.4
Madison	955,035	2.6	12.4	2.9	168.7	69.1	98.7
Marshfield	362,544	3.0	10.9	2.9	174.5	68.2	105.2
Milwaukee	2,457,959	2.7	12.4	3.0	190.3	64.4	124.9
Neenah	218,296	2.7	12.2	3.3	163.7	57.0	105.9
Wausau	184,306	2.0	10.9	2.5	168.4	65.0	102.5
Wyoming							
Casper	171,849	4.0	15.6	4.4	177.3	69.6	106.6
United States							
	269,442,661	2.8	13.2	3.3	188.9	65.0	122.9

Variations, Patient Need, Practice Style and Hospital Capacity

Variations, Patient Need, Practice Style and Hospital Capacity

Medical science provides clear guidelines about the need to hospitalize patients with some conditions. For patients with these conditions, the need for specific kinds of care determines what will be done, and the use of medical resources is not influenced by either the physician's practice style or the per capita supply of hospital beds in the region. For example, patients with hip fractures are almost always hospitalized, because of the severity of their pain and the need for inpatient operative repair. Similarly, patients with newly diagnosed colorectal cancers are almost always hospitalized, because major bowel surgery is the universally-accepted method of treating the disease.

But for many other conditions, medical science and theory are weak, and the rules of clinical practice are not nearly so clear cut. In the majority of cases of pneumonia, relapses of chronic pulmonary obstructive disease, or episodes of congestive heart failure, patients might be treated either in the hospital or in another setting (at home or in a nursing home, for example). When medical science is unclear, physicians must be guided by their subjective opinions about the effectiveness of admitting such patients to hospitals, rather than providing treatment in another setting. The variations among regions in admission rates of patients with these conditions can be ascribed to differences in clinical decision making, rather than to differences in underlying illness rates.

When science-based guidelines are weak, physicians' decisions are also influenced by a largely invisible factor: the capacity of the acute care hospital environment in which they practice. There is strong evidence that for the majority of conditions, decisions about hospitalization are dependent on physicians' opinions, which are influenced by local hospital capacity (although physicians are not aware of the per capita bed supply). The result is that variations in the rates of hospitalization for most conditions are driven by supply, rather than need.

The Patterns of Hospitalization for Treatment of Hip Fracture and Colorectal Cancer

Rates of hospitalization for hip fracture reflect the actual incidence of disease for several reasons. First, people with hip fractures are virtually certain to seek care, because the condition is extremely painful, and the need for medical attention is easily recognized. Second, once the patient reaches medical care, it is virtually certain that the fracture will be diagnosed correctly. Third, it is virtually certain that the attending physician will admit the patient to a hospital bed, because there is unanimity within the medical profession about the necessity of hospitalization.

The geographic pattern of variation in rates of hip fracture is, however, somewhat surprising (Map 3.1). People who lived in northern parts of the United States, where hip fracture rates might be expected to be higher because of the wintertime risk of slipping on ice and snow, actually had lower rates of hip fractures than people in the broad band stretching across the mid-South from North Carolina to New Mexico. This phenomenon is unexplained.

Variations in rates of hospitalizations for colectomy reflect variations in the incidence of colorectal cancer, rather than differences in treatment strategies. As with hip fractures, there is agreement among physicians on the need for immediate treatment. For patients with no evidence of metastasis, colon resection is performed in the hope of a long-term cure. For those whose cancers have spread to distant sites, tumors are removed to keep them from obstructing or perforating the colon.

There were some regional differences in the incidence of colectomy for colorectal cancer (Map 3.2). Colectomy was more common among people living in the East and parts of the Midwest; it was less common among residents of some areas of Southern and Western states.

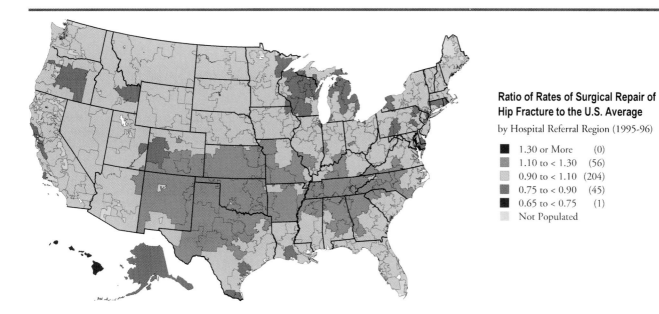

Ratio of Rates of Surgical Repair of Hip Fracture to the U.S. Average

by Hospital Referral Region (1995-96)

- ■ 1.30 or More   (0)
- ■ 1.10 to < 1.30   (56)
- ▨ 0.90 to 1.10   (204)
- ▨ 0.75 to < 0.90   (45)
- ■ 0.65 to < 0.75   (1)
- ▨ Not Populated

Map 3.1. Rates of Surgical Repair of Hip Fracture (1995-96)

There was little variation in rates of surgery to repair hip fractures or to treat colorectal cancers. Only a few hospital referral regions had rates of either procedure more than 30% higher than the national average, or more than 25% below the average. Differences in rates of the procedures, which closely reflect rates of underlying disease, appear to be related to environmental factors or other causes which resulted in higher than average rates of hip fracture in the mid-United States and lower than average rates of colorectal cancers in the Western states.

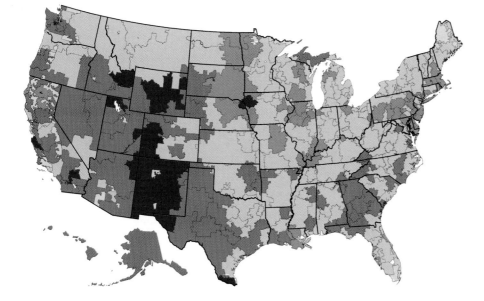

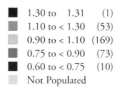

Ratio of Rates of Colectomy for Colorectal Cancer to the U.S. Average

by Hospital Referral Region (1995-96)

- ■ 1.30 to 1.31   (1)
- ■ 1.10 to < 1.30   (53)
- ▨ 0.90 to 1.10   (169)
- ▨ 0.75 to < 0.90   (73)
- ■ 0.60 to < 0.75   (10)
- ▨ Not Populated

Map 3.2. Rates of Colectomy for Colorectal Cancer (1995-96)

Need, Not Hospital Capacity, Drives Hip Fracture and Colectomy Hospitalization Rates

In the early 1960s, Milton Roemer proposed that hospital beds, once built, will be used, no matter how many there are. But Roemer's law does not apply equally to all conditions. Hospital capacity has no influence on the rate of hospitalization for hip fractures; the decision is based on professional consensus. Likewise, there is consensus that patients with newly-diagnosed colorectal cancer should be admitted to the hospital for colectomy. When all diagnosed cases are hospitalized, and the diagnosis itself is codified in an easily applied and highly specific set of rules, need drives hospitalization, and hospitalization rates are independent of the available supply of hospital beds. For these conditions, and for a handful of others, there would be a correlation between hospitalization rates and hospital beds per capita only if the number of hospital beds in a community had been determined by, among other things, the known population-based incidence rates of very low variation conditions such as colon cancer and hip fracture.

There is, in fact, little relationship between actual acute care hospital bed capacity and the incidence of colon cancer and hip fracture (Figure 3.1).

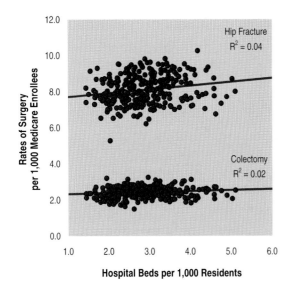

Figure 3.1. The Relationship Between the Supply of Acute Care Hospital Beds (1996) and Rates of Surgery for Hip Fracture and Rates of Colectomy for Colorectal Cancer (1995-96)

There was little relationship between regional supplies of acute care hospital beds and rates of surgery for the repair of hip fractures (R^2 = .04) or rates of colectomy for colorectal cancer (R^2 = .02).

Variations in Discharges for Medical Conditions

An important question is whether rates of admissions for repair of hip fractures and for colectomy, which are based on the rates of the conditions themselves, are the exception or the rule. Traditionally, small area analysis has approached this question by looking at the variations in Medicare hospitalization rates for modified diagnostic-related groups, or M-DRGs (see the Appendix on Methods for an explanation of the methods and codes used to construct M-DRGs). For the Atlas, this method was used to calculate hospitalization rates for each of 60 medical (non-surgical) conditions. The range of variation was estimated using the systematic component of variation, or SCV. The conditions were then put into four groups:

■ SCV less than hip fracture: low variation conditions

■ SCV between hip fracture and peripheral vascular disorders: moderate variation conditions

■ SCV between peripheral vascular disorders and biliary disorders: high variation conditions

■ SCV greater than biliary disorders: very high variation conditions

None of the 60 medical M-DRGs had hospitalization rates that were less variable than hip fracture. Only six M-DRGs, representing 13.8% of medical hospitalizations, were moderately variable conditions. Twenty-five M-DRGs (49.2% of all medical hospitalizations) were high variation conditions, and 29 (37.0% of medical hospitalization) were very high variation conditions.

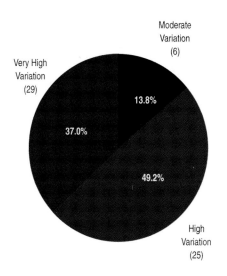

Figure 3.2. Percent of Hospitalizations for Medical Major Diagnosis-Related Groups According to Degree of Variation in Discharge Rates (1994-95)

The figure shows the proportion of medical M-DRGs according to the degree of variation in their discharge rates. Most causes of hospitalization have high or very high patterns of variation. The number of M-DRGs in each group is given in parentheses.

Variations in the Rates of Discharges for Medical Conditions

Discharges for all medical (non-surgical) conditions — that is, for all 60 medical M-DRGs, taken as a group — varied by a factor of almost 2.5, even after adjustment for age, sex race and illness differences among populations. Discharge rates ranged from 134 discharges per 1,000 Medicare enrollees in the Salem, Oregon hospital referral region to 330 per 1,000 enrollees among residents of the hospital referral region in Meridian, Mississippi.

Among the hospital referral regions where there were more than 300 discharges for medical conditions per 1,000 Medicare residents were Monroe, Louisiana (328); Slidell, Louisiana (321); Hattiesburg, Mississippi (311); and Alexandria, Louisiana (307). Rates were substantially lower than the national average of 227 discharges per 1,000 Medicare residents in Ogden, Utah (152); Bend, Oregon (156); Tacoma, Washington (157); Medford, Oregon (160); and San Mateo County, California (161).

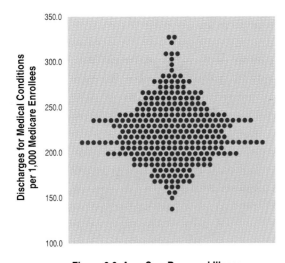

Figure 3.3. Age, Sex, Race and Illness Adjusted Discharges for All Medical Conditions (1995-96)

Rates of discharges for medical conditions ranged from fewer than 150 per 1,000 Medicare enrollees to more than 325. Each point represents one of the 306 hospital referral regions in the United States.

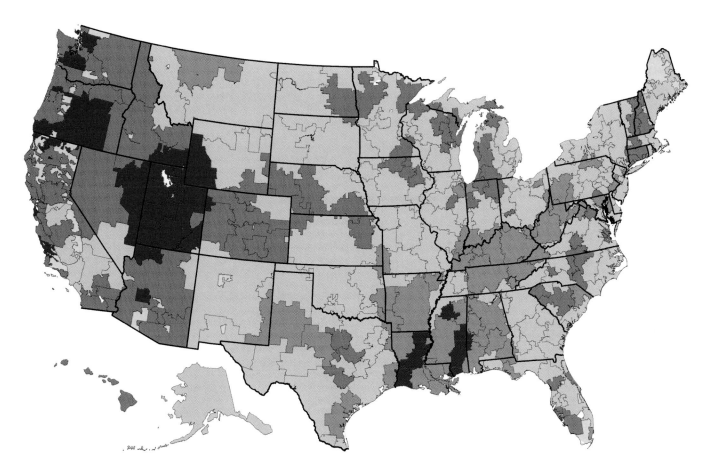

Map 3.3. Discharges for All Medical Conditions (1995-96)

Medical discharges were higher than the national average in hospital referral regions in much of the South. Rates were lower than the national average, generally, in the West and in parts of New England and the Great Lakes states.

Ratio of Rates of Discharges for All Medical Conditions to the U.S. Average

by Hospital Referral Region (1995-96)

■	1.30 to 1.46 (8)
▨	1.10 to < 1.30 (52)
▨	0.90 to < 1.10 (155)
▨	0.75 to < 0.90 (79)
■	0.59 to < 0.75 (12)
▢	Not Populated

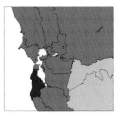

San Francisco

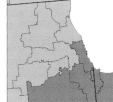

Chicago

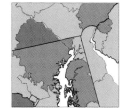

New York

Washington-Baltimore

Detroit

Rates of Medical Discharges
Are Not Adequately Explained by Variations in Rates of Illness

Although some rates of hospital admissions are influenced by local incidence of disease (as in areas which have higher than average rates of hip fracture or colon cancer), at the level of hospital referral regions, less than 30% of the variation in medical discharges can be explained by differences in population age, sex, race or illness. It is possible to demonstrate this phenomenon by making statistical adjustments to population rates to take into account differences in population age, sex, race, and illness, and then to look at how much such adjustments change the overall pattern of variation in rates.

In Figure 3.4, the left-hand distribution is the crude, or unadjusted, rate of discharges for medical conditions among the 306 hospital referral regions in the United States. The distribution in the center is the age, sex, race and illness adjusted distribution of the discharge rates. Adjustment for these factors has a modest effect on the pattern of variation.

The column on the right in Figure 3.4 gives a visual representation of what the variation would look like if utilization were based solely on age, sex, race and illness in hospital referral regions.

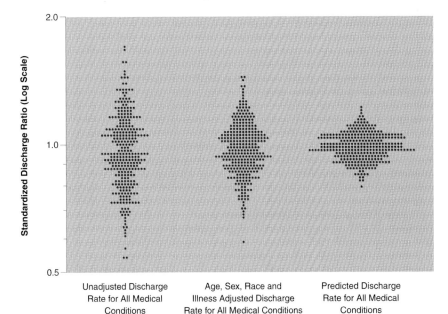

Standardized Discharge Ratio (Log Scale)

2.0

1.0

0.5

Unadjusted Discharge Rate for All Medical Conditions

Age, Sex, Race and Illness Adjusted Discharge Rate for All Medical Conditions

Predicted Discharge Rate for All Medical Conditions

Figure 3.4. Rates of Discharges for All Medical Conditions: Unadjusted, Adjusted for Differences in Age, Sex, Race, and Illness, and Predicted, Compared to the U.S. Average (1995-96)

Adjustment for differences in population age, sex, race, and illness characteristics has little effect on the variation. The range of variation is hardly changed, and the numbers of hospital referral regions with high and low rates remain about the same. The right-hand column estimates what the variation in rates of utilization for medical conditions would look like, if utilization were based on age, sex, race and illness rates alone.

Table 3.1. Statistical Measures of Variation of Rates of Medical Discharges, Unadjusted; Age, Sex and Race Adjusted; and Age, Sex, Race and Illness Adjusted (1995-96)

	Unadjusted Rate	Age, Sex and Race Adjusted Rate	Age, Sex, Race and Illness Adjusted Rate
Minimum	121.9	121.9	134.3
Maximum	390.2	359.9	330.3
Extremal Ratio	3.2	3.0	2.5
1st Quartile	190.2	192.1	201.2
3rd Quartile	248.6	251.9	242.4
Interquartile Ratio	1.3	1.3	1.2
Coefficient of Variation	20.6	19.6	14.7

Statistical measures of variation confirm that most of the variation is due to other factors (Table 3.1). The coefficient of variation shows little change after the adjustment for age, sex, and race; the range of variation is hardly changed, and the numbers of hospital referral regions with high and low rates remain about the same. The coefficient of variation of the unadjusted rate is 20.6; age, sex and race adjustment only reduces the coefficient of variation to 19.6, or about 4.9%. The ratio of the rates in the highest region to rates in the lowest region is reduced from 3.20 to 3.0. The additional adjustment for illness reduces the coefficient of variation to 14.7, or about 28.9% below the coefficient of variation for the unadjusted rate. The ratio of the highest to the lowest region is reduced to 2.5.

Maps 3.4a and 3.4b demonstrate the same information in another way. Map 3.4a is the actual distribution of discharges for medical conditions, and Map 3.4b predicts what the distribution would be expected to be if utilization were determined by illness (both are compared to the United States average).

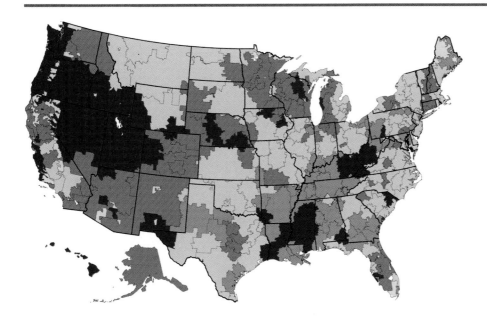

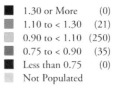

Ratio of Unadjusted Discharge Rates for All Medical Conditions to the U.S. Average

by Hospital Referral Region (1995-96)

- 1.30 to 1.72   (20)
- 1.10 to < 1.30   (54)
- 0.90 to < 1.10 (120)
- 0.75 to < 0.90   (77)
- 0.53 to < 0.75   (35)
- Not Populated

Map 3.4a. Actual Discharge Rates for All Medical Conditions (1995-96)

There is substantial variation among hospital referral regions in actual rates of Medicare discharges for medical conditions, from 47% below the national average to 72% above it. The range of variation predicted on the basis of age, sex, race and illness rates varies much less, from 20% below the United States average to 23% above it.

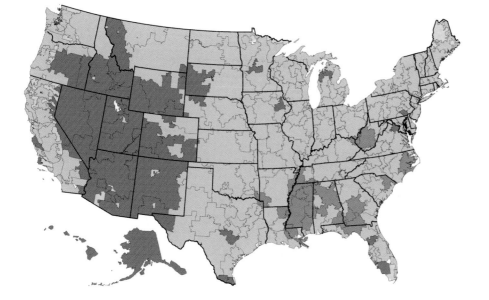

Ratio of Predicted Discharge Rates for All Medical Conditions to the U.S. Average

by Hospital Referral Region (1995-96)

- 1.30 or More   (0)
- 1.10 to < 1.30   (21)
- 0.90 to < 1.10 (250)
- 0.75 to < 0.90   (35)
- Less than 0.75   (0)
- Not Populated

Map 3.4b. Predicted Discharge Rates for Medical Conditions, If Utilization Were Determined by Illness (1995-96)

Hospital Capacity Matters

Roemer's law connecting hospital supply to hospital utilization accurately predicts the association between hospital beds and hospitalization rates for all medical conditions (R^2 = .56).

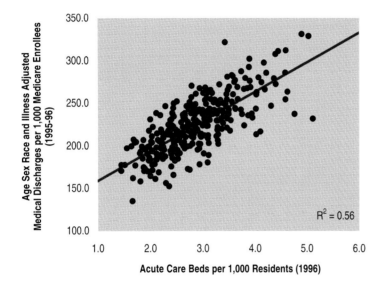

Figure 3.5. The Association Between Hospital Beds per 1,000 Residents and Age, Sex, Race and Illness Adjusted Hospitalization Rates for Medical Conditions per 1,000 Medicare Enrollees

More than half of the variability in rates of hospitalization for medical conditions can be attributed to differences in local supplies of acute care hospital beds (R^2 = .56).

Self-Reported Health Status
Does Not Predict Hospital Use or the Supply of Hospital Beds

Are the numbers of hospital beds per 1,000 residents determined by illness rates? One way of testing whether capacity follows demand is to ask whether the patients' own assessments of illness predict the level of bed supply. To test this hypothesis, we divided the Medicare Current Beneficiary Sample into five roughly equal groups, according to the number of hospital beds per 1,000 residents in the 306 hospital referral regions. Self-reported health status was used to predict hospitalization rates for residents living in each quintile (see the Appendix on Methods for further details). The actual use of hospitals, measured in patient days per person, was also calculated (Table 3.2).

The results indicate that utilization follows supply. Residents of regions with higher per capita supplies of hospital beds had higher rates of hospitalization than residents of regions with lower per capita supplies of hospital beds. Residents of the region with the lowest per capita supply of hospital beds used, on average, 1.6 hospital bed days per year; those living in the region with the highest per capita supply of beds used 2.6 hospital days per person per year.

The research failed to find evidence that greater numbers of hospital beds (and the associated increase in hospitalization rates) occurred because residents of high rate areas were sicker — there was no evidence, in other words, that the supply of acute care hospital resources has developed in response to demand for medical hospital-izations. Predicted demand for hospital days based on self-reported health status was the same in the regions in the lowest quintile of per capita supply of hospital beds as in the region in the highest quintile — about 2.2 days per person per year.

While health needs (at least those reflected by self-reported illness) are a powerful predictor of the demand for health care at the level of the individual patient, health needs do not explain the distribution of hospital beds, nor are they an important factor in determining variations in the rates of hospital utilization among hospital referral regions.

Table 3.2. Actual and Predicted Days in Hospitals (1993)

Rates of hospitalizations do not reflect population health status; predicted demand, based on self-reported health status, was the same in the regions in the lowest quintile of per capita supply of hospital beds as in the region in the highest quintile — about 2.2 days per person per year.

(1) Quintile of Beds	(2) Beds/1,000 (Range)	(3) Actual Hospital Days	(4) Hospital Days as Predicted by Health Status
1 Bottom 20%	<2.9	1.6	2.2
2 Second 20%	2.9–3.2	1.8	2.1
3 Middle 20%	3.2–3.5	2.0	2.2
4 Fourth 20%	3.5–3.9	2.6	2.2
5 Highest 20%	>3.9	2.6	2.2

Data Source: Medicare Current Beneficiary Survey, Atlas Data

The Effect of Capacity on Clinical Decision Making

Intuitively, it makes sense that illness determines the use of health care — that sicker people use more care than those who are less sick — and research confirms that this is true. For example, in a survey conducted by the Medicare program, Medicare enrollees who reported their health status as "poor" spent 2.8 times as many days in hospitals as those who reported their health to be "excellent" (Figure 3.6a).

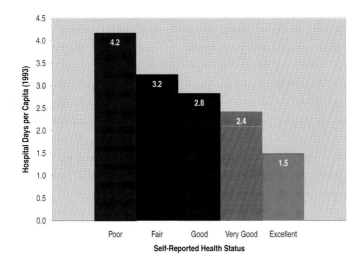

Figure 3.6a. Average Hospital Days Stratified by Self-Reported Health (1993)
The average number of hospital days corresponds to Medicare enrollees' self-reported health status; enrollees who report themselves to have better health status use fewer days of hospital care.

Yet while illness is indeed important in determining who receives care, differences in illness rates between communities have very little to do with the relative per capita amounts of hospital care that residents of a given community consume. The amount of hospital care consumed is determined by something that neither the physician nor the patient is even aware of: the per capita supply of hospital beds in the community in which the physician practices.

How does acute care hospital bed capacity affect clinical decision making? It is commonly assumed that physicians work under some standard set of rules of practice, and that their decisions about whether or not to admit a given patient to the hospital are made according to a set of rules which dictate that the sickest, most needy patient is the first to be hospitalized, the second most needy is the second to be hospitalized, and so on.

But the sorting processes are not nearly so rational, and the influence of capacity is not solely on the low end of the severity continuum. Capacity actually has an effect on physicians' decisions to admit patients with a broad spectrum of demographic characteristics, clinical conditions and severity of illness. The effect of capacity in setting the thermostat for hospitalization can be illustrated in several ways:

■ **Demographic characteristics.** The capacity effect is independent of race and income (Figure 3.6b).

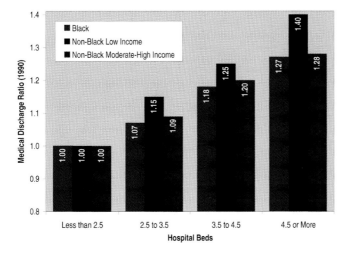

Figure 3.6b. Relative Odds of Discharge for Medical Conditions According to Race and Income and Hospital Bed Capacity in Region of Residence (1990)

For each race and income group, the rates of discharges are standardized to the rate in the hospital referral regions with the lowest supply of hospital beds. Greater capacity results in more hospitalizations for all demographic groups. For example, for non-black, low income populations, the medical discharge rate is 40% higher for those living in the hospital referral regions with the highest supplies of hospital beds per 1,000 residents than for residents of regions with the lowest supplies of hospital beds. (For further details, see the Endnote.)

■ **Illness levels.** The capacity effect influences risk of hospitalization across all levels of reported health status (Figure 3.6c).

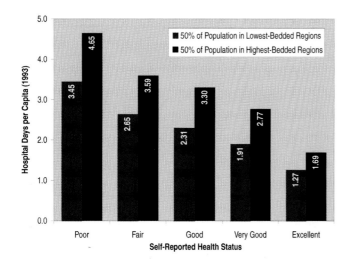

Figure 3.6c. Self-Reported Health Status Segmented by Hospital Referral Regions with High and Low Supplies of Hospital Beds (1993)
The left-hand (red) bars represent the populations living in the hospital referral regions with low supplies of hospital beds; the right-hand (black) bars represent those in hospital referral regions with high supplies of hospital beds per 1,000 residents. The vertical axis is the average number of days spent in hospitals; the horizontal axis is self-reported health status. Medicare enrollees living in hospital referral regions with higher numbers of beds per 1,000 residents had higher hospitalization rates, independent of reported health status.

■ **The proportion hospitalized.** The capacity effect influences the proportion of the population exposed to hospitalization (suggesting that the less seriously ill are admitted more often in regions with more hospital beds) (Figure 3.6d).

Figure 3.6d. Percent of Population Hospitalized at Least Once, According to Race and Income and Hospital Bed Capacity in the Hospital Referral Region of Residence (1990)
For each race and income group, the percent hospitalized is an increasing function of hospital bed capacity. (For further details, see the Endnote.)

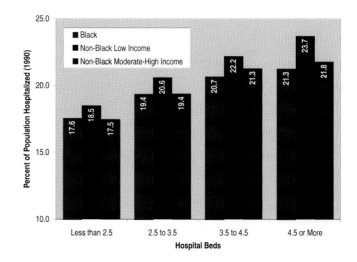

■ **The intensity of treatment of the very sick.** Capacity influences the intensity of terminal care for Medicare enrollees (Figure 3.6e). Medicare residents of areas with high per capita supplies of acute care beds are more likely to die as inpatients in hospitals (Figure 3.6e) and are more likely to be admitted to intensive care units during their last six months of life (Chapter Six).

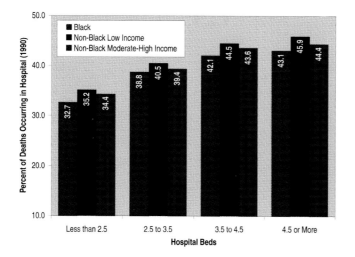

Figure 3.6e. Percent of All Deaths Among Medicare Enrollees That Occurred in Hospitals, According to Race and Income and Hospital Bed Capacity in the Hospital Referral Region of Residence (1990)
For each race and income group, the percent who died in hospitals is an increasing function of hospital bed capacity. (For further details, see the Endnote.)

Variation Among Regions Served by Academic Medical Centers

Another common assumption concerning geographic variations is that they occur because some physicians fail to practice according to the dictates of scientific medicine. Yet the pattern of hospitalizations in communities served primarily by academic medical centers provides no evidence of an underlying scientific consensus on "best practices," raising the question of whether there is such a thing as a scientific standard. Figure 3.7 shows the pattern of variation in hospitalizations for medical conditions among the 96 communities in the United States containing at least one medical school.

The discharge rates in these communities span the range of variation seen in the United States as a whole. The academic hospital referral region with the highest discharge rate for medical conditions is Lexington, Kentucky, home of the University of Kentucky College of Medicine, where the rate is 2.2 times higher than the academic hospital referral region in Salt Lake City, Utah, which comprises the University of Utah School of Medicine. The Baltimore hospital referral region, home of the Johns Hopkins and University of Maryland medical schools, has discharge rates 48% higher than the hospital referral region in Seattle, home of the University of Washington School of Medicine. The Birmingham, Alabama hospital referral region, which is home of the University of Alabama School of Medicine, has a medical discharge rate 30% higher than the rate in the New Haven hospital referral region, home of Yale Medical School. The hospital referral region in Nashville, Tennessee, home of Vanderbilt University School of Medicine, had a medical discharge rate more than 35% higher than the rate in the Columbia, South Carolina hospital referral region, home of the University of South Carolina School of Medicine.

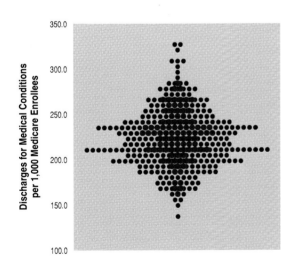

Figure 3.7. Age, Sex, Race, and Illness Adjusted Rates of Discharges for Medical Conditions in Hospital Referral Regions With One or More Medical Schools (1995-96)

Red points represent hospital referral regions that contain academic medical centers. Blue points represent hospital referral regions without medical schools.

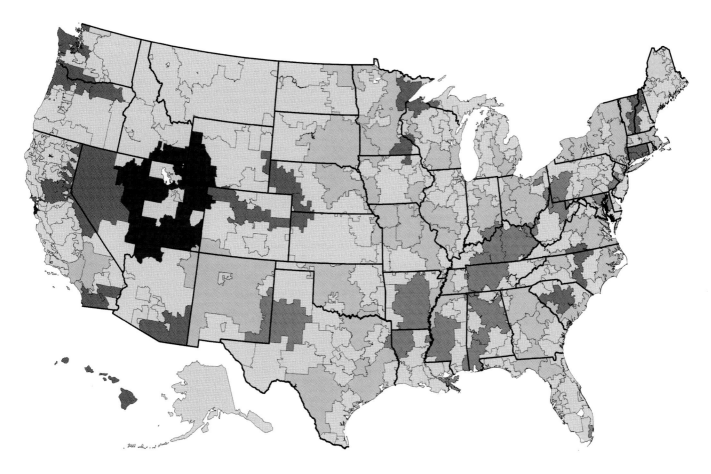

Map 3.5. Rates of Medical Discharges in Hospital Referral Regions With One or More Medical Schools (1995-96)

The table at the end of the chapter includes rates of discharges for medical conditions in communities with one or more medical schools.

Ratio of Rates of Discharges for Medical Conditions in HRRs With One or More Medical Schools to the U.S. Average (1995-96)

- 1.30 or More (0)
- 1.10 to < 1.30 (19)
- 0.90 to < 1.10 (59)
- 0.75 to < 0.90 (16)
- 0.59 to < 0.75 (2)
- No Medical School
- Not Populated

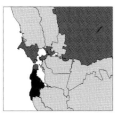

San Francisco

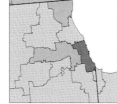

Chicago

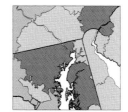

New York

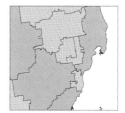

Washington-Baltimore

Detroit

The Threshold for Hospitalizing Residents of Boston and New Haven

The populations living in the Boston and New Haven hospital service areas are remarkably similar in demographic features and other factors that predict the need for care. Most Bostonians and New Havenites, when they are hospitalized, are admitted to hospitals associated with some of the nation's most prestigious medical schools. Such an advantage would seem to assure that residents of these communities are treated in the best, most scientific, high-quality way. Yet, in reality, "high quality" is defined very differently in the two communities.

For decades, and perhaps longer, the per capita amount of care provided to residents of Boston has been about 60% higher than the per capita amount provided to residents of New Haven. The most consistent differences between Boston and New Haven are in their per capita supplies of hospital beds, and the rates at which residents of the two communities are admitted to hospitals for medical conditions. Capacity, not medical science, drives the rates of hospitalizations, even in regions served by distinguished teaching hospitals.

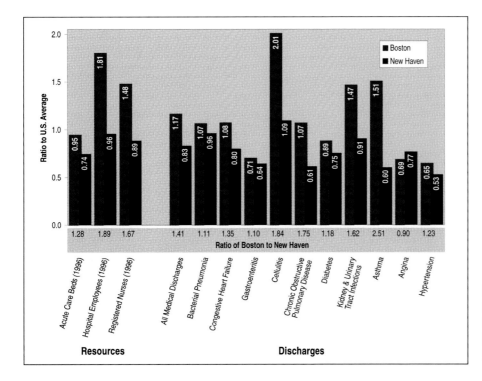

Figure 3.8. Acute Care Hospital Resources and the Medical Signatures of the Boston and New Haven Hospital Service Areas (1995-96)

Hospitalization Rates for Cohorts Living in Boston and New Haven

Another way of characterizing the threshold effect of capacity is to examine the patterns of hospitalization among patient cohorts with similar diseases. A cohort study of patients living in Boston and New Haven looked at all patients who were hospitalized with those few conditions for which need, not hospital capacity, is the major determinant of hospitalization. Five cohorts were formed: those with hip fracture, colectomy for colorectal cancer, stroke, heart attack (acute myocardial infarction) and bleeding from the gastrointestinal tract. Beginning at the moment of discharge for the need-driven hospitalization, the subsequent re-hospitalizations of members of these cohorts were recorded for up to three years. The risk of rehospitalization was about 60% higher for patients living in Boston than for those in New Haven. The readmissions were for a broad spectrum of conditions. The cohort study method yields essentially the same result as traditional small area analysis, with an added, important advantage: comparisons can be made according to patient illness characteristics.

We used this advantage to further characterize the effect of capacity on the propensity to hospitalize. The differences in readmission rates occurred in all illness groups, in all age groups, for men as well as women and for blacks as well as non-blacks. Patients living in Boston were hospitalized 60% more often than patients in New Haven.

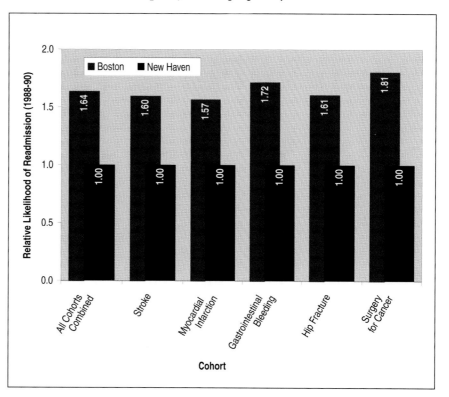

Figure 3.9. The Relative Likelihood of Readmission for Any Reason After Index Admission to Hospitals in the Boston and New Haven Hospital Service Areas (1988-90)
Source: "Hospital Readmission Rates for Cohorts of Medicare Beneficiaries in Boston and New Haven," Fisher, Wennberg, Stukel, Sharp, NEJM 10/13/94

The Propensity to Hospitalize at Specific Academic Medical Centers

Cohort methodology has an additional advantage: it can be used to study the practice patterns of the medical staffs of individual hospitals. This is possible because in fee-for-service medicine, most Medicare patients are loyal to a particular hospital. For example, it was determined that the hospitals to which patients were readmitted in the Boston-New Haven cohort study were most often the same hospitals where the patients were hospitalized for the initial (index) need-driven condition. This hospital loyalty — the tendency to be re-admitted, for whatever reason, to the hospital to which one was first admitted — makes it possible to compare hospitals' readmission ratios.

Application of the cohort method to individual hospitals reveals remarkable differences between Boston and New Haven hospitals in the propensity to hospitalize, and, just as strikingly, among the academic medical centers within Boston (Figure 3.10). The likelihood of readmission for any cause among patients initially admitted to the Massachusetts General Hospital was 50% higher than the likelihood that a patient who was initially admitted to Yale-New Haven hospital would be readmitted for any cause during any interval. The risks of readmission among those admitted to New England Medical Center and Boston University Hospital were 86% and 98% higher than among those initially admitted to Yale-New Haven Hospital.

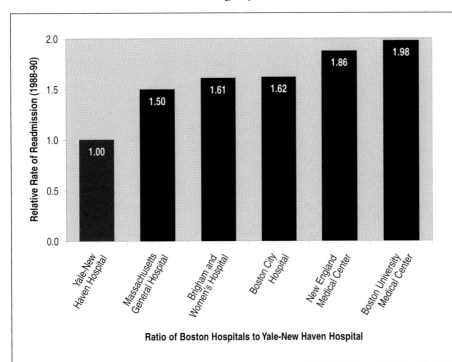

Figure 3.10. The Relative Likelihood of Readmission for Any Reason Following Index Admission to Yale-New Haven Hospital and to Selected Academic Medical Centers in Boston (1988-90)

Framing the Question of Hospital Efficiency: The Population-Based Perspective

Traditional efforts to improve the efficiency of hospital care have focused on reducing the resources allocated to treat a given case, for example by reducing length of stay or cost per case. The efforts of Medicare's Professional Standards Review Organizations were devoted almost exclusively to the task of reducing length of stay. The Diagnosis-Related Groups (DRG) program was implemented in the belief that a fixed payment per case would lead to overall improvement in efficiency, reducing escalations in Medicare spending.

When need drives the decision to hospitalize, as with hip fracture or surgery for colorectal cancer, then efforts to contain the costs of acute hospital care must concentrate on the processes of care, seeking more efficient strategies for accomplishing what must be done.

But for supply-sensitive conditions — those conditions for which physician practice style and the supply of hospital beds play important roles in determining the rates of hospitalization — the range of variation in per capita reimbursements is much greater than the range of need-driven conditions, and the discharge rate, not the cost per case, accounts for most of that variation. For example, per capita reimbursements for chronic pulmonary obstructive disease, a condition which accounts for about 4.5% of all hospitalizations for medical conditions, vary by a factor of seven. Seventy-five percent of the variation in reimbursements per capita is explained by differences in discharge rates (Figure 3.11a), and only 3% by differences in cost per capita (Figure 3.11b).

This is a critical consideration for managed care companies interested in finding efficient providers, and for providers trying to assess their own efficiency. Unit price is not a good predictor of the bottom line — the per person (illness adjusted) cost. Bargaining for discounts in unit prices without understanding the importance of propensity to treat is a serious source of error in predicting costs.

There is a strong correlation between the rate at which Medicare enrollees are admitted to hospitals for treatment of chronic obstructive pulmonary disease and the aggregate cost of COPD discharges (left-hand figure; R^2 = .75). By contrast, there is very little association between the cost per case and aggregate costs for treating patients with COPD in hospitals (right-hand figure; R^2 = .03). Addressing the issue of spending for hospital treatment of patients with COPD in a meaningful way requires attention to the fact that overall admission rates, not the unit cost of care, are the most important factor in aggregate spending.

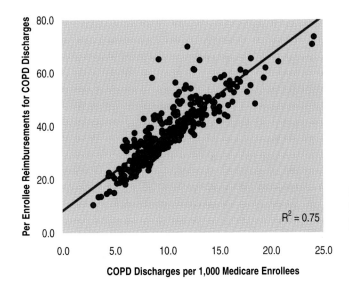

Figure 3.11a. The Association Between COPD Discharges per 1,000 Enrollees and Reimbursements per Capita for COPD Discharges (1994-95)

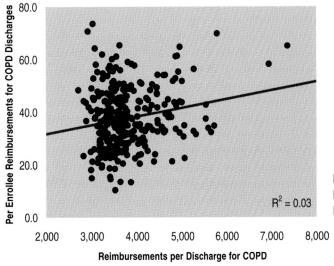

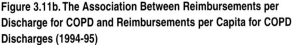

Figure 3.11b. The Association Between Reimbursements per Discharge for COPD and Reimbursements per Capita for COPD Discharges (1994-95)

Is More Acute Hospital Care Better?

The fundamental question is whether more acute hospital care inputs result in better health outcomes. The Minneapolis and Manhattan hospital referral regions provide important natural experiments for looking at this question. Sick people in Minneapolis are more likely to be treated outside the hospital than similarly sick patients who live in Manhattan. For example, in 1995-96, 48.4% of deaths among Manhattan Medicare enrollees occurred in hospitals. Only 24.2% of Minneapolis Medicare enrollees who died were in the hospital at the time of death. If the rate of use of resources of Minneapolis prevailed throughout the United States, money available for other sectors of care — providing ambulatory care, for example — could be increased without increasing overall Medicare outlays.

It is then important to ask whether patients living in areas with lower hospital capacity and less utilization receive adequate levels of care. There are three arguments that suggest patient populations exposed to less acute hospital care are not being harmed:

■ **First,** there is no scientific evidence that more is always better. There are few studies of the outcomes of hospitalization versus less intense ways of treating patients with the same disease profiles; and those that have been done show no advantage from more intensive care (see the Endnote).

■ **Second,** the influence of supply on utilization occurs without clinicians' explicit knowledge of the relative level of available resources. Clinicians serving populations in hospital referral regions where the supply of acute care hospital resources is relatively low do not appear to be aware of constraints on their practice of medicine.

■ **Third,** hospitalization itself is intrinsically risky and populations exposed to lower rates of hospitalization are less likely to experience untoward medical events associated with hospitalization. The magnitude of contemporary risks associated with hospitalization is not certain. The most comprehensive study of the risk of hospitalization, the Harvard Medical Practice Study, published in 1991, found that

3.7% of Medicare hospitalizations (i.e., people 65 and older) involved some form of complication, and in about 1% of Medicare hospitalizations complications resulted in death from an "untoward event."

How should the debate over whether more is better be framed? The first step is to understand the impact of increased supply on population-based utilization and outcomes. Most of the marginal resources in the acute care hospital sector appear to be invested in admitting patients to medical units in the hope of reducing mortality. The important question is population mortality: Do populations living in regions with greater hospital capacity live longer than those in regions with less?

Outcomes in terms of life expectancy are not different for populations living in Boston and New Haven. In the years since these studies began, the mortality rates of residents of Boston and New Haven have been essentially the same. This pattern is repeated across the United States: areas with greater hospital capacity, and with more inpatient days per capita, do not have lower mortality rates, even after controlling for a wide variety of health indicators. In other words, the United States might be on the "flat of the curve" in terms of mortality. If this is true, achieving for all areas the level of bed capacity in regions with fewer beds per capita would not affect life expectancy.

Chapter Three Table   Rates are adjusted for differences in age, sex, and race compositions of areas' populations. The rates represent the medical utilization of persons living in the specified area, regardless of where services were obtained. Hospital discharge rates are per 1,000 enrollees and are for the years 1995-96. Data exclude Medicare enrollees who were members of risk bearing health maintenance organizations. Specific codes used to define the numerator for rates and methods of age, sex, and race adjustment are given in the Appendix on Methods.

CHAPTER THREE TABLE

Rates of Medicare Discharges for Medical Conditions by Hospital Referral Regions (1995-96)

Hospital Referral Region	Medicare Population (1995 plus 1996)	All Medical Discharges per 1,000 Medicare Enrollees (1995-96)	All Surgical Discharges per 1,000 Medicare Enrollees (1995-96)	Bacterial Pneumonia per 1,000 Medicare Enrollees (1995-96)	Congestive Heart Failure per 1,000 Medicare Enrollees (1995-96)	Gastroenteritis per 1,000 Medicare Enrollees (1995-96)	Cellulitis per 1,000 Medicare Enrollees (1995-96)	Chronic Obstructive Pulmonary Disease per 1,000 Medicare Enrollees (1995-96)	Diabetes per 1,000 Medicare Enrollees (1995-96)	Kidney & Urinary Tract Infections per 1,000 Medicare Enrollees (1995-96)	Asthma per 1,000 Medicare Enrollees (1995-96)	Angina per 1,000 Medicare Enrollees (1995-96)	Hypertension per 1,000 Medicare Enrollees (1995-96)
Alabama													
Birmingham*	531,198	259.4	113.6	13.7	22.8	1.4	2.5	12.9	2.8	8.0	1.5	2.2	1.1
Dothan	91,261	291.6	102.3	17.7	28.3	2.8	3.8	17.4	3.0	7.7	3.5	3.5	1.7
Huntsville	110,797	236.2	101.9	10.8	27.5	1.0	1.8	11.0	2.6	7.2	1.4	1.9	0.9
Mobile*	164,496	268.2	113.3	15.8	27.3	1.6	2.9	13.9	3.1	7.3	1.8	3.7	1.1
Montgomery	98,631	250.9	106.8	11.0	24.5	1.8	2.5	14.6	2.6	5.7	1.4	3.2	1.0
Tuscaloosa	57,021	264.5	105.1	17.2	22.8	2.6	3.4	12.8	3.4	9.1	1.6	2.5	1.3
Alaska													
Anchorage	56,265	230.4	82.6	19.2	21.7	1.1	2.8	11.3	2.4	5.9	2.5	4.3	0.8
Arizona													
Mesa	107,378	176.6	91.9	14.9	16.6	0.6	1.3	8.0	1.2	4.3	1.3	2.3	0.5
Phoenix	372,696	196.0	94.9	14.2	17.2	0.9	2.0	8.7	2.0	5.4	1.7	3.2	0.8
Sun City	94,285	163.7	104.5	9.6	13.3	0.4	1.2	7.1	0.9	3.8	1.6	2.3	0.4
Tucson*	148,037	194.5	88.0	13.1	17.3	1.1	1.9	7.3	2.0	5.8	2.1	3.1	0.8
Arkansas													
Fort Smith	88,931	252.9	90.3	16.0	28.9	1.7	1.9	11.4	2.7	5.8	1.6	4.3	1.1
Jonesboro	62,053	271.3	106.2	19.3	27.5	3.0	2.2	16.0	3.9	8.6	0.9	4.8	1.7
Little Rock*	388,744	254.0	99.9	16.1	24.8	1.8	2.0	11.4	3.0	7.1	1.7	3.1	1.2
Springdale	95,202	221.3	90.5	16.2	24.2	1.2	1.4	7.7	2.2	5.5	1.0	2.4	1.2
Texarkana	69,646	271.5	97.6	19.0	26.5	1.5	2.5	13.6	3.2	8.0	2.2	3.9	1.3
California													
Orange Co.*	270,153	214.9	92.1	13.4	20.2	0.8	2.0	9.0	1.9	6.6	1.5	2.5	0.9
Bakersfield	117,982	218.2	100.7	22.3	21.9	0.8	1.8	9.5	2.4	7.7	1.8	3.7	0.7
Chico	71,355	198.7	100.8	16.1	19.5	0.6	1.7	7.7	1.4	6.0	1.8	4.1	0.5
Contra Costa Co.	114,631	176.5	85.3	12.8	15.3	0.6	1.4	6.3	1.4	4.3	1.6	2.1	0.4
Fresno	153,777	189.2	89.8	16.7	20.4	0.5	1.4	6.8	1.8	6.5	1.3	3.7	0.5
Los Angeles*	945,004	245.7	101.4	15.3	23.6	0.9	2.8	11.0	2.6	7.7	2.1	3.6	1.1
Modesto	112,858	212.6	91.9	18.8	19.1	0.6	1.7	10.4	1.5	6.1	1.4	3.6	0.7
Napa	68,998	199.1	110.8	16.1	17.7	0.6	2.2	7.5	1.7	4.3	1.0	2.9	0.4
Alameda Co.	187,366	193.9	89.8	12.3	20.4	0.6	1.7	6.1	1.4	3.5	1.9	2.2	0.3
Palm Spr/Rancho Mir	59,194	204.2	112.7	13.9	18.7	0.8	1.8	8.5	1.6	6.0	0.9	2.4	0.6
Redding	85,742	193.2	106.0	15.0	16.0	0.6	1.6	8.2	1.6	5.6	1.2	1.8	0.5
Sacramento*	330,362	198.7	87.1	15.9	18.0	0.6	1.9	8.1	1.5	4.4	1.5	2.9	0.4
Salinas	63,756	177.8	106.9	12.2	16.6	1.5	1.5	7.3	1.8	4.4	1.2	3.7	0.8
San Bernardino*	174,341	237.6	98.9	18.0	20.3	1.0	2.5	12.2	2.8	7.9	2.0	7.1	1.0
San Diego*	325,134	190.2	92.6	12.5	18.1	0.7	1.9	8.5	1.8	5.6	1.5	2.5	0.6
San Francisco*	216,897	183.9	78.8	11.9	17.6	0.6	1.9	5.3	1.4	3.8	1.9	2.2	0.3
San Jose	173,605	181.8	84.8	13.1	17.7	0.6	1.6	5.5	1.7	4.2	2.0	1.9	0.4
San Luis Obispo	42,298	169.6	89.4	11.5	13.8	0.7	1.5	6.2	1.4	3.7	0.8	3.9	
San Mateo Co.*	109,067	161.2	81.9	10.9	16.2	0.3	1.7	4.0	1.4	3.1	1.2	1.2	0.3
Santa Barbara	62,804	174.9	99.4	10.6	16.0	0.7	1.8	6.0	1.5	5.5	1.3	1.8	0.2

Indicates HRR with one or more medical schools

Hospital Referral Region	Medicare Population (1995 plus 1996)	All Medical Discharges per 1,000 Medicare Enrollees (1995-96)	All Surgical Discharges per 1,000 Medicare Enrollees (1995-96)	Bacterial Pneumonia per 1,000 Medicare Enrollees (1995-96)	Congestive Heart Failure per 1,000 Medicare Enrollees (1995-96)	Gastroenteritis per 1,000 Medicare Enrollees (1995-96)	Cellulitis per 1,000 Medicare Enrollees (1995-96)	Chronic Obstructive Pulmonary Disease per 1,000 Medicare Enrollees (1995-96)	Diabetes per 1,000 Medicare Enrollees (1995-96)	Kidney & Urinary Tract Infections per 1,000 Medicare Enrollees (1995-96)	Asthma per 1,000 Medicare Enrollees (1995-96)	Angina per 1,000 Medicare Enrollees (1995-96)	Hypertension per 1,000 Medicare Enrollees (1995-96)
Santa Cruz	43,356	184.1	93.4	12.1	17.2	0.8	1.4	6.6	1.1	4.5	1.5	4.5	
Santa Rosa	75,196	192.4	87.2	12.2	17.9	0.4	1.7	8.1	1.4	3.3	1.4	1.1	0.4
Stockton	73,773	204.5	98.0	14.5	20.9	0.9	1.9	9.9	1.6	4.8	1.9	2.6	0.6
Ventura	84,070	192.8	102.4	11.6	16.0	1.2	1.6	7.2	1.3	5.3	1.8	3.3	0.4
Colorado													
Boulder	29,397	196.4	89.6	12.1	16.0	1.4	1.9	14.4	1.5	3.5	1.7	3.7	(0.8)
Colorado Springs	117,647	202.9	87.9	17.3	15.6	1.5	1.7	8.1	1.8	4.8	1.2	3.9	0.6
Denver*	291,391	199.6	87.5	14.4	15.7	1.1	2.1	8.9	1.8	4.6	1.7	2.8	0.7
Fort Collins	49,776	198.4	101.9	12.7	14.2	1.6	1.8	8.8	2.0	4.6	1.6	2.6	0.6
Grand Junction	61,540	189.9	89.1	11.4	15.0	1.2	1.0	7.9	1.6	4.9	1.3	5.2	0.7
Greeley	59,056	211.1	98.2	16.1	16.7	1.4	1.8	11.1	1.7	4.7	1.5	4.6	1.1
Pueblo	34,804	201.2	100.0	15.4	16.8	1.4	1.7	7.7	2.2	4.0	1.9	2.2	(0.8)
Connecticut													
Bridgeport	176,155	188.7	91.8	13.0	20.4	0.7	2.4	6.0	2.0	3.9	2.2	4.0	0.4
Hartford*	379,442	188.4	92.5	13.6	18.4	0.6	2.2	7.3	1.9	3.9	1.4	5.5	0.3
New Haven*	354,500	198.7	93.8	15.0	19.5	0.7	2.6	7.4	1.9	4.9	1.2	3.6	0.4
Delaware													
Wilmington	148,958	217.0	93.4	14.5	23.2	1.0	2.0	10.7	2.6	5.5	1.8	3.0	0.9
District of Columbia													
Washington*	432,068	232.2	96.8	15.3	23.1	0.9	2.6	9.9	2.5	6.6	2.4	5.2	0.9
Florida													
Bradenton	95,601	181.7	96.8	8.9	17.1	0.7	1.0	7.4	1.2	3.7	1.1	3.1	0.6
Clearwater	179,366	210.0	103.4	7.8	19.9	0.8	1.5	8.1	1.7	4.1	2.0	1.8	0.7
Fort Lauderdale	626,104	210.5	98.6	7.6	21.1	0.6	2.3	7.8	1.6	3.9	1.7	2.6	0.6
Fort Myers	337,451	194.4	102.6	9.2	20.3	0.6	1.3	9.5	1.5	4.1	1.0	2.0	0.6
Gainesville*	101,489	226.8	88.5	16.9	24.3	1.1	1.8	11.8	2.2	7.0	1.5	3.7	1.0
Hudson	160,882	243.6	110.3	9.7	26.1	1.2	1.8	12.4	2.4	5.2	2.9	2.9	1.0
Jacksonville	230,794	246.9	98.9	13.5	26.0	1.2	2.6	13.0	2.3	8.2	1.8	2.2	1.0
Lakeland	86,654	213.7	96.4	12.0	20.8	0.7	1.4	10.8	1.4	6.0	1.4	2.1	0.5
Miami*	428,445	252.8	93.8	10.1	24.8	1.0	3.3	13.1	3.6	5.8	3.0	5.2	1.0
Ocala	165,671	197.3	96.4	8.4	20.5	0.8	1.2	10.7	1.9	4.4	1.7	3.0	0.7
Orlando	717,162	212.0	96.5	10.6	21.0	0.8	1.7	9.6	1.6	4.9	1.3	3.1	0.7
Ormond Beach	92,249	184.1	88.9	7.5	17.8	0.7	1.1	7.8	1.1	4.1	0.9	2.3	0.4
Panama City	45,564	261.2	103.0	16.9	27.2	1.3	2.9	16.3	3.0	8.8	1.5	1.3	0.8
Pensacola	155,000	245.2	100.4	12.2	23.3	0.9	2.4	12.8	2.4	5.8	1.3	2.6	1.0
Sarasota	192,292	181.3	99.2	8.4	16.8	0.7	1.4	7.5	1.3	3.1	0.9	1.9	0.4
St Petersburg	132,217	213.1	105.3	9.0	23.0	0.6	1.7	10.6	1.8	5.1	1.5	2.1	0.7
Tallahassee*	146,930	231.3	94.7	15.5	21.4	2.1	2.7	11.2	2.7	6.1	2.2	3.8	1.0
Tampa*	181,305	209.4	94.5	9.7	19.6	0.9	1.9	10.0	1.9	5.1	1.9	1.9	0.6
Georgia													
Albany	44,327	234.9	101.1	17.2	24.9	1.4	3.0	12.6	2.7	6.1	1.7	4.4	1.0
Atlanta*	724,634	237.5	93.8	16.2	21.8	1.4	2.4	11.8	2.3	7.9	1.9	3.4	0.8
Augusta*	126,511	236.7	98.0	20.2	21.3	1.8	2.6	9.4	2.6	7.6	1.4	2.9	1.2
Columbus	68,275	215.9	99.8	14.4	21.4	1.2	2.3	8.4	3.8	5.5	1.2	3.0	0.8
Macon*	146,073	241.7	101.0	17.0	22.5	1.9	2.5	10.5	2.8	8.3	1.6	4.3	1.0
Rome	61,522	239.3	101.3	14.5	22.6	1.4	2.2	13.2	2.7	8.4	1.6	1.7	1.0

Indicates HRR with one or more medical schools

Hospital Referral Region	Medicare Population (1995 plus 1996)	All Medical Discharges per 1,000 Medicare Enrollees (1995-96)	All Surgical Discharges per 1,000 Medicare Enrollees (1995-96)	Bacterial Pneumonia per 1,000 Medicare Enrollees (1995-96)	Congestive Heart Failure per 1,000 Medicare Enrollees (1995-96)	Gastroenteritis per 1,000 Medicare Enrollees (1995-96)	Cellulitis per 1,000 Medicare Enrollees (1995-96)	Chronic Obstructive Pulmonary Disease per 1,000 Medicare Enrollees (1995-96)	Diabetes per 1,000 Medicare Enrollees (1995-96)	Kidney & Urinary Tract Infections per 1,000 Medicare Enrollees (1995-96)	Asthma per 1,000 Medicare Enrollees (1995-96)	Angina per 1,000 Medicare Enrollees (1995-96)	Hypertension per 1,000 Medicare Enrollees (1995-96)
Savannah	144,045	249.4	99.7	19.4	23.6	1.7	2.3	11.8	2.5	6.5	1.4	3.4	1.0
Hawaii													
Honolulu*	187,844	170.5	67.6	10.3	15.4	0.9	1.8	4.9	2.2	3.5	2.1	2.1	0.4
Idaho													
Boise	141,914	185.7	100.5	14.6	14.6	0.9	1.5	7.8	1.4	4.2	1.6	3.0	0.6
Idaho Falls	34,038	172.0	98.0	15.3	11.6	0.7	2.1	4.1	1.4	5.3	1.0	1.7	(0.9)
Illinois													
Aurora	33,873	210.4	98.3	16.5	21.0	1.0	2.5	8.8	2.5	6.3	1.2	2.8	1.0
Bloomington	38,683	203.5	100.9	11.8	18.8	1.0	1.9	8.8	2.4	3.6	1.4	3.6	0.9
Blue Island	187,921	250.5	100.0	17.3	25.4	1.0	3.2	8.8	2.6	7.0	2.1	2.5	1.0
Chicago*	462,058	278.2	100.4	17.2	29.2	1.3	3.9	10.1	3.4	8.1	3.4	4.4	1.3
Elgin	85,637	230.3	93.7	16.5	22.0	1.3	2.5	10.7	2.3	5.4	1.7	2.5	0.7
Evanston	223,326	237.0	94.6	15.3	22.5	1.6	3.1	6.0	2.3	6.2	2.0	2.7	0.7
Hinsdale	63,880	206.5	94.4	16.6	18.9	0.7	2.9	7.2	2.1	6.8	1.8	1.7	0.6
Joliet	99,391	264.6	104.0	19.0	26.0	1.8	3.9	14.0	3.6	7.4	2.0	2.5	1.3
Melrose Park*	262,951	229.3	96.6	14.3	23.7	1.3	2.7	8.6	2.5	6.2	2.2	3.1	0.7
Peoria	190,047	211.6	96.6	14.5	20.9	1.2	2.0	10.6	2.3	4.8	1.6	3.7	0.7
Rockford	173,322	217.8	93.9	16.1	21.6	1.4	2.5	9.2	2.3	5.5	2.2	4.8	1.0
Springfield*	257,715	238.2	101.4	19.1	22.8	1.8	2.5	11.1	3.0	5.7	2.5	4.1	1.0
Urbana	113,172	221.1	92.8	18.3	23.3	1.8	2.2	11.2	2.3	6.1	2.2	6.1	0.8
Indiana													
Evansville	197,504	253.7	89.4	16.8	24.3	2.1	2.2	14.5	3.1	8.7	1.9	4.8	1.2
Fort Wayne	198,790	190.5	86.6	12.9	20.7	1.3	1.9	7.5	1.7	4.9	1.6	4.6	0.7
Gary	115,440	266.7	107.5	16.8	29.2	1.7	2.9	13.3	3.6	6.5	2.4	4.0	1.7
Indianapolis*	581,059	228.8	89.7	16.6	23.5	1.3	2.2	11.2	2.7	6.8	2.1	4.1	0.9
Lafayette	46,183	188.2	82.0	14.6	17.7	0.8	1.2	9.6	2.3	3.5	0.8	2.9	0.6
Muncie	46,075	241.0	93.6	18.5	24.9	1.7	2.3	11.9	4.1	7.7	2.8	5.1	1.1
Munster	81,110	276.0	107.7	16.1	32.9	2.4	3.4	11.8	4.0	6.6	2.8	4.2	1.9
South Bend	167,946	198.4	89.7	13.3	21.6	1.1	2.0	9.9	2.5	5.0	1.3	3.1	0.7
Terre Haute	53,927	224.7	100.1	14.8	24.2	0.9	2.3	10.1	3.0	5.6	1.8	2.5	0.7
Iowa													
Cedar Rapids	71,240	188.2	98.5	16.0	17.3	1.1	2.1	8.6	1.8	4.5	1.7	2.3	0.4
Davenport	139,617	210.5	92.9	17.8	20.1	1.4	1.6	9.8	2.5	4.8	1.8	5.4	0.6
Des Moines	280,952	229.3	99.6	19.2	21.4	1.6	2.4	9.3	2.2	5.3	1.6	3.8	1.0
Dubuque	43,877	205.6	96.9	11.8	20.1	1.2	1.8	7.6	2.0	2.8	1.1	2.9	0.7
Iowa City*	84,691	229.6	89.8	18.6	18.4	1.9	2.7	8.1	2.5	5.0	1.8	7.2	1.0
Mason City	53,653	177.4	97.6	14.0	15.5	1.3	2.2	6.2	1.2	3.7	0.7	2.9	0.5
Sioux City	80,240	213.2	102.6	20.9	18.6	1.6	1.9	7.5	2.3	4.4	1.7	3.2	1.0
Waterloo	63,821	201.7	95.0	16.0	18.7	1.6	2.5	7.9	1.8	4.4	2.8	3.3	0.6
Kansas													
Topeka	111,600	190.2	93.3	16.3	18.5	1.4	1.8	7.9	2.3	4.6	1.3	3.1	0.8
Wichita	353,253	236.5	105.7	20.0	21.3	1.9	2.2	8.9	3.3	5.2	1.4	3.7	1.4
Kentucky													
Covington	74,350	251.2	91.2	21.2	26.2	1.6	1.8	11.9	3.0	6.5	1.2	1.1	0.8
Lexington*	306,484	280.2	81.6	20.1	25.1	1.8	2.2	21.6	3.7	9.1	2.0	4.6	1.6
Louisville*	373,678	255.3	94.6	19.7	25.6	1.5	2.2	14.0	3.0	8.0	2.3	2.6	1.2

Hospital Referral Region	Medicare Population (1995 plus 1996)	All Medical Discharges per 1,000 Medicare Enrollees (1995-96)	All Surgical Discharges per 1,000 Medicare Enrollees (1995-96)	Bacterial Pneumonia per 1,000 Medicare Enrollees (1995-96)	Congestive Heart Failure per 1,000 Medicare Enrollees (1995-96)	Gastroenteritis per 1,000 Medicare Enrollees (1995-96)	Cellulitis per 1,000 Medicare Enrollees (1995-96)	Chronic Obstructive Pulmonary Disease per 1,000 Medicare Enrollees (1995-96)	Diabetes per 1,000 Medicare Enrollees (1995-96)	Kidney & Urinary Tract Infections per 1,000 Medicare Enrollees (1995-96)	Asthma per 1,000 Medicare Enrollees (1995-96)	Angina per 1,000 Medicare Enrollees (1995-96)	Hypertension per 1,000 Medicare Enrollees (1995-96)
Owensboro	36,335	266.7	104.5	22.9	27.1	1.1	1.9	12.0	3.4	6.8	3.1	6.6	1.1
Paducah	113,236	282.2	104.3	20.1	24.8	2.5	2.4	14.5	3.1	6.3	3.4	4.7	1.9
Louisiana													
Alexandria	68,645	307.0	107.8	24.3	32.6	2.2	4.3	13.7	3.7	11.6	1.6	5.8	1.8
Baton Rouge	125,996	254.1	95.3	18.6	24.4	1.1	3.1	11.2	2.4	9.9	1.7	3.5	1.0
Houma	46,172	278.8	125.3	16.9	32.1	1.5	3.8	14.8	3.1	8.6	5.6	4.5	1.4
Lafayette	119,008	262.1	110.2	18.8	27.0	1.8	2.5	11.9	3.4	9.6	2.4	3.5	1.1
Lake Charles	53,138	296.8	106.8	23.9	33.0	1.5	3.2	10.1	3.3	13.9	2.1	3.5	1.7
Metairie	84,026	275.4	109.8	19.0	33.3	1.1	3.7	12.9	3.7	10.1	2.2	4.7	1.7
Monroe	68,197	327.9	96.0	22.6	30.9	3.7	4.9	18.1	4.7	10.7	2.6	7.3	2.5
New Orleans*	157,397	253.6	103.0	14.2	31.4	0.9	3.6	11.3	2.3	8.2	1.8	3.1	1.4
Shreveport*	169,234	265.9	102.2	21.2	24.3	1.9	3.5	11.8	2.6	8.1	1.8	3.7	1.7
Slidell	31,604	320.8	113.5	23.4	35.5	2.0	4.8	16.6	3.2	11.4	2.4	6.4	2.0
Maine													
Bangor	111,529	248.0	95.5	17.4	21.8	1.2	2.3	12.1	2.9	5.1	2.1	10.3	0.6
Portland	261,069	215.9	91.1	13.3	20.1	1.1	1.9	9.6	2.2	4.5	1.4	5.2	0.5
Maryland													
Baltimore*	545,455	260.2	106.9	15.9	24.6	0.9	2.8	10.2	2.2	7.3	1.7	5.9	0.6
Salisbury	106,147	223.9	98.2	14.9	25.3	1.1	2.1	9.7	2.8	3.9	1.2	5.0	0.9
Takoma Park	131,825	213.7	97.2	13.3	20.1	0.8	2.2	6.1	1.9	6.1	1.2	3.8	0.5
Massachusetts													
Boston*	1,090,114	237.7	91.7	15.4	23.8	0.9	3.4	10.8	2.1	6.2	2.4	2.8	0.5
Springfield	197,790	202.3	83.9	17.8	22.0	1.3	2.5	8.3	2.7	5.4	2.2	6.5	0.5
Worcester*	136,618	235.2	94.9	18.7	23.7	0.8	3.4	11.1	2.7	7.2	1.8	3.5	0.5
Michigan													
Ann Arbor*	267,884	230.5	98.5	14.4	23.2	0.8	2.6	10.9	2.3	6.4	1.9	4.1	0.7
Dearborn	146,494	240.4	104.5	14.9	30.2	0.9	3.4	11.6	2.4	7.4	1.4	5.8	0.8
Detroit*	461,527	240.7	101.6	15.8	27.6	0.9	3.2	10.8	2.4	7.0	2.7	6.1	0.8
Flint	117,933	240.9	111.3	16.1	26.7	1.3	2.4	12.8	2.9	6.1	2.1	5.6	0.9
Grand Rapids	228,224	185.6	90.2	14.8	20.0	0.7	2.0	7.2	1.9	4.7	1.4	3.6	0.7
Kalamazoo	156,012	196.4	104.7	15.2	19.8	0.9	2.0	8.7	2.1	4.8	1.2	2.9	0.7
Lansing*	128,215	216.3	105.3	14.1	22.3	1.0	2.3	9.6	2.4	4.7	1.6	5.3	0.7
Marquette	65,828	219.2	98.7	15.4	21.1	1.4	2.7	7.2	2.1	4.3	1.9	7.3	1.0
Muskegon	69,589	171.0	96.8	12.4	18.7	0.8	1.7	5.7	1.4	4.4	0.8	2.1	0.3
Petoskey	50,748	196.0	98.6	13.0	20.4	0.9	1.9	6.2	1.6	3.9	1.3	4.8	0.6
Pontiac	74,704	249.0	101.1	14.7	26.8	1.4	2.8	12.1	2.3	6.7	2.5	4.5	0.9
Royal Oak	165,149	223.9	103.5	11.8	23.7	0.5	2.8	7.9	2.2	6.2	1.8	3.2	0.7
Saginaw	191,457	242.8	111.7	14.6	26.8	1.4	2.0	10.4	2.8	5.4	2.4	5.0	1.1
St Joseph	39,623	201.8	99.9	14.2	20.8	1.3	2.1	8.3	2.4	3.4	1.2	2.8	0.9
Traverse City	64,232	221.9	104.8	12.5	23.1	1.0	1.5	8.1	2.2	4.5	1.4	2.5	0.9
Minnesota													
Duluth*	109,464	202.4	99.2	13.2	17.4	1.3	1.8	6.5	2.3	4.7	1.5	5.3	0.5
Minneapolis*	571,687	205.9	93.4	15.6	17.9	1.4	1.9	6.8	1.8	4.0	1.7	4.0	0.7
Rochester*	111,509	202.2	91.4	17.2	19.7	1.0	3.0	6.6	1.9	4.6	1.4	5.2	0.7
St Cloud	51,664	215.9	91.3	18.6	18.8	1.7	2.4	7.5	2.0	3.9	2.2	4.4	0.9
St Paul	151,452	217.2	94.7	14.7	18.0	1.0	2.0	7.9	2.1	4.9	1.8	5.6	0.9

* Indicates HRR with one or more medical schools

Hospital Referral Region	Medicare Population (1995 plus 1996)	All Medical Discharges per 1,000 Medicare Enrollees (1995-96)	All Surgical Discharges per 1,000 Medicare Enrollees (1995-96)	Bacterial Pneumonia per 1,000 Medicare Enrollees (1995-96)	Congestive Heart Failure per 1,000 Medicare Enrollees (1995-96)	Gastroenteritis per 1,000 Medicare Enrollees (1995-96)	Cellulitis per 1,000 Medicare Enrollees (1995-96)	Chronic Obstructive Pulmonary Disease per 1,000 Medicare Enrollees (1995-96)	Diabetes per 1,000 Medicare Enrollees (1995-96)	Kidney & Urinary Tract Infections per 1,000 Medicare Enrollees (1995-96)	Asthma per 1,000 Medicare Enrollees (1995-96)	Angina per 1,000 Medicare Enrollees (1995-96)	Hypertension per 1,000 Medicare Enrollees (1995-96)
Mississippi													
Gulfport	38,727	301.4	110.9	12.6	38.7	1.7	2.5	14.8	3.3	9.6	1.3	1.1	1.3
Hattiesburg	64,370	311.3	107.0	21.8	28.3	3.4	3.3	17.6	4.0	10.5	2.2	6.8	1.8
Jackson*	239,395	285.0	89.9	17.4	26.6	3.4	3.3	13.8	3.5	8.1	2.4	6.2	1.3
Meridian	53,549	330.3	97.5	25.0	28.6	2.7	3.7	14.6	3.7	9.2	1.6	3.9	1.2
Oxford	34,480	310.3	100.8	21.9	28.1	4.1	3.3	17.1	3.7	7.9	1.2	4.1	1.5
Tupelo	90,693	273.7	91.4	20.7	24.4	3.2	3.2	18.2	3.3	8.2	1.1	5.9	1.1
Missouri													
Cape Girardeau	76,675	218.1	89.4	18.5	25.3	1.4	1.7	12.2	2.8	5.3	1.1	3.2	1.2
Columbia*	178,244	233.7	101.9	17.9	22.2	1.2	2.0	12.0	2.7	6.0	1.5	2.7	1.4
Joplin	104,566	259.6	104.6	19.6	22.6	2.5	2.2	12.9	3.4	7.6	2.0	2.8	1.5
Kansas City*	479,005	235.8	97.7	19.7	22.4	1.4	2.4	12.7	2.5	6.3	1.5	2.7	1.1
Springfield	218,568	210.6	96.7	12.8	21.6	1.2	1.6	9.5	2.2	4.8	1.2	2.3	1.0
St Louis*	807,992	231.3	98.5	17.0	24.5	1.2	2.5	9.8	2.5	5.7	1.5	3.1	0.9
Montana													
Billings	126,063	226.8	94.5	16.8	19.3	1.4	2.1	10.1	2.1	4.8	1.7	4.2	1.3
Great Falls	40,725	261.2	101.6	20.6	18.8	2.1	2.3	13.9	2.4	5.0	2.2	2.5	1.2
Missoula	86,069	232.5	98.8	17.1	18.2	2.3	1.8	10.3	2.2	4.8	2.2	3.9	1.3
Nebraska													
Lincoln	158,162	179.4	95.7	15.8	16.0	1.6	1.7	5.8	1.8	3.6	1.6	3.8	0.5
Omaha*	305,122	212.9	96.5	18.9	19.6	1.6	2.5	9.3	1.8	4.6	2.0	3.5	0.9
Nevada													
Las Vegas	167,674	206.1	94.6	13.8	22.1	0.7	1.8	13.0	1.6	5.0	1.6	2.0	0.8
Reno*	122,528	189.5	81.5	16.3	17.1	1.0	1.8	8.6	1.9	4.2	0.9	2.4	0.6
New Hampshire													
Lebanon*	109,382	201.5	78.7	16.6	17.8	1.0	2.2	8.1	2.6	4.4	1.2	6.1	0.4
Manchester	171,865	186.7	84.6	12.7	18.3	0.7	1.9	8.4	1.9	3.8	1.8	2.7	0.6
New Jersey													
Camden	697,067	240.1	98.8	13.8	26.3	1.5	2.3	10.1	3.2	5.2	1.7	5.6	1.1
Hackensack	310,809	228.8	100.9	12.3	24.8	1.6	2.5	9.0	2.9	5.2	2.3	6.2	1.2
Morristown	212,488	218.3	94.9	14.2	20.9	1.6	2.5	8.0	2.6	4.6	1.6	5.2	0.8
New Brunswick*	195,466	237.5	99.1	15.0	24.5	1.8	2.6	8.0	3.5	5.6	1.9	6.7	1.2
Newark*	344,765	262.7	102.6	14.5	28.6	2.0	3.3	11.3	4.7	5.3	2.2	7.4	1.5
Paterson	81,774	237.8	98.7	17.6	27.2	1.8	2.9	10.3	4.0	5.5	1.8	7.8	1.4
Ridgewood	87,608	234.9	94.9	18.4	23.8	1.9	3.1	8.4	2.5	6.0	1.6	4.6	1.0
New Mexico													
Albuquerque*	224,888	212.5	85.3	21.9	15.5	1.5	2.4	8.0	2.5	6.8	2.2	3.0	0.8
New York													
Albany*	482,105	223.1	89.0	18.0	22.7	1.4	2.8	11.0	2.5	5.0	1.5	5.0	0.7
Binghamton	111,256	224.2	84.4	18.5	23.9	1.3	2.5	10.6	2.8	4.8	1.7	5.4	1.0
Bronx*	197,752	246.1	93.0	19.9	26.1	1.3	3.7	7.2	4.1	6.3	5.3	6.3	1.3
Buffalo*	415,614	216.9	93.0	13.5	23.7	1.4	2.5	9.4	3.0	5.4	1.4	4.7	0.7
Elmira	109,738	238.3	92.3	14.8	22.6	1.5	2.8	13.4	2.9	5.1	2.7	3.4	1.1
East Long Island*	950,618	222.7	95.5	15.5	22.1	1.2	3.1	8.2	2.9	5.7	1.9	4.1	0.9
New York*	881,446	237.0	97.0	17.1	23.7	1.3	3.8	9.5	3.9	6.1	3.5	4.7	1.3
Rochester*	291,953	211.8	96.2	15.1	21.9	1.4	3.0	9.3	2.4	5.4	1.6	5.5	0.6

Hospital Referral Region	Medicare Population (1995 plus 1996)	All Medical Discharges per 1,000 Medicare Enrollees (1995-96)	All Surgical Discharges per 1,000 Medicare Enrollees (1995-96)	Bacterial Pneumonia per 1,000 Medicare Enrollees (1995-96)	Congestive Heart Failure per 1,000 Medicare Enrollees (1995-96)	Gastroenteritis per 1,000 Medicare Enrollees (1995-96)	Cellulitis per 1,000 Medicare Enrollees (1995-96)	Chronic Obstructive Pulmonary Disease per 1,000 Medicare Enrollees (1995-96)	Diabetes per 1,000 Medicare Enrollees (1995-96)	Kidney & Urinary Tract Infections per 1,000 Medicare Enrollees (1995-96)	Asthma per 1,000 Medicare Enrollees (1995-96)	Angina per 1,000 Medicare Enrollees (1995-96)	Hypertension per 1,000 Medicare Enrollees (1995-96)
Syracuse*	269,858	218.7	92.1	16.3	22.4	1.9	2.8	11.4	2.8	5.5	1.7	6.9	1.0
White Plains*	251,488	241.3	94.8	15.8	23.7	1.5	2.8	9.7	3.1	5.1	2.2	4.5	1.1
North Carolina													
Asheville	185,632	211.4	80.9	15.8	17.9	1.4	1.6	10.6	2.1	5.2	2.6	5.7	0.7
Charlotte	390,429	205.9	91.0	14.3	20.5	1.0	1.7	8.7	1.9	5.2	1.7	2.3	0.6
Durham*	292,501	199.1	86.6	12.5	18.4	1.0	1.6	9.0	1.7	5.2	2.1	3.2	0.5
Greensboro	128,316	202.5	93.3	13.6	20.3	0.7	1.6	9.4	2.0	5.7	1.8	3.9	0.6
Greenville*	169,580	222.5	92.7	14.7	22.2	1.6	1.9	10.3	2.1	5.6	2.3	5.7	0.6
Hickory	62,741	201.6	91.5	15.2	16.7	0.8	1.5	9.0	1.7	4.7	1.7	1.6	0.4
Raleigh	271,479	214.4	93.9	13.1	20.4	0.9	1.9	10.4	1.9	5.7	1.6	3.6	0.6
Wilmington	84,158	217.1	98.1	13.4	22.6	1.4	2.2	10.5	2.1	6.1	1.9	4.6	0.7
Winston-Salem*	249,303	223.8	93.1	16.0	19.8	1.3	1.7	11.1	2.4	5.7	1.8	3.8	0.6
North Dakota													
Bismarck	62,854	236.6	105.2	23.1	24.8	2.9	2.7	8.8	3.7	4.8	2.5	5.3	1.4
Fargo Moorhead -Mn	144,946	194.5	92.7	17.7	17.7	1.7	2.3	7.0	2.2	4.8	1.7	4.8	0.7
Grand Forks*	49,134	212.8	89.1	19.8	18.7	2.6	2.5	7.1	2.1	5.6	2.2	4.9	1.1
Minot	39,390	231.0	106.3	24.1	24.5	1.9	2.8	11.7	3.0	4.6	1.7	3.1	1.1
Ohio													
Akron*	179,066	256.1	95.9	19.7	28.7	1.1	3.3	11.5	2.5	10.2	1.6	3.0	1.1
Canton	174,748	209.9	92.1	14.2	22.3	1.1	2.2	11.0	2.2	5.0	1.8	2.7	0.8
Cincinnati*	366,415	216.4	92.3	19.3	22.8	0.9	2.1	9.5	2.3	6.3	1.6	2.6	0.6
Cleveland*	557,531	236.7	101.0	15.7	27.0	1.1	3.0	11.9	2.4	7.1	2.4	4.8	0.8
Columbus*	606,997	229.2	98.4	17.3	24.2	1.3	2.5	12.5	2.7	6.6	1.7	5.5	1.0
Dayton*	283,883	211.6	97.9	14.5	23.0	1.1	2.1	11.0	2.1	5.7	2.0	5.1	0.8
Elyria	59,452	236.5	116.9	17.2	27.6	1.4	2.8	12.2	3.1	6.5	2.3	3.9	0.6
Kettering	96,363	197.5	94.2	13.5	19.6	1.1	2.0	8.7	2.4	5.4	1.4	2.4	0.7
Toledo*	248,200	231.1	104.2	15.8	24.7	1.6	2.6	11.6	2.4	6.7	1.6	4.9	0.9
Youngstown	232,986	241.2	98.2	15.7	27.4	1.4	2.4	11.2	3.2	6.1	2.1	3.2	1.3
Oklahoma													
Lawton	48,926	225.9	91.4	15.3	20.0	1.5	2.4	7.1	2.3	7.7	1.9	3.0	1.5
Oklahoma City*	407,045	229.0	99.1	16.9	22.0	1.7	1.8	10.3	2.4	6.6	1.7	4.7	1.3
Tulsa	288,289	208.1	90.5	15.6	19.7	1.2	1.6	8.6	2.0	5.2	1.4	3.0	0.8
Oregon													
Bend	40,794	155.5	109.7	13.0	11.1	0.9	0.9	5.7	1.0	3.4	1.2	3.1	0.5
Eugene	164,058	173.9	89.0	11.8	17.8	0.8	1.5	6.0	1.4	4.0	1.8	4.0	0.3
Medford	119,321	160.3	85.2	13.7	13.5	0.6	1.6	5.7	1.0	3.6	1.6	2.5	0.3
Portland*	310,624	172.2	82.9	12.6	16.4	0.8	1.4	5.5	1.5	4.0	1.5	3.0	0.4
Salem	54,536	134.3	78.6	10.6	14.0	0.5	1.0	4.9	1.5	3.1	0.9	1.6	0.3
Pennsylvania													
Allentown	301,246	242.4	111.3	13.3	26.9	1.4	3.1	9.8	2.8	6.0	2.3	4.7	1.1
Altoona	94,974	242.3	94.9	13.2	29.5	2.0	2.5	11.1	2.5	5.0	2.0	7.8	1.0
Danville	143,082	230.3	94.6	16.6	23.5	1.2	2.6	10.7	3.0	5.6	1.4	6.5	1.1
Erie	227,568	241.4	93.9	16.9	24.7	1.5	2.8	11.5	2.8	5.3	2.3	6.3	1.2
Harrisburg*	251,207	208.3	94.9	12.9	24.0	1.1	2.2	8.1	2.7	4.2	1.6	2.5	0.6
Johnstown	88,969	286.7	111.8	16.1	32.5	1.5	2.3	13.8	3.4	7.0	2.3	5.8	1.1
Lancaster	139,571	206.0	101.2	12.9	21.0	0.9	2.1	8.9	2.7	4.5	1.6	2.1	0.9

Indicates HRR with one or more medical schools

Hospital Referral Region	Medicare Population (1995 plus 1996)	All Medical Discharges per 1,000 Medicare Enrollees (1995-96)	All Surgical Discharges per 1,000 Medicare Enrollees (1995-96)	Bacterial Pneumonia per 1,000 Medicare Enrollees (1995-96)	Congestive Heart Failure per 1,000 Medicare Enrollees (1995-96)	Gastroenteritis per 1,000 Medicare Enrollees (1995-96)	Cellulitis per 1,000 Medicare Enrollees (1995-96)	Chronic Obstructive Pulmonary Disease per 1,000 Medicare Enrollees (1995-96)	Diabetes per 1,000 Medicare Enrollees (1995-96)	Kidney & Urinary Tract Infections per 1,000 Medicare Enrollees (1995-96)	Asthma per 1,000 Medicare Enrollees (1995-96)	Angina per 1,000 Medicare Enrollees (1995-96)	Hypertension per 1,000 Medicare Enrollees (1995-96)
Philadelphia*	900,104	250.3	106.1	14.1	26.6	1.1	3.1	10.5	2.5	6.6	1.7	4.3	0.8
Pittsburgh*	975,984	268.5	109.8	16.7	30.1	1.4	3.2	13.6	3.2	7.3	2.8	4.4	1.0
Reading	163,121	221.3	102.3	12.9	25.6	1.2	2.5	8.7	3.1	4.6	3.1	3.3	1.0
Sayre	56,091	252.8	98.1	19.1	25.4	1.9	2.5	12.8	3.1	6.2	1.5	7.2	0.7
Scranton	110,662	236.6	95.8	14.9	26.6	1.1	3.2	9.9	2.6	6.0	2.0	3.3	0.9
Wilkes-Barre	90,912	229.2	97.6	11.1	27.2	1.2	2.9	10.4	3.5	4.4	1.8	2.4	0.7
York	97,457	197.8	93.6	12.0	21.1	0.6	2.5	6.8	2.3	4.9	1.6	3.5	0.7
Rhode Island													
Providence*	302,229	216.9	88.9	13.3	23.7	0.6	2.6	10.1	2.4	5.2	1.7	5.1	0.5
South Carolina													
Charleston*	167,086	221.2	98.8	9.6	23.0	1.2	1.8	9.3	2.4	5.5	1.8	1.5	0.7
Columbia*	225,786	196.0	89.4	14.5	18.8	1.1	2.0	7.8	2.2	5.5	1.4	2.5	0.6
Florence	79,509	259.5	100.2	15.7	25.8	1.7	2.8	10.5	3.1	6.9	2.4	2.4	1.5
Greenville	178,591	194.4	91.7	13.6	18.8	0.9	1.7	8.8	2.1	6.0	1.5	3.7	0.5
Spartanburg	85,807	211.0	84.7	14.4	20.1	1.3	2.2	9.0	2.4	5.6	2.4	3.6	0.7
South Dakota													
Rapid City	46,330	220.4	100.5	22.6	17.6	2.4	2.4	10.5	2.7	5.2	2.1	5.1	1.0
Sioux Falls*	234,742	223.1	104.5	22.6	17.6	2.2	2.8	8.2	2.4	4.5	1.6	4.5	0.9
Tennessee													
Chattanooga	151,930	248.4	94.1	14.4	24.1	1.9	2.1	11.7	3.2	8.6	1.3	3.5	0.9
Jackson	92,775	247.8	92.2	17.4	21.9	1.6	2.2	16.6	2.7	7.9	1.6	3.5	1.3
Johnson City*	62,541	239.9	86.8	16.9	22.0	1.3	2.0	11.5	2.1	6.5	1.6	1.6	0.7
Kingsport	134,555	280.9	78.3	19.5	26.0	1.9	2.5	20.8	3.1	8.7	2.1	4.3	1.4
Knoxville	308,599	259.9	89.8	17.9	24.9	1.8	2.0	14.7	2.8	8.6	2.2	3.7	1.2
Memphis*	368,719	242.5	95.5	15.3	25.1	2.1	2.4	13.3	2.7	6.9	1.4	4.0	1.1
Nashville*	493,251	267.5	93.0	15.7	25.9	1.4	2.3	13.4	2.5	7.8	1.9	2.2	1.3
Texas													
Abilene	88,733	253.3	96.8	18.1	22.2	2.1	2.3	12.5	2.9	6.7	2.1	2.8	1.7
Amarillo	105,473	232.3	99.4	17.5	18.8	2.0	2.4	11.4	2.7	7.3	1.3	3.5	2.0
Austin	158,656	203.7	90.7	13.6	19.4	1.1	2.0	8.3	2.3	6.9	2.0	2.8	0.9
Beaumont	118,418	284.8	105.8	20.3	27.3	1.2	2.6	14.3	3.3	10.7	1.8	3.9	1.8
Bryan*	37,939	208.8	84.9	18.1	20.4	1.5	2.3	8.9	3.0	9.0	1.7	2.8	0.7
Corpus Christi	99,580	264.2	108.0	13.8	34.0	2.1	4.1	12.9	3.5	9.2	2.3	5.5	1.4
Dallas*	571,236	213.3	92.9	15.5	22.8	0.9	1.9	9.3	2.0	6.8	1.7	2.5	1.0
El Paso	168,495	211.8	87.2	14.9	20.9	1.1	1.9	8.3	3.6	8.4	2.2	1.8	1.0
Fort Worth	249,518	197.8	85.3	13.9	20.0	0.9	1.7	9.1	1.8	6.3	1.4	3.1	0.8
Harlingen	84,587	235.8	104.6	14.9	28.0	2.2	2.5	8.6	4.4	11.1	2.4	4.6	1.7
Houston*	661,844	241.8	100.4	14.8	24.1	1.2	2.9	11.0	2.7	8.7	1.6	2.7	1.5
Longview	47,342	220.8	95.2	15.7	22.6	0.5	1.4	10.4	1.3	5.3	1.4	1.9	0.7
Lubbock*	154,500	265.2	116.2	21.7	27.4	1.5	2.1	11.2	2.9	7.3	2.6	2.3	1.9
McAllen	70,740	245.8	108.8	16.5	27.9	2.9	3.5	10.8	5.0	10.2	1.8	4.6	1.7
Odessa	66,030	249.3	107.5	19.1	22.6	1.8	1.7	15.7	2.8	9.0	1.9	1.8	1.8
San Angelo	42,868	243.4	93.7	22.2	23.2	1.8	2.9	13.8	3.6	9.4	3.5	4.0	1.1
San Antonio*	343,711	223.3	95.5	14.9	25.9	1.3	2.6	8.1	3.0	8.7	1.9	3.2	1.2
Temple	65,578	209.2	80.5	17.1	20.7	0.9	2.3	7.9	2.1	9.0	1.4	4.4	0.9
Tyler	138,956	235.6	100.7	18.1	24.0	0.7	2.0	10.1	2.3	8.0	1.6	2.1	1.0

Hospital Referral Region	Medicare Population (1995 plus 1996)	All Medical Discharges per 1,000 Medicare Enrollees (1995-96)	All Surgical Discharges per 1,000 Medicare Enrollees (1995-96)	Bacterial Pneumonia per 1,000 Medicare Enrollees (1995-96)	Congestive Heart Failure per 1,000 Medicare Enrollees (1995-96)	Gastroenteritis per 1,000 Medicare Enrollees (1995-96)	Cellulitis per 1,000 Medicare Enrollees (1995-96)	Chronic Obstructive Pulmonary Disease per 1,000 Medicare Enrollees (1995-96)	Diabetes per 1,000 Medicare Enrollees (1995-96)	Kidney & Urinary Tract Infections per 1,000 Medicare Enrollees (1995-96)	Asthma per 1,000 Medicare Enrollees (1995-96)	Angina per 1,000 Medicare Enrollees (1995-96)	Hypertension per 1,000 Medicare Enrollees (1995-96)
Victoria	39,186	279.5	101.1	17.8	28.1	2.0	4.0	11.1	5.9	8.0	3.0	3.4	2.4
Waco	85,123	189.3	85.0	16.7	20.1	1.3	2.0	7.1	1.7	6.5	1.7	3.5	0.9
Wichita Falls	57,700	234.7	88.8	21.1	22.7	1.3	3.2	7.7	2.6	6.6	1.6	5.0	1.8
Utah													
Ogden	58,586	151.7	89.4	9.8	14.0	0.3	1.4	3.8	1.6	3.7	1.1	0.8	0.3
Provo	54,192	168.0	103.4	16.1	15.5	0.6	1.8	3.4	1.6	4.2	1.3	2.4	0.4
Salt Lake City*	276,853	165.0	90.0	13.0	13.1	0.7	1.6	4.1	1.6	4.6	1.4	2.4	0.5
Vermont													
Burlington*	141,153	227.2	91.3	17.8	22.0	1.5	2.1	10.6	2.7	4.9	2.0	5.7	0.8
Virginia													
Arlington	217,532	202.9	85.3	11.4	18.7	0.9	2.0	7.7	1.5	5.1	1.7	3.9	0.7
Charlottesville*	119,093	233.7	84.9	14.8	21.2	1.0	2.2	9.7	2.0	4.9	2.3	2.2	0.7
Lynchburg	63,252	199.4	86.7	13.2	18.4	0.9	1.8	8.7	2.7	5.4	2.1	1.0	0.5
Newport News	100,986	203.6	100.1	12.3	20.9	0.9	1.7	7.6	1.7	4.3	1.3	1.4	0.4
Norfolk*	223,741	216.8	98.4	13.8	20.8	1.1	2.1	9.8	2.1	5.9	2.1	3.2	0.6
Richmond*	314,554	229.4	102.4	12.0	21.6	1.2	2.1	9.3	2.2	5.5	2.9	3.4	0.5
Roanoke	192,456	236.0	92.9	13.9	21.5	1.1	1.6	12.4	2.3	4.8	1.4	2.1	0.6
Winchester	81,227	269.5	95.2	19.5	30.3	2.2	3.1	14.7	3.0	6.7	2.8	6.0	1.2
Washington													
Everett	81,205	169.8	81.5	11.7	14.7	0.5	1.1	5.4	1.5	3.1	1.1	2.5	0.3
Olympia	67,206	169.3	90.7	14.4	16.0	0.6	1.3	7.7	1.4	3.5	1.4	4.2	0.3
Seattle*	405,155	176.1	86.9	12.6	16.1	0.8	1.7	6.3	1.4	4.0	1.6	2.9	0.3
Spokane	289,363	184.8	91.9	14.2	15.4	0.9	1.4	7.6	1.7	3.8	1.6	3.4	0.6
Tacoma	112,312	157.4	85.0	11.8	14.6	0.6	1.1	7.0	1.2	3.4	1.2	1.3	0.2
Yakima	57,239	183.1	82.6	13.3	18.4	1.1	1.4	6.1	1.9	4.2	1.6	1.8	0.4
West Virginia													
Charleston	254,827	274.2	95.6	17.1	24.4	1.6	2.3	18.1	3.3	7.4	1.8	7.1	1.5
Huntington*	100,854	268.1	89.2	18.0	26.0	1.5	2.3	15.1	3.2	9.4	2.2	5.4	1.1
Morgantown*	114,046	262.0	94.6	20.4	27.6	1.0	2.7	14.6	3.2	7.5	2.3	6.7	1.2
Wisconsin													
Appleton	77,833	176.8	91.6	11.9	19.1	1.2	1.6	6.6	2.0	3.2	1.3	2.2	0.6
Green Bay	132,406	192.4	94.4	11.0	19.3	1.1	1.7	7.1	2.0	3.6	1.2	3.4	0.5
La Crosse	96,697	208.9	83.2	14.7	17.2	1.4	2.4	6.3	2.1	3.6	1.4	6.6	0.6
Madison*	228,077	208.8	90.2	13.4	18.1	1.2	2.1	8.0	2.1	4.7	1.4	4.2	0.8
Marshfield	108,937	211.4	92.9	14.3	20.8	1.3	2.0	8.1	2.1	4.6	1.6	5.6	0.6
Milwaukee*	574,765	209.6	99.3	12.5	22.4	1.0	2.4	7.5	2.3	4.7	1.7	3.4	0.6
Neenah	60,821	198.2	103.6	14.3	19.4	1.2	2.0	7.4	2.3	3.2	1.2	2.7	0.5
Wausau	54,206	185.1	95.1	13.3	19.7	1.4	1.9	5.7	2.4	4.4	1.3	3.2	0.6
Wyoming													
Casper	44,566	242.6	101.5	19.7	19.7	1.6	2.5	10.9	2.9	5.0	2.3	4.1	1.3
United States													
	57,875,844	227.1	96.2	15.3	22.6	1.2	2.4	10.1	2.5	6.1	1.9	3.9	0.9

Indicates HRR with one or more medical schools

Quality of Care: The Use of Ambulatory Care

The Use of Ambulatory Care

The quality of ambulatory care was examined from the perspective of the use of preventive services and rates of hospital discharges which might have been prevented through better use of ambulatory care. Primary prevention (the prevention of harm from disease through immunization or early detection of disease) and secondary prevention (the prevention of complications of established disease) are among the most important goals of medicine. This chapter looks at selected immunizations and screening tests that are known to be effective in order to evaluate the underuse of care.

The quality of preventive care was highly variable in 1995-96:

■ The rate at which Medicare enrollees received vaccinations for pneumococal pneumonia varied by a factor of more than four; the rate at which female Medicare enrollees received annual mammograms varied by a factor of more than four; and the rate at which Medicare enrollees received fecal occult blood tests or sigmoidoscopy examinations varied by a factor of almost ten.

■ The rate at which diabetic Medicare enrollees received annual eye examinations vaired by a factor of more than two and one-half; the rate at which they received routine monitoring of HgbA1c, a marker of glucose, varied by a factor of almost eight, and the rate at which diabetics were tested for LDL blood lipid levels varied by a factor of ten.

Ambulatory care was also examined, by looking at the quality of care for Medicare enrollees with "ambulatory care-sensitive conditions" (including such diseases as chronic obstructive pulmonary disease and asthma). Regions with high rates of hospitalizations for these conditions are frequently thought to have poor access to care and poor continuity of care, or to suffer from shortages of primary care physicians. The findings call these conclusions into question:

■ Rates of discharges for ambulatory care-sensitive conditions — reflecting hospitalizations which, it has been postulated, might have been prevented through better
use of ambulatory care — varied by a factor of almost three.

■ Although rates of discharges for these conditions were highly variable, the variations did not relate to access to or continuity of care, or to the supply of primary
care physicians. Most of the variation was related to the supply of hospital beds.

Immunizations and Screening Examinations Recommended by the United States Preventive Services Task Force

The United States Preventive Services Task Force (1996) used an evidence-based
approach to arrive at recommendations for immunizations and screening tests. In
order to recommend immunizations, the Task Force required evidence of biological
effectiveness — that is, in order to be recommended, immunizations must reduce
or eliminate the diseases they are designed to prevent. The Task Force had three
major requirements for screening tests. First, they had to accurately detect
conditions earlier than would be possible without screening. Second, there had to
be effective treatments available for the diseases being detected. Third, those
treatments had to be more effective when used at the preclinical stages of disease
than after disease has become clinically apparent.

This section examines the quality of preventive care as measured by the frequency
of use of three preventive services recommended by the Task Force for routine use
among Medicare enrollees:

■ Immunization to reduce the risk of pneumococcal pneumonia

■ Mammography to detect early-stage breast cancer

■ Fecal occult blood tests or sigmoidoscopy to detect early-stage colon cancer

Vaccination for Pneumococcal Pneumonia

The United States Preventive Services Task Force recommends that people over age 65 be vaccinated against pneumococcal pneumonia because of the high mortality and morbidity associated with the infection in older people. In the judgment of the Task Force, the vaccination's effectiveness has been established by a number of clinical trials, and there is little evidence of serious side effects. The protection provided by the vaccine is, moreover, becoming increasingly important as antibiotic-resistant strains of the bacteria emerge.

The Task Force does not make a specific recommendation on the frequency of vaccination. The duration of protection is unknown, but there is evidence that protection lasts at least five years, and perhaps as many as ten. To achieve a minimum compliance with the intent of the Task Force's recommendation, Medicare enrollees should be re-immunized at least every ten years (10 to 20% of the population should be vaccinated in every two calendar years).

The actual frequency of immunization fell substantially below the recommendation in 1995-96. Compliance ranged from 7.5% to less than 1.8%. Immunization rates were 7.0% or higher in only five hospital referral regions, three of which were in North Carolina: Raleigh (7.5%); Greenville (7.4%); and Greensboro (7.0%).

The frequency of immunization was lower than the national average of 4.3% in the hospital referral regions in Napa, California (1.7%); the Bronx, New York (1.9%); Redding, California (2.0%); Palm Springs-Rancho Mirage, California (2.0%); and El Paso, Texas (2.1%).

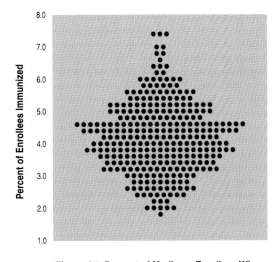

Figure 4.1. Percent of Medicare Enrollees Who Received Immunization Against Pneumococcal Pneumonia at Least Once in a Two-Year Period (1995-96)

The target immunization rate of the U.S. Preventive Services Task Force is 10-20% in each two-year period; actual rates ranged from less than 2% to about 7.5%. Each point represents one of the 306 hospital referral regions in the United States.

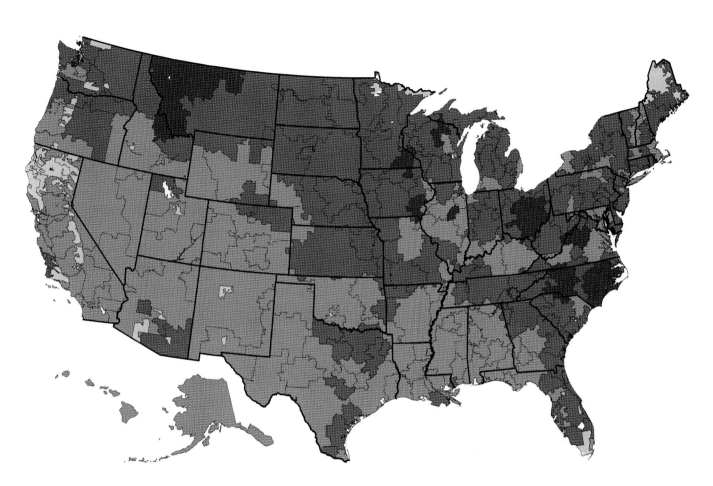

Map 4.1. Immunization Against Pneumococcal Pneumonia (1995-96)

Rates of immunization against pneumococcal pneumonia were generally higher in the North and East than in the South and West.

Percent of Medicare Enrollees Who Received Immunization Against Pneumococcal Pneumonia

by Hospital Referral Region (1995-96)

■	8 or More	(0)
▦	6 to < 8	(16)
▦	4 to < 6	(154)
▦	2 to < 4	(133)
░	Less than 2	(3)
░	Not Populated	

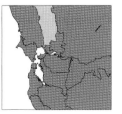

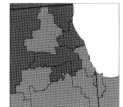

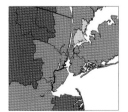

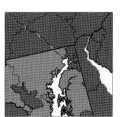

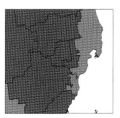

| San Francisco | Chicago | New York | Washington-Baltimore | Detroit |

Screening for Breast Cancer

The United States Preventive Services Task Force recommends routine mammographic screening every one or two years for women age 50 to 69. Clinical trials provide convincing evidence of the effectiveness of this screening in reducing mortality from breast cancer. The Task Force found that there was not enough evidence to recommend universal screening for women over age 69, but opined that healthy women age 70 and over might benefit from routine mammography.

The frequency of mammography among female Medicare enrollees between 65 and 69 fell considerably short of the Task Force's recommendation in 1995-96. The two year rate of mammography in the United States was 28.3%, and varied by a factor of more than four, from less than 12.5% to over 50%.

There were interesting regional patterns of variation: women in the Northeast, Florida and Michigan were much more likely to receive mammography than women elsewhere. In every hospital referral region in Michigan, the mammography rate was substantially higher than the national average. Rates were higher than 40% in ten hospital referral regions, six of them in Michigan, including Traverse City (50.1%); Petoskey (45.2%); and Flint (43.1%). The higher than average rates of mammographic screening in all Michigan hospital referral regions might be the result of local outreach efforts spearheaded by the Centers for Disease Control's National Breast and Cervical Cancer Early Detection Program, in which a principal aim was to increase the use of mammography among the elderly.

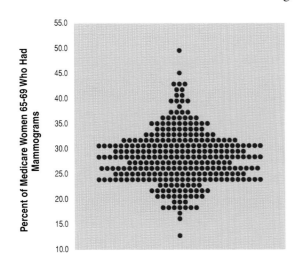

Figure 4.2. Percent of Medicare Women Age 65-69 Who Had Mammograms at Least Once in a Two-Year Period (1995-96)

The target screening rate of the U.S. Preventive Services Task Force is one mammogram every one to two years for women between 65 and 69. Actual rates of screening ranged from less than 15% to 50%. Each point represents one of the 306 hospital referral regions in the United States.

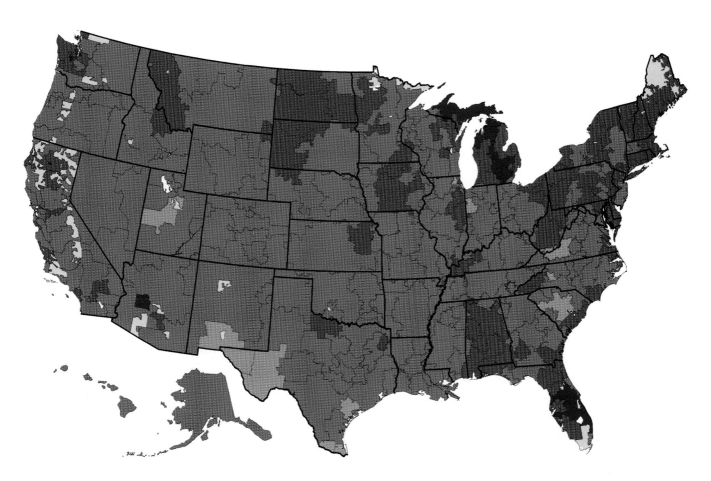

Map 4.2. Percent of Medicare Women Who Had Mammograms (1995-96)

Rates of mammography were high among female Medicare enrollees in Michigan, in the Northeast, and in Alabama and Florida. Rates of mammography among eligible women were lower in parts of the Southeast and in several areas in the Southwest.

Percent of Medicare Women Age 65-69 Who Had Mammograms

by Hospital Referral Region (1995-96)

■	40 or More	(10)
■	30 to < 40	(99)
■	20 to < 30	(184)
■	10 to < 20	(13)
░	Less than 10	(0)
░	Not Populated	

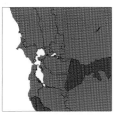

San Francisco

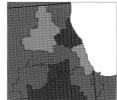

Chicago

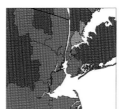

New York

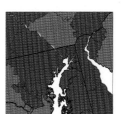

Washington-Baltimore

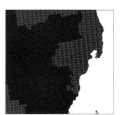

Detroit

Screening for Colorectal Cancer

The United States Preventive Services Task Force recommends annual fecal occult blood testing or sigmoidoscopy for all Americans over age 50. The fecal occult blood screening recommendation is based on the outcomes of randomized clinical trials, and the recommendation for sigmoidoscopy arose from the results of carefully conducted case-control studies. Both screening tests have demonstrated effectiveness in reducing mortality from colorectal cancer (although the Medicare program did not pay for these screening tests until 1997). Compliance with the colorectal cancer screening guideline varied by a factor of almost ten, from 2.4% of Medicare enrollees in the Terre Haute, Indiana hospital referral region, to 22.2% in Takoma Park, Maryland.

Annual screening for colorectal cancer was more common than the national average of 12.3% among residents of the hospital referral regions in Fort Lauderdale, Florida (22.0%); Salinas, California (22.0%); White Plains, New York (21.6%); Ridgewood, New Jersey (21.4%); and Sun City, Arizona (21.2%).

The two screening procedures were used less frequently than the national average among residents of the hospital referral regions in Lafayette, Indiana (2.5%); Colorado Springs, Colorado (2.7%); Grand Junction, Colorado (3.1%); Muncie, Indiana (3.3%); and Lake Charles, Louisiana (3.4%).

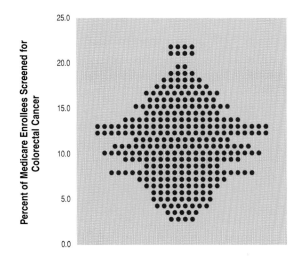

Figure 4.3. Percent of Medicare Enrollees Receiving Annual Screening for Colorectal Cancer (1995-96)

The U.S. Preventive Services Task Force recommends annual screening for colorectal cancer for Medicare enrollees. Compliance with the guideline ranged from less than 3% to more than 20%. Each point represents one of the 306 hospital referral regions in the United States.

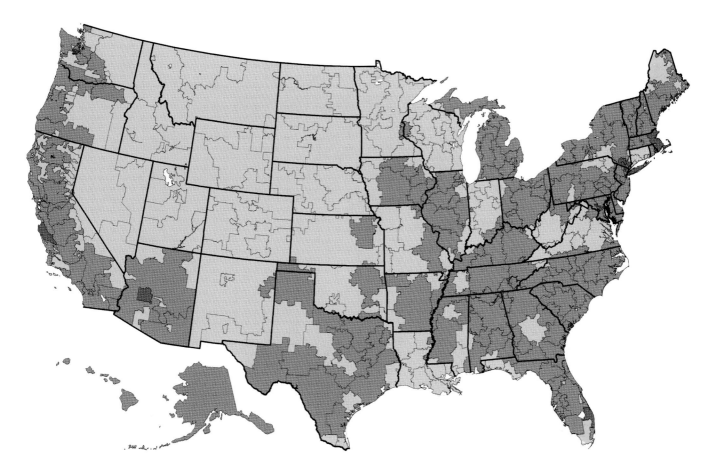

Map 4.3. Percent of Medicare Enrollees Receiving Annual Screening for Colorectal Cancer (1995-96)

Compliance with the guidelines for screening for colorectal cancer was lower in the Midwest and West than in the East and South, with the exception of much of Texas and the West Coast. Compliance was generally low; no hospital referral regions had rates greater than 30%.

**Percent of Medicare Enrollees
Receiving Annual Screening
for Colorectal Cancer**

by Hospital Referral Region (1995-96)

40 or More	(0)
30 to < 40	(0)
20 to < 30	(8)
10 to < 20	(185)
Less than 10	(113)
Not Populated	

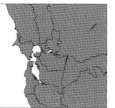

San Francisco

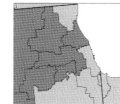

Chicago

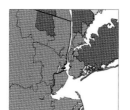

New York

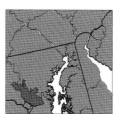

Washington-Baltimore

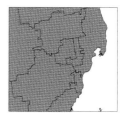

Detroit

Secondary Prevention Services for Diabetics

Concern over the quality of secondary preventive services in managed care organizations has led to the wide adoption of practice guidelines for such services, as well as the development of performance measures to evaluate adherence to the guidelines. Recognizing the serious risk of complications associated with diabetes, and the fact that several studies have suggested that the care of diabetic patients in the United States is sub-optimal, a coalition of private and public organizations sponsored the Diabetes Quality Improvement Project. Members included the American Diabetes Foundation, the American College of Physicians, the American Academy of Family Physicians, the Department of Veterans Affairs, the Health Care Financing Administration, the Foundation for Accountability, and the National Center for Quality Assurance.

Diabetes is a chronic illness that affects over 16 million Americans. There are two basic types of diabetes: insulin-dependent and non-insulin-dependent. Patients with insulin-dependent diabetes have lost their ability to make insulin, the major regulatory hormone for glucose control. Patients with non-insulin-dependent diabetes, the most common form of the disease among Medicare enrollees, have developed resistance to insulin.

People with both forms of diabetes are at significant risk of morbidity and mortality, including retinal disease that can lead to blindness and kidney disease that can lead to renal failure. Diabetics also develop coronary artery disease at a much higher rate than non-diabetics. Recent randomized trials have shown that better glucose control in people with insulin-dependent diabetes can decrease the risk of these complications. These findings have been extrapolated to people with non-insulin-dependent diabetes; several studies are now underway to directly assess this relationship.

The Diabetes Quality Improvement Project recommends annual eye examinations, annual measurement of glucose markers, and semiannual measurement of LDL blood lipid levels. The Project also developed a set of diabetes-specific performance measures with which individual physicians, plans and systems can be evaluated. In this section we report on the care of Medicare diabetics, using three quality measures (the proportion of diabetics receiving the test): dilated eye exam, measurement of long term glucose control, and measurement of LDL lipid levels.

Annual Eye Examinations for Diabetics

In people with both insulin-dependent and non-insulin-dependent diabetes, randomized trials have confirmed that yearly retinal exams and treatment of eye disease reduce the risk of blindness. The Diabetes Quality Improvement Project recommends annual eye exams. In 1995-96, all hospital referral regions fell well short of the guideline recommendation for annual eye examinations for Medicare enrollees who were diabetics. Compliance with the guideline varied by a factor of more than 2.5, from 25.1% to 66.1%.

Among the hospital referral regions with higher than average rates of annual eye examinations for diabetic Medicare enrollees were Fort Lauderdale, Florida (66.1%); Worcester, Massachusetts (62.1%); Ormond Beach, Florida (60.2%); Hudson, Florida (59.9%); and Sarasota, Florida (59.6%).

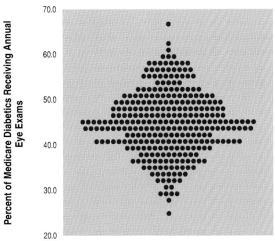

Among the hospital referral regions with lower than average rates of annual eye exams for diabetic Medicare enrollees were Terre Haute, Indiana (25.1%); Johnson City, Tennessee (27.5%); Portland, Oregon (28.5%); Bloomington, Illinois (28.5%); and Petoskey, Michigan (28.9%).

Figure 4.4. Percent of Diabetic Medicare Enrollees Receiving Annual Eye Examinations (1995-96)

The Diabetes Quality Improvement Project recommends annual eye exams for all diabetics. Actual rates of compliance with the guideline ranged from 25% to 66%. Each point represents one of the 306 hospital referral regions in the United States.

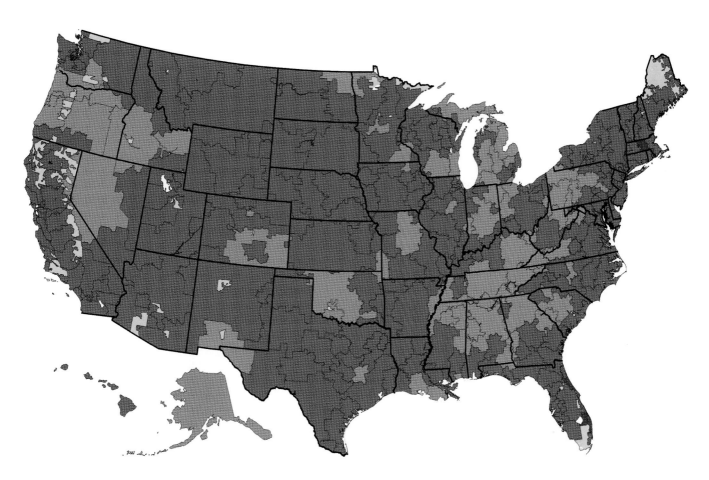

Map 4.4. Percent of Diabetic Medicare Enrollees Receiving Annual Eye Examinations (1995-96)

Compliance with the guideline for annual eye examinations was less than 60% in all but three hospital referral regions. Compliance was lowest in the East South Central states, parts of the Midwest and Texas, and in Oregon and Western Nevada.

Percent of Diabetic Medicare Enrollees Receiving Annual Eye Examinations

by Hospital Referral Region (1995-96)

■	80 or More	(0)
■	60 to < 80	(3)
▦	40 to < 60	(232)
▦	20 to < 40	(71)
▢	Less than 20	(0)
▢	Not Populated	

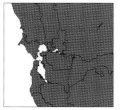

San Francisco

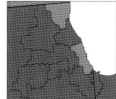

Chicago

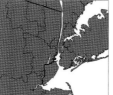

New York

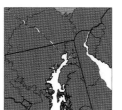

Washington-Baltimore

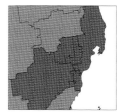

Detroit

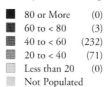

Annual HgbA1c Monitoring for Diabetics

The Diabetes Quality Improvement Project recommends routine monitoring of HgbA1c, a marker of glucose; tight control of glucose levels results in decreased complications. While definitive results have not been found for patients with non-insulin-dependent diabetes, the Project has expanded this recommendation to all diabetics. Overall, compliance with this guideline fell far short of the recommendation, varying from 8.9% of eligible Medicare enrollees to 70.2%.

Among the hospital referral regions with the highest levels of annual HgbA1c testing were Idaho Falls, Idaho (70.2%); Sun City, Arizona (67.2%); Salem, Oregon (66.7%); Wausau, Wisconsin (63.5%); Mesa, Arizona (62.3%); and Duluth, Minnesota (61.0%).

Among the hospital referral regions where Medicare enrollees with diabetes were less likely than average to receive annual glucose testing were York, Pennsylvania (8.9%); Muskegon, Michigan (13.0%); Great Falls, Montana (13.5%); Lafayette, Louisiana (14.3%); and Johnstown, Pennsylvania (14.5%).

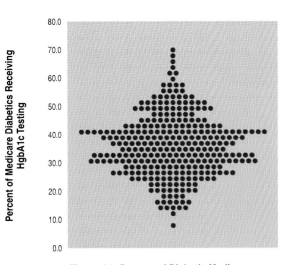

Figure 4.5. Percent of Diabetic Medicare Enrollees Receiving Annual HgbA1c Testing (1995-96)

The Diabetes Quality Improvement Project recommends annual HgbA1c testing for all diabetics. Compliance with the guideline ranged from less than 10% to about 70%. Each point represents one of the 306 hospital referral regions in the United States.

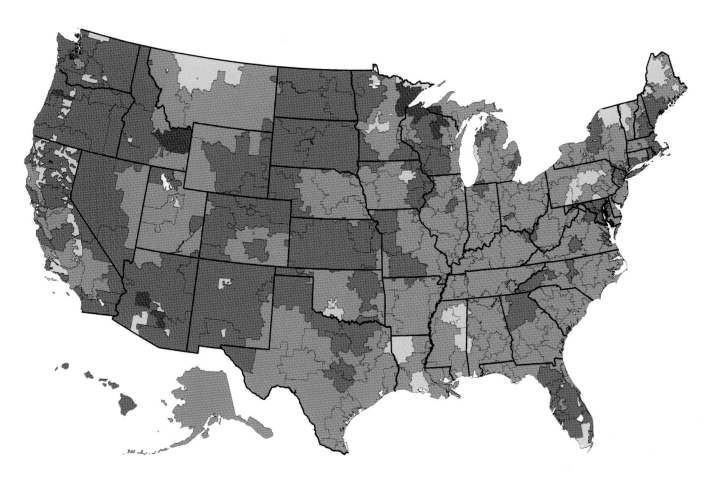

Map 4.5. Percent of Diabetic Medicare Enrollees Receiving Annual HgbA1c Testing (1995-96)

Glucose monitoring of diabetics was less common among Medicare residents of the East, Midwest, and Mountain states than among residents of the Great Plains states and those living in Arizona, New Mexico, Nevada and the Northwest.

Percent of Diabetic Medicare Enrollees Receiving Annual HgbA1c Testing

by Hospital Referral Region (1995-96)

■	80 or More	(0)
■	60 to < 80	(6)
■	40 to < 60	(104)
■	20 to < 40	(177)
	Less than 20	(19)
	Not Populated	

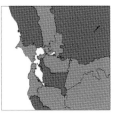

San Francisco

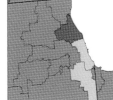

Chicago

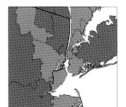

New York

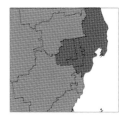

Washington-Baltimore

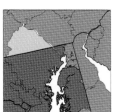

Detroit

Annual Blood Lipids Testing for Diabetics

Cardiac disease occurs at a much higher rate in diabetics than in the non-diabetic population, and the most common cause of death in diabetics is cardiovascular disease. Some, although not all, of this excess incidence is related to lipid abnormalities. Because of this excess risk, the Diabetes Quality Improvement Project recommends aggressive management of lipid abnormalities in diabetics, including monitoring of LDL blood lipids. Compliance with the guideline (at least one blood lipids test every two years) fell short of this recommendation; the percent of diabetic enrollees who received one or more tests in 1995-96 varied by a factor of ten, from 6.8% to 68.9%.

Among the hospital referral regions where rates of blood lipids testing for Medicare diabetics were higher than average were Bradenton, Florida (68.9%); Paterson, New Jersey (65.5%); Miami (64.4%); New Brunswick, New Jersey (63.8%); Ridgewood, New Jersey (63.2%); and Hackensack, New Jersey (62.4%).

Among the hospital referral regions where Medicare enrollees with diabetes were less likely than average to receive blood lipids testing were York, Pennsylvania (6.8%); La Crosse, Wisconsin (9.0%); Lawton, Oklahoma (9.0%); Muskegon, Michigan (10.3%); Muncie, Indiana (10.7%); Bangor, Maine (11.4%); and Burlington, Vermont (11.5%).

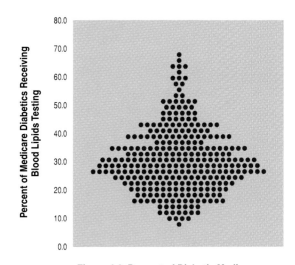

Figure 4.6. Percent of Diabetic Medicare Enrollees Receiving One or More LDL Blood Lipids Tests (1995-96)

The Diabetes Quality Improvement Project recommends blood lipids testing for all diabetics at least once every two years. The percent of Medicare diabetics who had one or more tests in the two-year period ranged from less than 7% to almost 70%. Each point represents one of the 306 hospital referral regions in the United States.

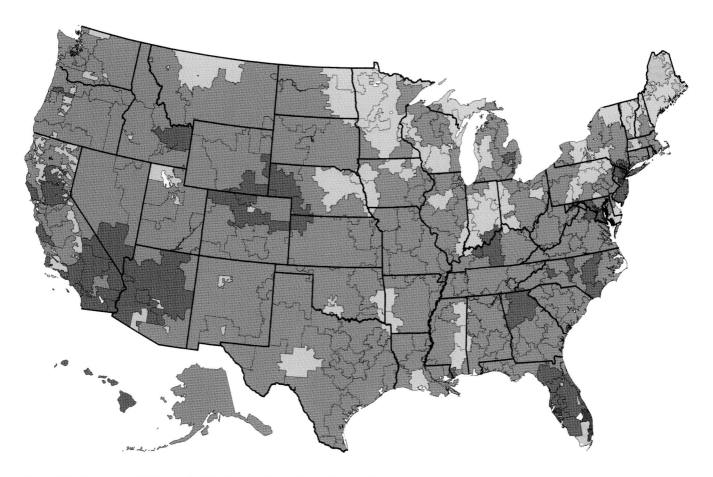

Map 4.6. Percent of Diabetic Medicare Enrollees Receiving One or More Blood Lipids Tests (1995-96)

Compliance with the guideline for blood lipids testing was higher in Florida and Arizona than in other states. No hospital referral region had a rate of compliance of more than 80%, and only a few had rates as high as 60%.

Percent of Diabetic Medicare Enrollees Receiving Annual Blood Lipids Testing

by Hospital Referral Region (1995-96)

- 80 or More   (0)
- 60 to < 80   (8)
- 40 to < 60   (52)
- 20 to < 40   (193)
- Less than 20   (53)
- Not Populated

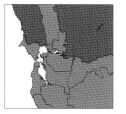

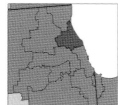

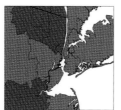

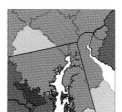

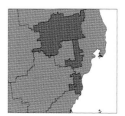

| San Francisco | Chicago | New York | Washington-Baltimore | Detroit |

The Preventive Care Profiles of Hospital Referral Regions

If measures of the use of immunizations, screening tests, and preventive care reflect the overall performance of health care delivery systems, there should be an association between the rates of use of services. For example, areas with high-quality care of one or more kinds would be expected to have higher than average rates for all quality of care measures. But in reality, the patterns of provision of screening and preventive services are essentially unrelated to one another. In 1995-96, there was little or no correlation between the pattern of use of the six measures of the quality of preventive care (Table 4.1).

Moreover, profiles of the propensity of given regions to use appropriate and recommended screening and diagnostic tests illustrate the idiosyncratic, non-systematic patterns of delivery of preventive services. A region that does well with regard to use of one service might do very poorly with regard to another, although some hospital referral regions did (relatively) well on all measures.

	Immunization for Pneumococcal Pneumonia	Screening for Breast Cancer (Age 65-69)	Screening for Colorectal Cancer	Eye Examination (Diabetics)	HgbA1c Testing (Diabetics)	Blood Lipids Testing (Diabetics)
Immunization for Pneumococcal Pneumonia	1.00					
Screening for Breast Cancer (Age 65-69)	0.08	1.00				
Screening for Colorectal Cancer	0.01	0.21	1.00			
Eye Examination (Diabetics)	0.00	0.07	0.07	1.00		
HgbA1c Testing (Diabetics)	0.00	0.03	0.01	0.05	1.00	
Blood Lipids Testing (Diabetics)	0.01*	0.01	0.18	0.07	0.23	1.00

*Indicates inverse association (negative correlation coefficient)

Table 4.1. The Relationships Between the Use of Selected Preventive Services (R^2 Values) (1995-96)
There was little relationship between receiving any given recommended preventive service and the likelihood of receiving any other. For example, although diabetics who received one of the recommended tests were slightly more likely to have the other diabetic screenings and to be screened for colon cancer, there were virtually no other correlations among preventive services.

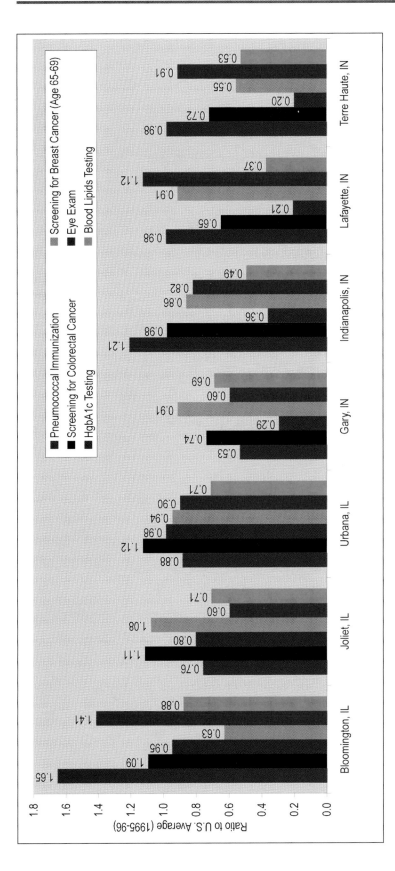

Figure 4.7. The Preventive Services Signatures of Seven Hospital Referral Regions (1995-96)

These seven hospital referral regions are contiguous, but they had distinctly different preventive services profiles. Medicare enrollees in Bloomington, Illinois, for example, were 65% more likely than the national average to receive the pneumococcal pneumonia vaccine, but diabetic residents were almost 40% less likely than the national average to have annual eye exams. By contrast, enrollees in Urbana, Illinois, were 12% less likely than the national average to receive the pneumonia vaccine, but diabetics were only 6% less likely to have annual eye exams. Women age 65-69 in Urbana were 12% more likely than the national average to have mammograms; women of the same age are Lafayette, Indiana, were 35% less likely than the national average to receive this cancer screening test.

Capacity of the Health Care System and Use of Screening and Preventive Services

What is the relationship between the capacity of the health care system to provide preventive services and the outcomes of care, measured by the use of services of known effectiveness? What is the relationship between measures of access, continuity of care, and outcomes?

The supply of primary care physicians in 1996 varied from fewer than 34 physicians per 100,000 residents of the McAllen, Texas hospital referral region, to more than 105 per 100,000 residents of White Plains, New York. But the supply of generalist physicians was essentially uncorrelated with the frequency of use for any of the screening and preventive services recommended by the United States Preventive Services Task Force and the Diabetes Quality Improvement Project (Table 4.2). In simple correlation analysis, there was virtually no association between the level of the generalist physician workforce and use of mammography (R^2 = .06); pneumococcal vaccination against pneumococcal pneumonia (R^2 = .00); or eye examinations for diabetics (R^2 = .05); and little relationship with screening for colorectal cancer (R^2 = .13).

The supply of specialist physicians in 1996 ranged from 53 per 100,000 residents of the McAllen, Texas hospital referral region, to 227 per 100,000 residents of White Plains, New York. As with generalist physicians, the supply of specialists was generally uncorrelated with the frequency of use of preventive services recommended by the United States Preventive Services Task Force and the Diabetes Quality Improvement Project. There was virtually no association between the level of the specialist physician workforce and use of mammography (R^2 = .03), pneumococcal vaccinations (R^2 = .00), or eye examinations for diabetics (R^2 = .08); and only a modest relationship between the supply of specialists and rates of colorectal screening (R^2 = .19).

Access to care, as measured by the percent of Medicare enrollees living in a region who had one or more visits to a doctor in calendar year 1995, was only weakly related to use of mammograms (R^2 = .18) and pneumococcal vaccinations (R^2 = .14), and had very little correlation with the frequency of eye examinations among diabetics (R^2 = .03).

An index of the continuity of ambulatory care measures the proportion of patients who see a single physician for the majority of their ambulatory care visits. Continuity of care, measured by the percent of patients in a region who receive at least 50% of their ambulatory care visits from one physician, also bore little relationship to the rates of use of preventive services. There was an inverse relationship between continuity of care and use of mammography, screening for colorectal cancer, and blood lipids testing for diabetics.

	Primary Care Physicians (1996)	Specialist Physicians (1996)	Access to Care (1996)	Continuity of Ambulatory Care (1996)
Immunization for Pneumococcal Pneumonia (1995-96)	0.00	0.00*	0.14	0.00
Screening for Breast Cancer (Age 65-69) (1995-96)	0.06	0.03	0.18	0.07*
Screening for Colorectal Cancer (1995-96)	0.13	0.19	0.09	0.20*
Eye Examination (Diabetics) (1995-96)	0.05	0.08	0.03	0.13*
HgbA1c Testing (Diabetics) (1995-96)	0.03	0.04	0.01*	0.05*
Blood Lipids Testing (Diabetics) (1995-96)	0.05	0.21	0.02	0.30*

*Indicates inverse association (negative correlation coefficient)

Table 4.2. The Relationships Between the Supply of Generalist and Specialist Physicians, Access to Care, and Continuity of Care and the Frequency of Use of Recommended Preventive Services (R^2 Values) (1995-96)
There was little relationship between the supply of specialist and generalist physicians and access to care, continuity of care, and the use of preventive services. The strongest positive correlation was between the supply of specialist physicians and the rate of blood lipids testing (R^2 = .21); no correlation at all was found between the supply of physicians (generalists or specialists) and the rate of compliance with guidelines for pneumococcal pneumonia vaccination (R^2 = .00). There was a moderately strong inverse correlation between measures of continuity of care and the rate at which diabetics received recommended blood lipids testing (R^2 = .30).

Hospitalizations for Ambulatory Care-Sensitive Conditions

Health services researchers have used the incidence of hospitalization for certain conditions as an indicator of the quality of ambulatory care. The theory is that when the access to or the quality of ambulatory care are poor, patients with diseases such as asthma, pneumonia, chronic pulmonary obstructive disease and congestive heart failure are inadequately treated in the clinic or outpatient department; this sub-optimal care results in higher rates of hospitalization compared to similar patients with high quality care. Several researchers have suggested that the regions with high rates of hospitalization for these "ambulatory care-sensitive conditions" should be targeted for special interventions to improve the quality of primary care.

Discharge rates for ambulatory care-sensitive conditions among Medicare enrollees varied by a factor of three among hospital referral regions in 1995-96. Among residents of the Ogden, Utah hospital referral region, there were fewer than 42 discharges per 1,000 enrollees; among residents of the Monroe, Louisiana hospital referral region, the rate was almost 120.

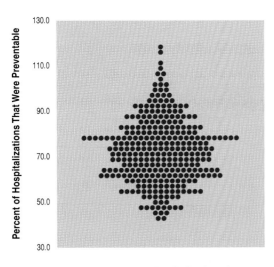

Figure 4.8. Rates of Hospitalizations for Ambulatory Care-Sensitive Conditions (Preventable Hospitalizations) (1995-96)
Rates of discharges for ambulatory-care sensitive conditions ranged from about 40 to 120 per 1,000 Medicare enrollees. Each point represents one of the 306 hospital referral regions in the United States.

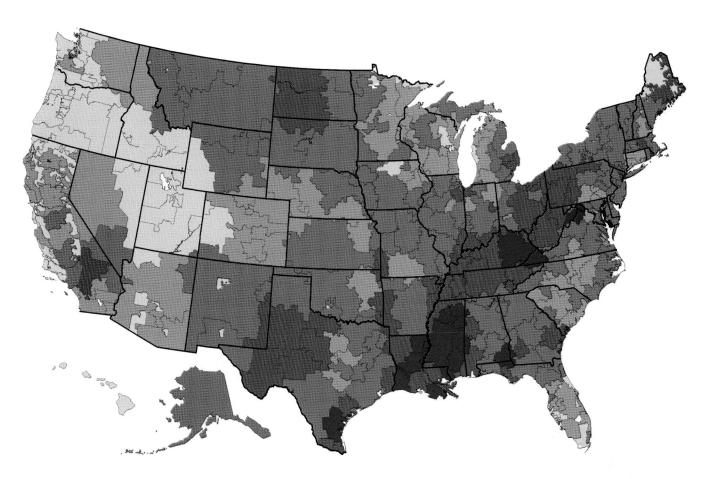

Map 4.7. Rates of Hospitalizations for Ambulatory Care-Sensitive Conditions (1995-96)

Rates of hospitalizations for ambulatory care-sensitive conditions were higher in the East, particularly in the Southeast, than in the Western United States. Rates were particularly low among Medicare residents of Utah, Idaho, and Oregon.

Ratio of Rates of Hospitalization for Ambulatory Care-Sensitive Conditions to the U.S. Average

by Hospital Referral Region (1995-96)

- 1.30 to 1.63   (17)
- 1.10 to < 1.30   (62)
- 0.90 to < 1.10   (116)
- 0.75 to < 0.90   (79)
- 0.56 to < 0.75   (32)
- Not Populated

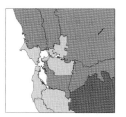

San Francisco

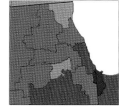

Chicago

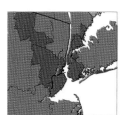

New York

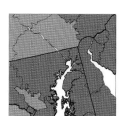

Washington-Baltimore

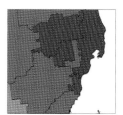

Detroit

Supply of Resources, Access to Care, Continuity of Care, and Hospitalizations for Ambulatory Care-Sensitive Conditions

Is there an association between the capacity of a region's health care system and rates of discharges for ambulatory care-sensitive conditions? Do regions with fewer physicians have higher rates of admissions to hospitals for ambulatory care-sensitive conditions? Do communities with fewer primary care physicians or specialists have higher rates of such admissions? Does better access to care, and more continuity of ambulatory care, help avoid preventable hospitalizations?

Apparently not (Table 4.3). Rates of discharges for ambulatory care-sensitive conditions were not related to the supply of primary care physicians per 100,000 residents (R^2 = .04); the supply of specialists (R^2 = .02); measures of access (R^2 = .01) or measures of continuity of care (R^2 = .01).

	Primary Care Physicians (1996)	Specialist Physicians (1996)	Access to Care (1996)	Continuity of Ambulatory Care (1996)	Outpatient Visits (1996)
Discharges for Ambulatory Care Sensitive Conditions (1995-96)	0.04*	0.02*	0.01	0.01	0.01

*Indicates inverse association (negative correlation coefficient)

Table 4.3. The Relationship Between the Supply of Generalist and Specialist Physicians, Access to Care, and Continuity of Care and Rates of Discharges for Ambulatory Care-Sensitive Conditions (R^2 Values) (1995-96)
There was virtually no relationship between the supply of physicians, access to care, and continuity of care, and the rates of discharges for ambulatory care-sensitive conditions.

What about the supply of hospital beds? Rates of hospitalizations for ambulatory care-sensitive conditions were highly correlated with local hospital bed capacity (Figure 4.9) and with discharges for all other medical conditions (Figure 4.10). The acute care hospital bed capacity of the local environment explained about half the variation in rates of hospitalizations for ambulatory care-sensitive conditions (R^2 = .55), but there was an even stronger relationship with "all other medical condition" discharge rate, which explained three-quarters of the variability in the ambulatory care-sensitive conditions discharge rate (R^2 = .74).

It appears that ambulatory care-sensitive conditions are not "special case" conditions. Rather, a particular aspect of the local health care system, the supply of hospital beds, has the same influence on general medical admissions and on admissions for ambulatory care-sensitive conditions. Further, there is no evidence that either the size of the physician workforce or access to outpatient care is a strong influence on rates of discharges for ambulatory care-sensitive conditions. The capacity of the acute care hospital system has a dominating influence on rates of hospitalizations for all medical conditions. At least for the Medicare population, discharges for ambulatory care-sensitive conditions appear to be a measure of hospital bed capacity, not the quality of ambulatory care or the illness of the population.

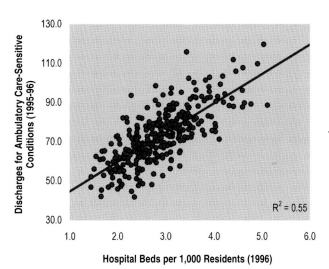

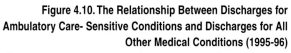

Figure 4.9. The Association Between Allocated Acute Care Hospital Beds and Rates of Discharges for Ambulatory Care-Sensitive Conditions (1995-96)

The acute care hospital bed supply explained about half the variation in rates of hospitalization for ambulatory care-sensitive conditions. Residents of regions with more beds per 1,000 residents were more likely to be hospitalized for conditions such as pneumonia, congestive heart failure, and chronic obstructive pulmonary disease; residents of regions with lower supplies of hospital beds per 1,000 residents were more likely to be treated for these conditions in another setting.

Figure 4.10. The Relationship Between Discharges for Ambulatory Care- Sensitive Conditions and Discharges for All Other Medical Conditions (1995-96)

There was a strong positive correlation (R^2 = .74) between the rates of hospitalizations for all medical conditions and the rates of discharges for ambulatory care-sensitive conditions. Higher supplies of acute care hospital beds resulted in more frequent hospitalizations for almost all categories of medical admissions.

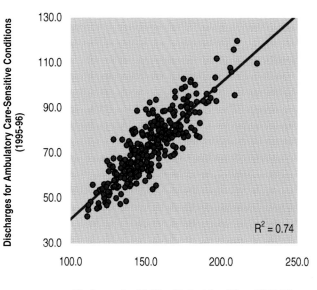

Chapter Four Table   All measures of screening (columns two through seven) are unadjusted, and are expressed as percents of Medicare enrollees receiving the preventive service. Percents are calculated using a two year "person-year" denominator, which varies according to the specific measure, e.g., all Medicare enrollees, women between the ages of 65 and 69, and diabetic Medicare enrollees. The measures in columns eight and nine are expressed in rates per 1,000 Medicare enrollees, and are adjusted for differences in the age, sex, race, and illness level of the population. Data exclude Medicare enrollees who were members of risk bearing health maintenance organizations.

Specific codes used to define the numerators for rates, and methods of age, sex, race and illness adjustment are included in the Appendix on Methods.

CHAPTER FOUR TABLE

Rates of Common Surgical Procedures Among Non-HMO Medicare Enrollees by Hospital Referral Region (1995-96)

Hospital Referral Region	Percent of Medicare Enrollees Receiving Immunization Against Pneumococcal Pneumonia (1995-96)	Percent of Medicare Women Age 65-69 Having Mammograms (1995-96)	Percent of Medicare Enrollees Receiving Screening for Colorectal Cancer (1995-96)	Percent of Diabetic Medicare Enrollees Receiving Eye Examination (1995-96)	Percent of Diabetic Enrollees Receiving HgbA1c Testing (1995-96)	Percent of Diabetic Enrollees Receiving One or More Blood Lipids Tests (1995-96)	Hospitalizations for Ambulatory Care Sensitive Conditions per 1,000 Medicare Enrollees (1995-96)	Hospitalizations for All Other Medical Conditions per 1,000 Medicare Enrollees (1995-96)
Alabama								
Birmingham	3.8	32.0	13.6	32.1	28.2	26.7	77.5	184.0
Dothan	2.9	33.3	11.1	31.3	30.7	21.3	97.8	195.6
Huntsville	3.4	29.9	16.0	30.6	34.1	29.8	74.0	164.1
Mobile	3.7	30.9	11.8	41.4	32.8	26.6	87.9	182.8
Montgomery	3.2	37.5	17.2	42.8	38.0	26.9	76.8	175.6
Tuscaloosa	2.7	34.7	17.7	35.2	29.1	30.9	87.2	179.0
Alaska								
Anchorage	2.9	25.1	10.3	36.2	39.7	39.3	78.4	153.7
Arizona								
Mesa	4.4	31.3	13.5	47.8	62.3	44.0	55.7	122.2
Phoenix	3.9	29.5	12.3	42.5	51.5	50.8	61.7	136.0
Sun City	4.2	40.1	21.2	58.4	67.2	57.7	45.6	118.9
Tucson	4.4	25.7	13.1	41.1	40.2	32.2	59.6	136.1
Arkansas								
Fort Smith	4.2	23.4	7.7	41.2	38.4	15.3	82.3	172.6
Jonesboro	2.8	27.8	8.5	51.8	32.4	26.4	95.0	178.5
Little Rock	3.1	25.0	11.4	50.9	29.7	27.9	78.8	177.1
Springdale	4.3	26.3	12.8	56.4	31.6	24.9	68.6	154.0
Texarkana	2.7	25.4	7.1	42.8	23.9	15.9	87.7	185.8
California								
Orange Co.	3.3	33.3	17.9	48.1	49.9	51.9	65.1	151.4
Bakersfield	2.4	29.0	12.9	45.7	38.6	38.9	79.7	140.8
Chico	2.5	36.0	14.4	58.4	49.8	46.6	65.5	135.2
Contra Costa Co.	2.9	26.3	15.9	43.6	37.2	35.1	51.8	125.9
Fresno	2.3	29.2	17.4	47.1	40.1	32.3	64.5	125.8
Los Angeles	2.9	23.6	15.0	44.1	36.3	53.3	78.0	170.2
Modesto	2.1	27.9	13.2	45.7	35.3	36.3	70.3	143.8
Napa	1.7	30.0	12.1	52.7	30.4	21.5	60.2	139.9
Alameda Co.	2.5	20.9	14.1	47.3	40.7	36.5	56.3	138.9
Palm Springs/Rancho Mirage	2.0	30.5	18.4	45.8	28.0	29.4	60.8	145.4
Redding	2.0	33.9	12.5	54.5	49.2	34.0	58.4	135.9
Sacramento	3.5	28.3	15.7	45.8	45.1	43.6	60.7	139.2
Salinas	2.5	28.8	22.0	46.6	41.6	40.8	55.4	124.1
San Bernardino	2.4	24.2	10.4	43.0	35.8	41.1	81.8	157.8
San Diego	3.9	25.9	16.4	46.8	45.9	50.0	58.8	133.0
San Francisco	3.3	22.3	15.5	43.0	32.0	31.3	51.4	133.6
San Jose	3.0	21.4	13.1	43.9	37.3	38.4	54.6	128.2
San Luis Obispo	4.2	30.9	15.6	51.4	33.6	27.4	47.8	122.9
San Mateo Co.	2.6	26.2	15.3	49.7	35.8	35.3	45.0	117.5
Santa Barbara	5.2	29.7	19.2	50.8	51.2	45.3	50.9	125.4

Hospital Referral Region	Percent of Medicare Enrollees Receiving Immunization Against Pneumococcal Pneumonia (1995-96)	Percent of Medicare Women Age 65-69 Having Mammograms (1995-96)	Percent of Medicare Enrollees Receiving Screening for Colorectal Cancer (1995-96)	Percent of Diabetic Medicare Enrollees Receiving Eye Examination (1995-96)	Percent of Diabetic Medicare Enrollees Receiving HgbA1c Testing (1995-96)	Percent of Diabetic Enrollees Receiving One or More Blood Lipids Tests (1995-96)	Hospitalizations for Ambulatory Care Sensitive Conditions per 1,000 Medicare Enrollees (1995-96)	Hospitalizations for All Other Medical Conditions per 1,000 Medicare Enrollees (1995-96)
Santa Cruz	4.0	36.6	13.7	48.3	51.1	39.7	54.3	130.9
Santa Rosa	3.7	28.4	14.8	56.7	47.2	40.3	55.7	137.7
Stockton	3.2	31.1	11.2	44.9	22.0	23.8	65.9	140.2
Ventura	3.4	29.3	19.8	51.1	51.1	55.0	55.0	139.5
Colorado								
Boulder	3.9	28.0	4.2	39.0	52.0	17.0	62.3	136.0
Colorado Springs	3.0	22.3	2.7	33.6	33.9	22.0	61.9	142.4
Denver	4.0	27.2	5.2	47.0	52.6	43.8	59.1	142.2
Fort Collins	5.5	27.8	9.7	43.4	42.3	42.9	56.2	143.8
Grand Junction	2.7	28.8	3.1	43.8	42.3	30.8	54.5	136.3
Greeley	5.7	29.7	4.5	50.2	51.1	27.3	66.0	146.4
Pueblo	3.2	20.7	4.1	43.6	52.5	29.1	59.2	143.5
Connecticut								
Bridgeport	3.9	27.9	8.8	50.4	39.2	46.8	61.2	129.7
Hartford	4.7	33.2	7.8	53.0	35.4	29.2	61.1	129.2
New Haven	4.2	31.1	8.7	55.5	46.3	36.6	62.7	138.0
Delaware								
Wilmington	4.7	31.6	12.4	47.5	34.6	35.1	72.4	147.2
District of Columbia								
Washington	4.0	30.0	16.6	43.4	41.5	40.2	77.2	157.4
Florida								
Bradenton	4.8	42.9	14.8	57.2	54.6	68.9	49.6	130.2
Clearwater	6.0	34.5	19.1	57.9	50.9	49.0	53.6	154.6
Fort Lauderdale	5.5	41.8	22.0	66.1	54.4	60.5	55.3	156.7
Fort Myers	4.7	34.7	16.4	50.7	43.0	42.2	55.5	140.1
Gainesville	5.3	33.3	11.1	51.9	40.0	43.0	77.7	150.8
Hudson	5.0	40.1	15.2	59.9	52.1	58.7	72.2	170.2
Jacksonville	5.8	33.2	12.2	42.5	33.2	37.2	79.3	169.9
Lakeland	3.7	35.7	10.2	47.8	36.1	40.9	63.5	152.0
Miami	3.1	28.4	12.2	49.8	44.6	64.4	77.3	178.3
Ocala	3.8	39.1	11.8	56.3	41.8	46.0	58.0	139.7
Orlando	4.5	33.3	12.6	51.2	49.5	50.8	61.9	151.3
Ormond Beach	5.4	29.8	13.9	60.2	34.9	43.3	48.3	137.0
Panama City	2.6	29.8	5.7	41.6	32.2	37.3	86.0	177.7
Pensacola	3.7	30.4	9.2	47.8	28.7	29.5	71.9	174.7
Sarasota	3.9	35.7	17.5	59.6	47.4	52.0	47.0	133.1
St Petersburg	4.7	30.3	14.0	57.4	38.1	42.5	62.0	153.2
Tallahassee	3.4	26.5	11.1	45.1	33.7	35.1	75.7	157.0
Tampa	4.4	30.8	10.1	49.8	40.1	48.9	59.4	152.3
Georgia								
Albany	2.7	31.9	10.9	41.9	38.9	24.9	82.9	153.3
Atlanta	4.2	24.9	13.2	39.6	41.9	45.3	77.5	161.9
Augusta	4.2	24.3	13.8	34.2	20.0	26.7	78.0	160.4
Columbus	3.8	23.9	12.2	37.0	27.5	29.7	71.1	147.1
Macon	3.4	26.8	9.1	40.9	26.1	32.4	80.2	163.1
Rome	4.6	28.6	10.1	41.6	29.8	32.0	76.0	165.4

Hospital Referral Region	Percent of Medicare Enrollees Receiving Immunization Against Pneumococcal Pneumonia (1995-96)	Percent of Medicare Women Age 65-69 Having Mammograms (1995-96)	Percent of Medicare Enrollees Receiving Screening for Colorectal Cancer (1995-96)	Percent of Diabetic Medicare Enrollees Receiving Eye Examination (1995-96)	Percent of Diabetic Enrollees Receiving HgbA1c Testing (1995-96)	Percent of Diabetic Enrollees Receiving One or More Blood Lipids Tests (1995-96)	Hospitalizations for Ambulatory Care Sensitive Conditions per 1,000 Medicare Enrollees (1995-96)	Hospitalizations for All Other Medical Conditions per 1,000 Medicare Enrollees (1995-96)
Savannah	5.1	25.1	12.5	40.0	32.3	38.6	81.5	169.9
Hawaii								
Honolulu	3.2	26.3	13.3	40.6	43.8	41.7	49.7	122.3
Idaho								
Boise	3.7	25.2	5.0	31.8	48.2	30.5	54.9	131.8
Idaho Falls	4.5	24.4	5.2	32.3	70.2	47.8	47.9	124.9
Illinois								
Aurora	3.3	24.5	10.0	41.2	33.3	33.9	71.0	140.9
Bloomington	7.0	31.0	11.6	28.5	50.3	29.1	61.3	143.7
Blue Island	3.2	24.2	9.1	45.6	16.1	23.4	78.6	174.4
Chicago	2.6	18.3	8.2	37.7	18.3	27.0	91.9	190.0
Elgin	3.5	18.9	10.2	46.6	31.3	33.8	72.7	159.5
Evanston	4.3	31.7	16.8	56.2	41.5	45.3	69.6	169.7
Hinsdale	4.1	30.8	13.4	48.9	34.3	34.5	65.0	143.7
Joliet	3.2	31.5	9.8	48.7	21.2	23.4	89.4	177.9
Melrose Park	4.0	26.5	10.2	46.8	27.3	29.5	72.3	159.7
Peoria	3.6	29.5	10.5	45.6	29.4	19.6	68.4	145.3
Rockford	4.4	28.0	10.8	41.1	35.8	23.6	73.4	146.4
Springfield	4.0	26.1	13.4	48.5	33.5	26.3	80.0	160.5
Urbana	3.7	31.8	12.1	42.7	31.9	23.5	80.3	142.6
Indiana								
Evansville	4.0	24.3	4.3	43.2	20.5	18.5	86.8	168.7
Fort Wayne	4.6	23.3	6.4	39.4	27.5	14.4	63.8	127.9
Gary	2.3	20.9	3.6	41.3	21.2	22.8	92.0	178.0
Indianapolis	5.1	27.7	4.4	38.9	29.1	16.3	77.8	152.7
Lafayette	4.2	18.3	2.5	41.2	39.9	12.3	59.3	130.5
Muncie	5.1	25.0	3.3	40.2	37.6	10.7	88.6	154.5
Munster	3.1	22.4	4.9	41.3	23.8	21.6	96.2	183.8
South Bend	4.4	27.9	4.3	40.3	41.6	20.8	67.4	132.8
Terre Haute	4.2	20.3	2.4	25.1	32.4	17.4	73.2	153.4
Iowa								
Cedar Rapids	4.0	32.8	12.3	49.8	54.7	24.7	60.7	129.3
Davenport	3.9	29.0	12.8	41.4	43.2	28.4	71.5	140.8
Des Moines	4.4	31.4	11.2	49.7	31.0	20.8	74.0	157.4
Dubuque	3.8	26.5	9.3	52.9	56.6	26.5	57.3	149.6
Iowa City	6.3	27.6	12.9	54.4	41.6	28.9	72.5	158.5
Mason City	4.3	31.6	10.7	55.0	31.1	15.5	52.4	125.8
Sioux City	4.7	27.0	8.2	50.5	36.8	19.6	67.8	147.0
Waterloo	5.7	25.5	11.9	49.0	19.1	16.2	65.0	137.8
Kansas								
Topeka	4.0	30.2	13.0	51.8	48.4	31.7	63.4	128.0
Wichita	4.3	27.2	7.6	55.2	41.4	21.7	75.6	162.4
Kentucky								
Covington	5.5	23.9	10.6	44.6	23.4	16.3	81.7	172.1
Lexington	3.5	23.6	10.0	34.4	28.3	35.7	102.1	180.1
Louisville	3.7	27.3	10.5	43.4	33.6	42.8	88.2	169.4

Hospital Referral Region	Percent of Medicare Enrollees Receiving Immunization Against Pneumococcal Pneumonia (1995-96)	Percent of Medicare Women Age 65-69 Having Mammograms (1995-96)	Percent of Medicare Enrollees Receiving Screening for Colorectal Cancer (1995-96)	Percent of Diabetic Medicare Enrollees Receiving Eye Examination (1995-96)	Percent of Diabetic Enrollees Receiving HgbA1c Testing (1995-96)	Percent of Diabetic Enrollees Receiving One or More Blood Lipids Tests (1995-96)	Hospitalizations for Ambulatory Care Sensitive Conditions per 1,000 Medicare Enrollees (1995-96)	Hospitalizations for All Other Medical Conditions per 1,000 Medicare Enrollees (1995-96)
Owensboro	4.5	33.9	15.6	41.6	39.6	45.7	93.6	175.3
Paducah	4.9	32.0	10.3	45.1	31.9	30.8	92.7	191.7
Louisiana								
Alexandria	2.4	20.1	4.9	50.1	28.0	26.6	111.6	197.0
Baton Rouge	3.4	23.4	8.2	45.4	23.6	32.4	86.3	169.1
Houma	4.7	23.8	3.7	38.6	32.8	31.0	101.2	179.8
Lafayette	3.3	24.3	5.6	34.1	14.3	19.3	90.3	173.5
Lake Charles	3.2	23.0	3.4	44.3	27.2	28.9	103.2	196.0
Metairie	2.9	23.9	7.1	55.1	24.1	34.4	102.6	175.3
Monroe	3.6	23.7	4.8	51.3	22.3	30.6	119.4	210.2
New Orleans	2.8	24.0	5.6	47.0	26.4	32.8	87.5	168.3
Shreveport	2.6	21.9	6.5	44.7	14.7	26.3	90.7	176.8
Slidell	4.5	21.6	6.9	58.9	30.0	40.5	115.6	208.0
Maine								
Bangor	5.3	30.1	14.0	55.4	39.8	11.4	84.1	165.6
Portland	4.8	34.5	17.4	48.1	42.5	18.2	66.7	150.6
Maryland								
Baltimore	3.9	31.1	15.7	45.1	41.9	32.8	79.8	182.6
Salisbury	4.0	34.9	13.1	51.0	22.9	17.1	73.7	152.2
Takoma Park	4.7	30.6	22.2	44.0	59.6	60.0	62.5	153.4
Massachusetts								
Boston	3.7	34.5	20.9	56.6	40.9	26.7	76.6	163.2
Springfield	2.9	28.1	16.4	57.6	23.5	17.5	75.7	128.4
Worcester	4.2	32.7	14.7	62.1	38.6	24.8	81.9	155.9
Michigan								
Ann Arbor	5.1	40.9	15.9	46.6	35.4	33.5	74.5	158.4
Dearborn	3.6	35.7	12.5	42.6	31.9	43.2	85.9	157.7
Detroit	3.6	33.5	13.2	44.8	41.6	38.2	84.6	158.8
Flint	4.3	43.1	18.0	39.2	37.1	43.9	84.8	158.9
Grand Rapids	6.0	36.6	17.4	35.8	27.5	15.0	61.6	125.3
Kalamazoo	3.7	35.3	15.1	36.4	26.8	21.8	63.6	134.3
Lansing	4.7	41.2	18.8	39.8	22.7	21.4	69.1	148.9
Marquette	5.3	42.8	14.7	38.4	20.5	14.6	70.5	150.0
Muskegon	4.6	37.6	14.6	54.7	13.0	10.3	53.3	119.2
Petoskey	5.2	45.2	15.5	28.9	26.4	26.4	60.7	136.6
Pontiac	5.0	38.6	14.7	42.7	45.4	37.9	82.0	169.5
Royal Oak	5.3	37.5	19.1	49.4	48.7	49.6	67.3	158.7
Saginaw	4.7	37.8	12.2	34.1	28.5	27.9	78.8	166.1
St Joseph	3.3	30.1	12.5	37.8	22.2	22.2	62.9	140.4
Traverse City	5.6	50.1	16.7	48.4	40.3	25.6	64.1	158.7
Minnesota								
Duluth	4.7	29.6	6.2	40.3	61.0	21.0	60.2	143.3
Minneapolis	4.8	27.6	9.2	45.3	38.2	18.6	62.0	145.0
Rochester	6.4	34.5	9.3	39.8	52.1	20.0	66.6	136.6
St Cloud	5.4	33.4	9.8	36.4	19.5	16.9	68.8	148.2
St Paul	5.1	25.7	11.9	44.8	35.9	18.6	64.8	153.6

Hospital Referral Region	Percent of Medicare Enrollees Receiving Immunization Against Pneumococcal Pneumonia (1995-96)	Percent of Medicare Women Age 65-69 Having Mammograms (1995-96)	Percent of Medicare Enrollees Receiving Screening for Colorectal Cancer (1995-96)	Percent of Diabetic Medicare Enrollees Receiving Eye Examination (1995-96)	Percent of Diabetic Enrollees Receiving HgbA1c Testing (1995-96)	Percent of Diabetic Enrollees Receiving One or More Blood Lipids Tests (1995-96)	Hospitalizations for Ambulatory Care Sensitive Conditions per 1,000 Medicare Enrollees (1995-96)	Hospitalizations for All Other Medical Conditions per 1,000 Medicare Enrollees (1995-96)
Mississippi								
Gulfport	3.2	21.4	9.4	38.3	19.4	24.9	95.4	208.8
Hattiesburg	2.8	25.3	9.7	40.3	31.0	17.8	107.5	205.8
Jackson	3.2	24.8	10.2	43.6	23.5	21.0	96.0	190.5
Meridian	2.2	24.3	8.2	38.9	15.0	17.5	109.5	223.3
Oxford	3.2	22.0	7.3	35.8	16.8	27.2	105.7	206.6
Tupelo	3.6	20.2	11.3	34.6	16.3	18.9	99.1	176.3
Missouri								
Cape Girardeau	3.7	21.7	5.5	44.9	36.5	25.1	78.2	141.9
Columbia	3.8	25.1	7.3	36.1	32.2	22.1	76.5	159.2
Joplin	4.4	24.4	9.0	36.9	25.2	22.3	84.1	177.5
Kansas City	4.8	24.7	9.7	44.8	42.5	34.8	79.3	158.7
Springfield	4.9	25.8	9.4	43.0	40.3	28.9	64.0	148.0
St Louis	4.6	23.9	10.2	43.2	31.8	26.5	76.0	157.5
Montana								
Billings	4.7	25.1	7.5	50.1	33.2	25.2	69.7	158.2
Great Falls	6.7	26.4	6.2	48.1	13.5	17.9	76.9	185.8
Missoula	6.0	30.7	5.5	51.9	21.8	20.0	70.7	162.9
Nebraska								
Lincoln	4.8	26.4	8.1	56.1	38.5	26.9	56.0	124.7
Omaha	4.6	27.2	7.7	53.6	33.2	19.6	70.3	144.1
Nevada								
Las Vegas	3.5	24.2	8.4	41.3	57.0	45.0	68.7	139.7
Reno	3.1	23.4	8.6	33.2	47.0	32.0	60.3	130.7
New Hampshire								
Lebanon	3.7	32.1	13.6	45.3	35.4	13.5	66.7	136.2
Manchester	4.4	32.1	17.9	56.8	45.2	30.7	57.8	130.3
New Jersey								
Camden	5.2	29.8	15.1	47.7	39.6	47.1	78.3	164.8
Hackensack	3.0	26.7	15.2	45.7	43.8	62.4	75.5	156.9
Morristown	4.6	31.0	15.1	49.0	44.6	57.2	68.2	152.9
New Brunswick	3.6	24.8	16.7	46.2	41.4	63.8	78.2	162.8
Newark	2.4	24.7	10.6	44.7	29.0	50.5	89.5	177.7
Paterson	4.5	27.0	17.6	43.6	38.2	65.5	87.3	154.6
Ridgewood	4.3	30.7	21.4	47.7	52.5	63.2	79.8	158.5
New Mexico								
Albuquerque	3.1	20.6	7.2	41.2	42.3	24.4	71.5	142.4
New York								
Albany	4.7	29.4	16.3	52.2	36.0	30.0	77.4	148.1
Binghamton	3.2	33.3	7.9	51.2	22.5	14.0	78.9	147.3
Bronx	1.9	19.7	12.4	52.9	30.2	40.5	88.2	161.3
Buffalo	3.9	34.6	12.8	48.4	23.6	23.0	72.1	147.3
Elmira	4.4	39.2	14.7	53.8	32.8	22.7	79.0	161.3
East Long Island	3.6	32.1	20.9	58.0	42.6	50.1	72.9	152.8
New York	2.4	24.3	15.7	55.0	34.3	46.3	82.5	158.1
Rochester	4.5	28.5	11.7	49.2	24.4	15.8	71.8	142.1

Hospital Referral Region	Percent of Medicare Enrollees Receiving Immunization Against Pneumococcal Pneumonia (1995-96)	Percent of Medicare Women Age 65-69 Having Mammograms (1995-96)	Percent of Medicare Enrollees Receiving Screening for Colorectal Cancer (1995-96)	Percent of Diabetic Medicare Enrollees Receiving Eye Examination (1995-96)	Percent of Diabetic Enrollees Receiving HgbA1c Testing	Percent of Diabetic Enrollees Receiving One or More Blood Lipids Tests (1995-96)	Hospitalizations for Ambulatory Care Sensitive Conditions per 1,000 Medicare Enrollees (1995-96)	Hospitalizations for All Other Medical Conditions per 1,000 Medicare Enrollees (1995-96)
Syracuse	5.0	39.3	15.3	52.4	41.0	31.5	79.1	141.5
White Plains	3.5	34.1	21.6	53.8	38.6	53.0	76.7	167.5
North Carolina								
Asheville	5.3	30.0	13.9	48.3	40.4	38.2	68.4	144.3
Charlotte	6.4	23.5	11.2	43.7	30.8	39.3	63.3	144.5
Durham	6.0	28.6	10.5	45.3	29.6	34.8	60.5	140.1
Greensboro	7.0	28.4	15.9	39.5	40.3	40.9	65.3	138.7
Greenville	7.4	29.3	12.7	44.3	32.5	31.9	72.5	151.5
Hickory	4.6	16.7	14.5	43.4	40.6	43.2	59.1	144.2
Raleigh	7.5	29.5	11.0	46.3	32.0	41.5	65.6	150.5
Wilmington	6.7	31.1	13.4	49.5	36.4	48.6	71.5	147.2
Winston-Salem	6.0	23.8	12.1	41.1	26.8	33.0	70.1	155.7
North Dakota								
Bismarck	4.5	35.6	9.3	47.1	44.9	34.6	89.0	150.0
Fargo Moorhead -Mn	4.7	33.6	8.7	41.1	57.7	16.9	67.3	128.4
Grand Forks	5.1	29.0	5.9	39.6	45.3	11.7	74.9	138.9
Minot	4.5	35.2	8.0	57.1	40.8	32.1	88.4	144.1
Ohio								
Akron	5.6	35.1	12.6	45.1	29.0	21.8	90.8	168.0
Canton	6.2	31.8	13.3	46.1	21.5	16.2	69.2	142.9
Cincinnati	5.7	25.2	13.9	40.6	21.0	16.7	73.9	144.5
Cleveland	5.6	30.5	13.7	46.5	31.0	24.4	83.6	155.8
Columbus	6.0	25.7	10.8	43.0	29.7	27.1	81.3	149.9
Dayton	5.4	28.0	13.1	37.9	36.5	19.2	73.7	139.9
Elyria	4.4	26.1	12.1	36.9	26.1	20.4	83.7	155.6
Kettering	6.4	28.4	16.1	42.4	47.4	26.8	64.2	135.2
Toledo	4.7	25.9	10.8	37.5	25.4	25.3	80.0	153.2
Youngstown	5.7	31.9	12.2	42.1	26.9	24.3	81.9	161.6
Oklahoma								
Lawton	3.8	21.2	6.3	32.7	17.1	9.0	72.1	155.2
Oklahoma City	3.3	23.5	8.1	37.6	32.9	22.3	76.3	154.5
Tulsa	3.3	27.0	12.2	40.9	46.3	31.5	64.5	145.2
Oregon								
Bend	4.8	25.3	7.5	29.0	49.7	23.2	44.4	111.7
Eugene	3.8	25.2	13.4	34.9	47.7	21.7	53.7	121.0
Medford	3.5	25.3	12.8	48.1	51.6	35.3	47.9	113.3
Portland	4.3	26.6	11.3	28.5	44.6	32.0	51.3	121.9
Salem	3.1	22.4	8.4	39.6	66.7	43.2	41.8	93.8
Pennsylvania								
Allentown	5.6	30.4	15.4	47.6	32.4	31.2	78.8	166.6
Altoona	4.3	26.3	12.8	35.9	18.6	13.9	84.1	160.4
Danville	5.9	31.3	13.0	36.4	18.0	12.5	78.5	153.6
Erie	5.6	30.4	10.5	36.5	31.1	22.9	82.5	160.9
Harrisburg	4.8	31.9	14.0	44.0	31.3	26.5	65.5	144.8
Johnstown	3.4	28.0	6.1	32.9	14.5	13.1	92.8	196.8
Lancaster	5.7	29.9	17.0	45.8	25.6	27.9	63.8	144.3

Hospital Referral Region	Percent of Medicare Enrollees Receiving Immunization Against Pneumococcal Pneumonia (1995-96)	Percent of Medicare Women Age 65-69 Having Mammograms (1995-96)	Percent of Medicare Enrollees Receiving Screening for Colorectal Cancer (1995-96)	Percent of Diabetic Medicare Enrollees Receiving Eye Examination (1995-96)	Percent of Diabetic Enrollees Receiving HgbA1c Testing (1995-96)	Percent of Diabetic Enrollees Receiving One or More Blood Lipids Tests (1995-96)	Hospitalizations for Ambulatory Care Sensitive Conditions per 1,000 Medicare Enrollees (1995-96)	Hospitalizations for All Other Medical Conditions per 1,000 Medicare Enrollees (1995-96)
Philadelphia	5.6	30.2	14.0	44.0	35.1	39.7	80.1	173.0
Pittsburgh	4.7	30.3	12.6	38.6	26.4	23.3	91.5	180.1
Reading	5.1	29.4	13.0	35.6	27.3	23.6	72.5	151.3
Sayre	3.5	29.9	9.6	45.2	39.8	18.3	89.0	166.3
Scranton	4.8	28.1	8.3	51.6	28.7	15.8	78.6	160.4
Wilkes-Barre	3.8	24.8	7.6	40.6	16.9	12.4	73.8	157.8
York	5.7	34.0	12.8	43.5	8.9	6.8	61.4	138.4
Rhode Island								
Providence	4.6	30.1	18.0	58.7	43.7	25.6	71.6	147.1
South Carolina								
Charleston	5.4	30.1	16.8	53.1	25.5	28.7	64.2	158.7
Columbia	4.5	19.6	18.1	38.4	25.0	29.5	61.6	136.0
Florence	4.0	27.2	10.6	43.4	31.2	24.6	80.9	180.4
Greenville	5.1	23.0	17.0	44.6	25.1	30.0	63.0	133.4
Spartanburg	4.7	22.8	13.3	33.8	26.7	38.1	67.8	144.9
South Dakota								
Rapid City	4.4	33.2	7.7	44.9	40.4	30.8	79.1	143.0
Sioux Falls	4.4	27.7	9.1	50.1	41.4	21.0	73.3	151.1
Tennessee								
Chattanooga	5.0	29.1	11.3	35.1	30.0	30.4	78.0	172.0
Jackson	5.5	20.8	7.3	43.9	25.6	28.9	83.0	166.7
Johnson City	5.0	28.4	8.7	27.5	29.2	38.6	73.0	168.2
Kingsport	4.5	25.6	5.7	39.9	31.8	23.9	100.0	182.8
Knoxville	5.1	27.3	10.4	31.8	34.9	38.8	87.0	174.8
Memphis	3.8	21.0	12.3	39.9	29.3	30.3	81.8	162.8
Nashville	4.9	25.7	10.8	35.3	31.1	33.6	83.0	186.1
Texas								
Abilene	3.4	23.6	9.5	41.0	37.9	26.8	81.5	173.4
Amarillo	2.4	27.8	10.2	51.2	43.8	35.1	75.5	158.4
Austin	4.7	22.7	16.4	49.4	42.5	34.6	65.2	140.2
Beaumont	3.4	26.2	9.0	45.0	31.6	35.3	94.2	193.0
Bryan	3.8	28.7	14.0	34.9	29.7	34.3	75.6	134.3
Corpus Christi	5.4	28.7	11.9	44.7	29.7	28.3	97.1	169.6
Dallas	4.0	23.7	14.5	44.7	43.8	38.9	70.6	144.6
El Paso	2.1	12.2	8.0	36.9	40.7	29.1	71.0	142.8
Fort Worth	5.1	21.4	14.0	45.9	45.5	31.0	65.1	134.1
Harlingen	2.6	18.1	8.6	54.9	34.4	30.6	87.1	152.0
Houston	3.1	25.4	10.1	44.3	35.3	37.2	78.3	165.8
Longview	4.1	34.0	19.5	46.2	31.5	27.7	68.5	153.9
Lubbock	2.9	27.7	9.9	47.8	37.3	29.3	89.9	177.6
McAllen	4.0	18.2	7.4	50.3	30.6	37.4	93.4	156.6
Odessa	3.7	15.7	12.4	43.0	27.8	35.8	88.4	162.7
San Angelo	3.6	21.6	12.6	44.9	35.5	12.6	92.2	152.5
San Antonio	2.8	23.6	12.2	49.1	30.7	29.9	77.9	147.7
Temple	3.4	21.6	8.4	44.9	42.0	26.9	73.2	137.3
Tyler	4.1	26.0	14.3	41.2	39.3	32.2	76.9	160.1

Hospital Referral Region	Percent of Medicare Enrollees Receiving Immunization Against Pneumococcal Pneumonia (1995-96)	Percent of Medicare Women Age 65-69 Having Mammograms (1995-96)	Percent of Medicare Enrollees Receiving Screening for Colorectal Cancer (1995-96)	Percent of Diabetic Medicare Enrollees Receiving Eye Examination (1995-96)	Percent of Diabetic Enrollees Receiving HgbA1c Testing	Percent of Diabetic Enrollees Receiving One or More Blood Lipids Tests (1995-96)	Hospitalizations for Ambulatory Care Sensitive Conditions per 1,000 Medicare Enrollees (1995-96)	Hospitalizations for All Other Medical Conditions per 1,000 Medicare Enrollees (1995-96)
Victoria	5.5	18.5	9.8	45.8	37.0	26.0	92.8	188.3
Waco	3.4	25.7	10.2	40.2	28.5	26.5	66.1	124.1
Wichita Falls	5.2	30.9	17.1	49.3	41.4	25.5	81.8	154.4
Utah								
Ogden	4.6	25.9	4.5	48.7	54.9	19.4	41.6	111.1
Provo	2.5	18.8	3.9	46.9	37.7	21.3	52.0	117.0
Salt Lake City	3.6	22.1	5.2	42.2	38.9	25.3	47.4	118.5
Vermont								
Burlington	6.0	33.5	15.4	54.8	16.7	11.5	76.3	152.8
Virginia								
Arlington	5.1	26.6	15.4	42.6	53.4	48.1	61.0	143.7
Charlottesville	7.4	25.9	7.5	42.6	36.6	38.9	68.3	166.7
Lynchburg	5.4	24.5	4.8	57.6	48.7	28.9	61.9	139.2
Newport News	4.0	31.1	7.9	48.2	44.5	38.6	59.8	145.4
Norfolk	5.1	32.4	10.6	45.2	35.7	31.1	68.6	150.4
Richmond	3.9	26.9	7.7	44.6	36.6	37.4	68.8	162.7
Roanoke	3.8	18.8	6.8	37.0	38.8	33.4	69.0	168.8
Winchester	5.1	26.9	6.4	33.3	37.5	37.9	98.3	174.2
Washington								
Everett	4.1	28.2	7.9	47.6	49.5	31.5	46.6	123.9
Olympia	3.8	30.2	8.2	40.5	56.2	30.5	55.6	114.7
Seattle	4.3	30.4	10.4	47.5	54.2	31.3	52.5	124.6
Spokane	4.2	28.8	10.0	48.9	53.0	34.3	55.6	130.3
Tacoma	3.1	28.1	11.3	47.0	30.9	28.7	46.6	111.8
Yakima	5.1	26.5	10.5	35.3	49.4	34.9	54.9	129.2
West Virginia								
Charleston	4.1	30.0	9.4	43.6	27.4	27.9	92.5	183.9
Huntington	4.4	23.6	7.6	39.8	40.8	35.6	92.5	177.7
Morgantown	4.4	31.7	11.1	38.8	23.5	28.6	94.4	169.7
Wisconsin								
Appleton	4.0	27.6	4.2	43.3	39.9	21.2	54.5	123.5
Green Bay	4.3	32.1	7.0	50.2	25.8	18.8	56.0	137.7
La Crosse	5.4	26.4	6.6	44.2	49.5	9.0	62.9	147.1
Madison	4.5	28.0	5.4	37.6	49.0	18.3	62.6	147.6
Marshfield	5.1	28.6	6.5	49.2	57.9	24.1	67.9	144.7
Milwaukee	4.3	29.3	7.1	37.9	39.0	27.6	65.0	146.7
Neenah	5.4	32.7	5.9	45.6	43.4	15.4	60.3	139.8
Wausau	6.8	33.1	6.0	51.6	63.5	26.4	57.5	128.9
Wyoming								
Casper	3.9	24.7	6.1	50.3	41.0	28.6	78.9	165.4
United States								
United States	4.3	28.3	12.3	45.3	35.6	33.1	73.7	155.5

Practice Variations and the Quality of Surgical Care for Common Conditions

Practice Variations and the Quality of Surgical Care for Common Conditions

Quality in health care means doing the right things right. Traditional efforts to improve the quality of surgical care have concentrated on improving surgical performance — *doing things right*. Performance quality in surgery is usually measured in terms of mortality or complication rates, and problems are indicated by variations in outcome rates. Efforts to improve quality usually focus on improving processes of care, from how skillfully the operation is performed to how well patients are cared for after surgery.

Although performance quality is important, so too is the quality of clinical decision making — *doing the right thing*. To measure this aspect of quality, it is necessary to ask whether the initial decision to proceed with surgery was correct. Measuring decision quality is much more difficult than tracking mortality or complication rates. However, as with performance quality, variation is an important indicator of problems in the quality of decision making. From a population perspective, variation in surgical decision making becomes apparent from the large regional variations in the rates at which populations undergo specific surgical procedures. Population-based rates of many common procedures vary by as much as a factor of ten (sometimes even more) — that is, residents of some parts of the country are as much as ten times more likely to receive particular surgical procedures than people with the same disease profiles who live elsewhere.

This chapter explores how both these components of quality — decision making and performance — are reflected in the patterns of surgical care across the United States. The chapter first describes the current degree of regional variation of ten common surgical procedures, identifying the procedures in which there is the greatest opportunity for improving decision making. The chapter then profiles two procedures, surgery for stroke prevention (carotid endarterectomy) and invasive treatment of coronary artery disease, to describe the factors that determine quality in surgical decision making and the quality of the surgery being performed — the outcomes of surgery.

Variations in the Surgical Treatment of Common Diseases

Ten surgical procedures — repair of hip fracture, colectomy for colorectal cancer, cholecystectomy, angioplasty, coronary artery bypass surgery, hip replacement, lower extremity bypass surgery, carotid endarterectomy, back surgery, and radical prostatectomy — represented approximately 42% of Medicare inpatient surgery and accounted for 44% of reimbursements for surgical care in 1995-96.

The ten procedures had very different variation profiles. For example, rates of colectomy for colorectal cancer varied by only a factor of two, from 1.5 per 1,000 Medicare enrollees in the Harlingen, Texas hospital referral region to 3.2 per 1,000 Medicare residents of the Sioux City, Iowa hospital referral region. There were only ten hospital referral regions with rates of colectomy for colorectal cancer less than 25% lower than the national average, and only one with a rate more than 30% higher than the national average.

There was far more variation in rates of most other common surgical procedures. Rates of radical prostatectomy for prostate cancer varied by a factor of more than nine, from 0.5 per 1,000 Medicare enrollees in the Binghamton, New York hospital referral region to 4.7 in the Baton Rouge, Louisiana hospital referral region. There were 67 hospital referral regions which had rates of prostatectomy more than 25% lower than the national average, and 62 hospital referral regions where male Medicare residents underwent prostatectomy at rates more than 30% higher than the national average. According to the systematic component of variation, rates of radical prostatectomy were more than 12 times more variable than rates of colectomy for colon cancer (Table 5.1). Rates of lower extremity bypass surgery for Medicare enrollees with inadequate circulation to their legs, carotid endarterectomy for stroke prevention, and back surgery were also highly variable among hospital referral regions.

Why Procedures Vary to Different Degrees

Although regional variation in health care is ubiquitous, not all surgical procedures vary to the same degree. Procedures which are not very variable are generally applied to clinical conditions for which treatment is constrained to a single clinical approach. For example, there is wide consensus that surgery is the primary treatment for both hip fracture and colorectal cancer. The geographic variation in the use of surgery for these two conditions is largely due to variations in illness rates — for example, colorectal cancer is slightly more common among residents of the Mountain states and parts of the Southeast than among residents of other parts of the country (Chapter Three).

The amount of regional variation for most procedures, however, is too large to attribute to chance or variation in illness rates; the rates of surgery described in Table 5.1 and Figure 5.1 have been adjusted for regional differences in illness rates, but still vary substantially. Variations in the rates of the use of these procedures reflect variations in practice style and in how physicians diagnose and treat common clinical conditions.

Table 5.1. Quantitative Measures of Variability of Ten Common Surgical Procedures by Hospital Referral Region (1995-96)

	Hip Fracture Repair	Colectomy for Colorectal Cancer	Cholecystectomy	Coronary Artery Bypass Grafting	Hip Replacement	Back Surgery	Carotid Endarterectomy	Percutaneous Transluminal Coronary Angioplasty	Lower Extremity Bypass	Radical Prostatectomy
Index of Variation										
Systematic Component of Variation (SCV)	10.3	15.7	26.5	38.0	61.8	88.0	95.6	102.0	104.8	130.3
Ratio to SCV of surgical repair of hip fracture	1.0	1.5	2.6	3.7	6.0	8.6	9.3	9.9	10.2	12.7
Range of Variation										
Extremal Ratio (highest to lowest region)	2.0	2.2	2.7	3.7	4.5	5.7	7.7	6.9	9.0	9.4
Interquartile Ratio (75th to 25th percentile region)	1.2	1.2	1.3	1.3	1.4	1.5	1.5	1.5	1.5	1.6
Number of Regions with High and Low Rates										
Rates more than 25% below the national average	1	10	10	19	40	41	54	61	80	67
Rates 30% or more above the national average	0	1	19	21	46	63	53	54	29	62

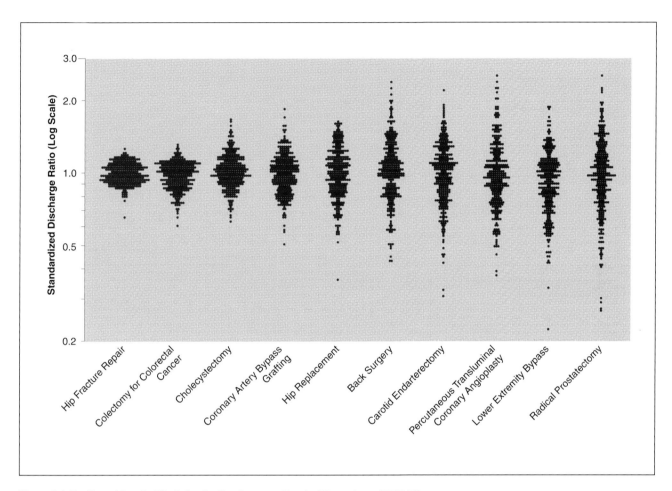

Figure 5.1. Profiles of Surgical Variation for Ten Common Surgical Procedures (1995-96)

■ **Variation in diagnostic intensity.** Surgery rates might vary because physicians in different regions vary in how aggressively they look for surgically treatable disease. For example, because early-stage prostate cancer frequently has no symptoms, the diagnosis is increasingly being made through a screening test for prostate-specific antigen. There is a great deal of regional variation in the frequency of use of this controversial screening test; as a result, there is also variation in the rate at which men are diagnosed (screening more men means that more men are diagnosed with early-stage disease) and variation in how often men undergo surgery (where more men are diagnosed with early-stage disease, more undergo surgical treatment for the condition).

■ **Problems with medical science.** For some procedures, regional variation in the use of surgery is due to gaps in medical science and professional uncertainty about the implications of alternative treatments. For example, variation in rates of radical prostatectomy might be partly attributable to the lack of controlled clinical trials comparing the risks and benefits of surgery, radiation therapy, and watchful waiting. For other procedures, even the best clinical trials are often not sufficient to eliminate variation in procedure rates: physicians vary in how they interpret and apply findings from the carefully controlled settings of clinical trials to decision making for individual patients in other settings.

■ **Failure to incorporate patient preferences into treatment decisions.** Although medical science is necessary for quantifying risks and benefits, some of the trade-offs involved in surgical decisions can only be assessed by patients. For example, the major risks of radical prostatectomy are urinary incontinence and impotence. Only patients themselves can weigh the importance of these side effects against the potential benefits of surgically removing the prostate cancer. Table 5.2 lists the treatment options available to patients and the clinical trade-offs patients face in terms of the risks and benefits for the ten conditions for which the procedures in Figure 5.1 are commonly performed.

Table 5.2. Trade-Offs, Risks and Benefits of Treatment Options for Selected Conditions

Clinical condition	Treatment Options	Trade-Offs Among Alternatives
Hip fracture	Surgical repair	No alternatives
Colorectal cancer	Colectomy	No alternatives
Chronic cholecystitis (intermittent abdominal pain from gallstones)	Watchful waiting	Avoids surgery, but carries a risk of a later serious attack (acute cholecystitis) and the need for urgent, open surgery
	Cholecystectomy (usually laparoscopic rather than open surgery)	Very effective, but there are small risks of serious complications
Chronic stable angina (chest pain or other symptoms from coronary artery disease)	Medical treatment	Avoids the downsides of interventions, but is less effective at improving symptoms and some patients have shorter survival
	Angioplasty	Lower procedure risks than surgery, but symptom relief is not as long lasting
	Bypass surgery	Effective and durable in relieving symptoms, but there are significant risks of mortality and disability, including stroke
Hip osteoarthritis	Medical treatment	Low risk, but not very effective in relieving symptoms
	Hip replacement	Very effective, but there are modest risks of mortality and complications, as well as a long recovery period
Claudication (exertional leg pain from peripheral vascular disease)	Medical treatment, exercise	Low risk, but only modestly effective
	Angioplasty	Effective at improving symptoms, but there are risks of complications and subsequent interventions are often necessary
	Bypass surgery	Very effective and durable, but there are significant risks of complications and death
Carotid stenosis (stroke risk from narrowing of carotid artery)	Aspirin	Lower short-term risks, but higher risks of stroke over the long term
	Carotid endarterectomy	Reduces overall stroke risks, but there are significant risks of mortality and of perioperative stroke
Herniated disc or Spinal Stenosis (causing back pain or other symptoms)	Medical treatment, chiropractic, other	Symptoms often resolve without surgery, but might not
	Back surgery	Frequently relieves symptoms, but has complication risks and is not always effective
Early-stage prostate cancer	Watchful waiting	Many prostate cancers never progress to affect quality of life or survival, but some do
	Radiation (conventional or implant seeds)	Shrinks or eliminates cancer in the prostate, but there are risks of side effects
	Radical prostatectomy	Removes prostate cancer entirely, but there are substantial risks of incontinence and impotence

Surgery for Preventing Stroke

Strokes are the third leading cause of death in the United States, and a major source of disability in the elderly. Most strokes are attributable to atherosclerosis and narrowing, or stenosis, of the carotid arteries, which supply blood to the brain. To reduce the risk of stroke associated with carotid stenosis, many patients undergo carotid endarterectomy, a surgical procedure in which plaque is removed from the artery. The procedure carries a relatively small risk of death, but a higher and more variable risk of perioperative stroke.

Although carotid endarterectomy has been widely available since the 1970s, the procedure was considered controversial until the 1990s, when the results of the first carefully controlled clinical trials of its risks and benefits began to be published. There was a dramatic increase in the use of carotid endarterectomy in the United States in the 1990s. Between 1988 and 1996, the number of procedures increased by more than 85%, from 70,000 to 130,000 per year. Particularly sharp increases were seen following publication of results of the North American Symptomatic Carotid Atherosclerosis Study (NASCET) and the Asymptomatic Carotid Artery Surgery (ACAS) trial.

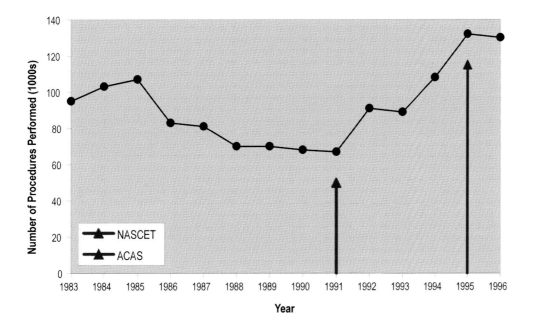

Figure 5.2. Increase in Number of Carotid Endarterectomy Procedures by Year, 1983-1996

The number of carotid endarterectomy procedures declined between 1985 and 1991, but rose sharply again after publication of the results of the NASCET trial in 1991. Publication of results of the NASCET (1991) and ACAS (1995) studies are indicated by arrows.

Source: The National Center for Health Statistics

The Quality of Medical Decision Making for Prevention of Stroke

Variation in the quality of medical decision making is reflected in the illness adjusted rates of carotid endarterectomy, which vary more than almost any other common inpatient procedure. In 1995-96, rates of carotid endarterectomy among Medicare enrollees ranged from 1.1 per 1,000 enrollees in the Idaho Falls, Idaho hospital referral region to 7.6 per 1,000 among Medicare residents of the Houma, Louisiana hospital referral region, a factor of almost seven. This variation indicates that there are persistent problems in the quality of medical decision making.

Among the hospital referral regions where rates of carotid endarterectomy were substantially higher than the United States average of 3.5 per 1,000 Medicare enrollees were Slidell, Louisiana (6.6); Lafayette, Louisiana (6.5); Gulfport, Mississippi (6.4); Albany, Georgia (6.2); St. Petersburg, Florida (6.1); and Wilmington, North Carolina (6.0).

Among the regions where rates of carotid endarterectomy per 1,000 Medicare enrollees were lower than average were Honolulu (1.1); Salt Lake City (1.5); La Crosse, Wisconsin (1.5); Charlottesville, Virginia (1.6); and Rochester, Minnesota (1.6).

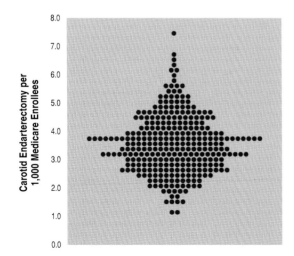

Figure 5.3. Rates of Carotid Endarterectomy Among Hospital Referral Regions (1995-96)

Rates of carotid endarterectomy ranged from 1.1 to 7.6 per 1,000 Medicare enrollees, even after adjustments for differences in the age, sex, race and illness rates of local populations. Each point represents one of the 306 hospital referral regions in the United States.

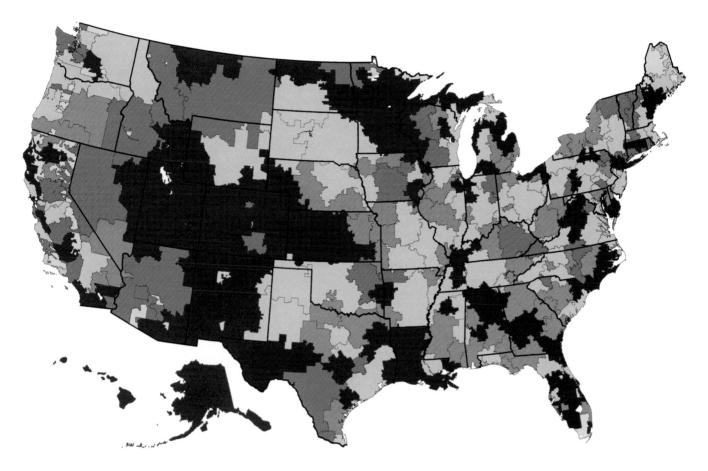

Map 5.1. Carotid Endarterectomy (1995-96)

Rates of carotid endarterectomy were highly variable among hospital referral regions; some regions in the highest quintile were contiguous with regions in the lowest quintile. Broadly, rates were lower in the Western part of the United States than in the East, although there were no clear patterns of use.

Ratio of Rates of Carotid Endarterectomy to the U.S. Average

by Hospital Referral Region (1995-96)

- 1.30 to 2.19 (53)
- 1.10 to < 1.30 (63)
- 0.90 to < 1.10 (86)
- 0.75 to < 0.90 (50)
- 0.30 to < 0.75 (54)
- Not Populated

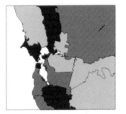

San Francisco

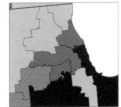

Chicago

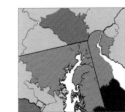

New York

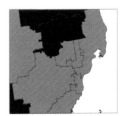

Washington-Baltimore

Detroit

Diagnostic Intensity as Source of Variation in Carotid Artery Surgery Rates

Surgery rates might also vary because physicians in some regions look harder for disease than do physicians elsewhere. An increasing proportion of carotid endarterectomies are being performed on asymptomatic patients — those in whom carotid stenosis can only be identified by diagnostic testing, usually with carotid duplex, or ultrasound. However, there is no consensus among physicians about which patients should be screened with carotid duplex, and as a result duplex rates vary widely among hospital referral regions. Rates of carotid duplex varied from fewer than 20 to more than 115 per 1,000 Medicare enrollees in 1995-96.

Moreover, carotid duplex rates are highly correlated with rates of carotid endarterectomy; the prevalence of screening explains about 40% of the variability in rates of carotid endarterectomy (Figure 5.5). The more carefully physicians look for surgically treatable carotid disease, the more they find, and the more likely asymptomatic people are to undergo surgery.

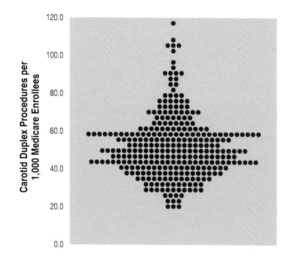

Figure 5.4. Rates of Carotid Duplex Diagnostic Procedures Among Hospital Referral Regions (1995-96)

Rates of carotid duplex diagnostic procedures ranged from fewer than 20 to almost 120 per 1,000 Medicare enrollees. Each point represents one of the 306 hospital referral regions in the United States.

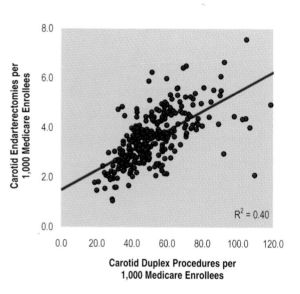

Figure 5.5. The Relationship between Rates of Carotid Duplex Diagnostic Procedures and Rates of Carotid Endarterectomy (1995-96)

The prevalence of screening was strongly correlated with the likelihood that Medicare enrollees would undergo carotid endarterectomy (R^2 = .40).

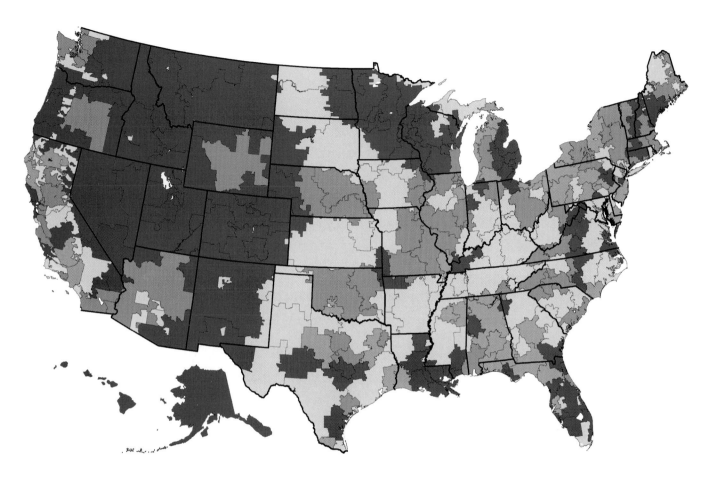

Map 5.2. Carotid Duplex Diagnostic Procedures (1995-96)

Carotid duplex imaging procedures were performed more frequently in Florida, Louisiana, and parts of Michigan and Texas than in most other regions in the United States; the procedure was, generally, far less frequently used among residents of the Western United States than in the South and Midwest.

Ratio of Rates of Carotid Duplex Diagnostic Procedures to the U.S. Average

by Hospital Referral Region (1995-96)

- 1.30 to 2.24 (42)
- 1.10 to < 1.30 (48)
- 0.90 to < 1.10 (84)
- 0.75 to < 0.90 (65)
- 0.35 to < 0.75 (67)
- Not Populated

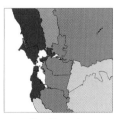

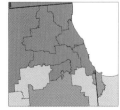

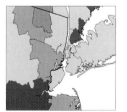

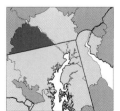

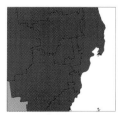

San Francisco   **Chicago**   **New York**   **Washington-Baltimore**   **Detroit**

The Quality of Medical Science and Importance of Patient Preferences

The quality of medical science concerning carotid endarterectomy is in some respects very good: few surgical procedures have been as closely scrutinized with carefully controlled clinical trials. Among the most influential trials was the North American Symptomatic Carotid Atherosclerosis Study (NASCET), in 1991, which focused on patients with severe stenosis (more than 70% narrowing of the carotid arteries) and pre-stroke symptoms, including transient blindness or weakness of an extremity. Patients in the study who were randomized to surgery had substantially lower rates of stroke than patients treated with aspirin alone (12% vs. 26% after two years of follow-up). The Asymptomatic Carotid Artery Surgery (ACAS) trial, for which results were published in 1995, demonstrated the effectiveness of surgery in asymptomatic patients with severe stenosis, but the benefit was substantially smaller (the risk of stroke was 5%, vs. 11%, after five years of follow-up).

Considerable uncertainty persists, however, about applying the results of the clinical trials to the everyday practice of medicine; there is substantial uncertainty about the outcomes of care among patients and institutions not included in the clinical trials. Although the clinical trials were based on relatively young, healthy patients undergoing surgery at hospitals with proven records of excellent results, only a minority of carotid endarterectomies performed in other settings meet these strict criteria. In 1996, more than 46,000 carotid endarterectomy procedures were performed on Medicare enrollees age 74 or older. Variations in surgery rates might be a reflection of physicians' different assumptions about the effectiveness of surgery in older, sicker patients receiving care in settings where outcomes are less certain.

The Quality of Surgical Performance: Carotid Endarterectomy

Since the reduction in stroke rates among asymptomatic patients who had carotid endarterectomy is relatively modest (slightly more than 1% per year), the value of surgery depends on surgery having even lower risks of morbidity and mortality than doing nothing. Hospitals participating in the NASCET and ACAS trials were selected carefully, based on their prior results and experience with the procedure. For example, only one of 825 patients (0.1%) in the ACAS trial died as a result of surgery.

Not all surgeons or hospitals have been able to achieve similar results. Among Ohio hospitals in 1993-94, for example, rates of stroke or death following carotid endarterectomy varied widely. One of the strongest predictors of stroke risk was hospital experience with the procedure: hospitals performing at least 70 carotid endarterectomies annually had stroke or death rates under 3.0%. Conversely, low-volume hospitals (those performing fewer than 40 procedures per year) had stroke or death rates exceeding 7.0%.

These observations are not unique to Ohio. Although surgical stroke rates are difficult to examine with claims data, mortality rates in Medicare patients undergoing carotid endarterectomy vary widely. In addition, hospital volume was strong correlated with performance quality. In 1992-93, mortality rates at low-volume hospitals (2.5%) were at least 50% higher than at high-volume centers (1.7%) and "centers of excellence" which participated in the clinical trials (1.5%).

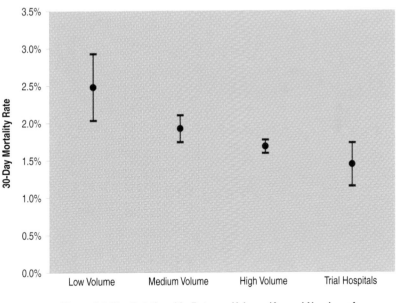

Figure 5.6. The Relationship Between Volume (Annual Number of Procedures Performed) and Outcomes (Mortality) of Carotid Endarterectomy (1992-93)

Death within 30 days of carotid endarterectomy was far more likely among patients at hospitals where the procedure was performed fewer than 40 times per year. Mortality was lower among patients at high-volume hospitals (those performing at least 70 procedures per year); but even high-volume hospitals were unable to achieve the lower mortality rates of the hospitals in which the clinical trials of the procedure took place. (The 95% confidence limits are given in brackets.)

Source: The Journal of the American Medical Association (see Endnote)

Invasive Treatment of Coronary Artery Disease

The leading cause of death in the United States, coronary artery disease is caused by atherosclerosis and blockage of the coronary arteries, which supply blood to the heart. Coronary artery disease can present for the first time with an acute event, such as a heart attack or sudden death. Alternatively, it can manifest as chronic symptoms, such as shortness of breath or chest pain (angina) with exertion. In some patients, coronary artery disease is "silent," detected only by a routine cardiogram or stress test. The severity of coronary artery disease (the number of artery blockages and the severity of narrowing of the arteries) is determined by coronary angiography, an imaging test in which dye is injected into the heart through a catheter.

Although most patients with coronary artery disease are treated with medications, a substantial number undergo invasive treatment. Coronary artery bypass grafting surgery was first developed in the 1960s. This surgery involves bypassing blocked arteries, usually with pieces of vein taken from the leg. Since the 1980s, angioplasty, in which coronary blockages are opened with a balloon inserted through a catheter, has been available as an alternative to bypass surgery. Clinical trials suggest that both of these procedures improve angina symptoms and, in a few specific patient subgroups, increase long-term survival.

The number of invasive procedures for the treatment of coronary artery disease has increased steadily. The number of angioplasty procedures among members of the Medicare population increased by a factor of more than 16 in a 12-year period, from fewer than 12,000 in 1984 to almost 200,000 in 1996. Angioplasty does not seem to be used as a substitute for bypass surgery, however; rates of bypass surgery in the same population actually increased 300% over the same time interval, from fewer than 60,000 procedures in 1984 to more than 180,000 in 1996.

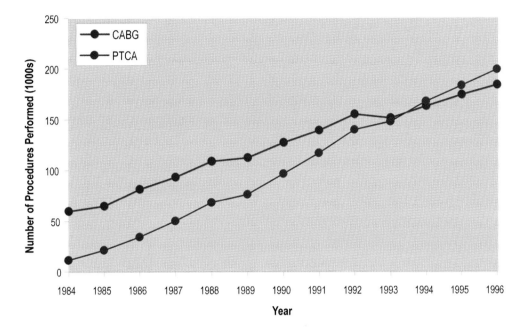

Figure 5.7. Growth in Number of Invasive Cardiac Procedures Among Medicare Enrollees (1984-96)

The number of invasive procedures for the treatment of coronary artery disease increased rapidly between 1984 and 1996, from about 70,000 per year to more than 380,000. Although balloon angioplasty was purported to be a substitute for more-invasive bypass surgery, the frequencies of both procedures grew at simultaneously rapid rates.

The Quality of Medical Decision Making

There was substantial regional variation in rates of invasive treatment of coronary artery disease in 1995-96. Rates of coronary artery bypass grafting among Medicare enrollees varied by a factor of more than 3.5, from 3.1 to 11.5 per 1,000 enrollees. Rates of coronary angioplasty (PTCA) were even more variable, ranging from 2.5 to 16.9 per 1,000 enrollees.

Among the hospital referral regions where rates of coronary artery bypass grafting per 1,000 Medicare enrollees were highest were Redding, California (11.5); Houma, Louisiana (10.6); Bloomington, Illinois (9.8); and Hudson, Florida (9.4).

Regions with rates lower than the national average of 6.2 bypass grafting procedures per 1,000 enrollees included Albuquerque, New Mexico (3.1); Grand Junction, Colorado (3.5); and Santa Rosa, California (3.6).

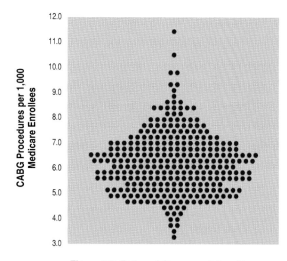

Figure 5.8. Rates of Coronary Artery Bypass Grafting Among Hospital Referral Regions (1995-96)

Rates of bypass surgery ranged from fewer than 3.5 to more than 11 per 1,000 Medicare enrollees, even after adjustments for differences in the age, sex, race and illness rates of local populations. Each point represents one of the 306 hospital referral regions in the United States.

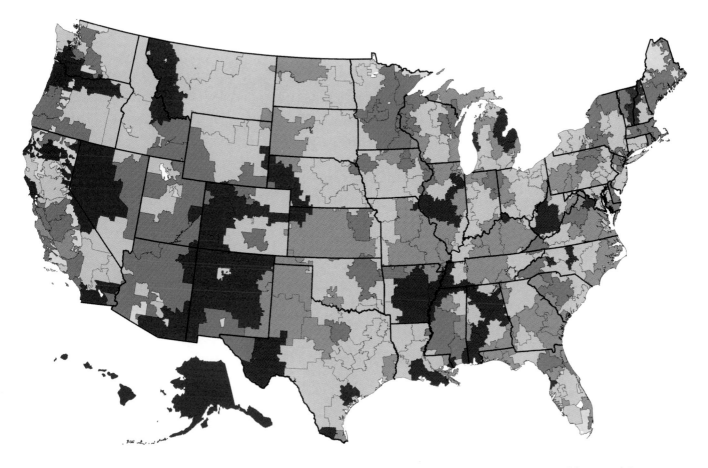

Map 5.3. Coronary Artery Bypass Grafting (1995-96)

The likelihood of undergoing bypass surgery was highly dependent on where the Medicare enrollee lived. Rates of bypass surgery were as much as 87% higher than the national average in some regions, and as low as 50% below the national average in others. Generally, rates were lower in the Mountain states and higher in the Midwest and mid-South.

Ratio of Rates of Coronary Artery Bypass Grafting Procedures to the U.S. Average

by Hospital Referral Region (1995-96)

- 1.30 to 1.87 (21)
- 1.10 to < 1.30 (69)
- 0.90 to < 1.10 (126)
- 0.75 to < 0.90 (71)
- 0.50 to < 0.75 (19)
- Not Populated

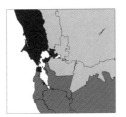

San Francisco

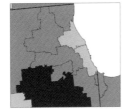

Chicago

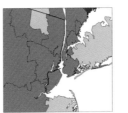

New York

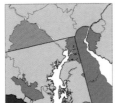

Washington-Baltimore

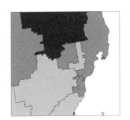

Detroit

Rates of PTCA were substantially higher than the national average of 6.6 procedures per 1,000 Medicare enrollees in the hospital referral regions in Elyria, Ohio
(16.9); Alexandria, Louisiana (15.9); and Jonesboro, Arkansas (15.0). Rates were
substantially lower than the national average among residents of the hospital referral
regions in York, Pennsylvania (2.5); Asheville, North Carolina (2.6); Buffalo, New
York (3.1) and Lebanon, New Hampshire (3.2).

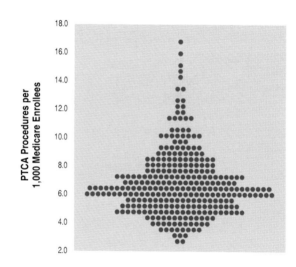

**Figure 5.9. Rates of Percutaneous Transluminal Coronary Angioplasty
Among Hospital Referral Regions (1995-96)**

*Rates of coronary angioplasty ranged from 2.5 to more than 16.5 per 1,000
Medicare enrollees, even after adjustments for differences in the age, sex, race and
illness rates of local populations. Each point represents one of the 306 hospital referral
regions in the United States.*

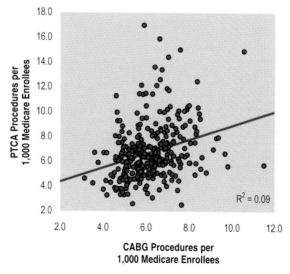

**Figure 5.10. The Relationship between Rates of Coronary Artery Bypass
Grafting and Rates of Percutaneous Transluminal Coronary Angioplasty
(1995-96)**

*Although PCTA is often considered a substitute for more invasive bypass surgery,
age, sex, race, and illness adjusted rates of the two procedures in fact have a
positive correlation (R^2 = .09). Each point represents one of the 306 hospital
referral regions in the United States.*

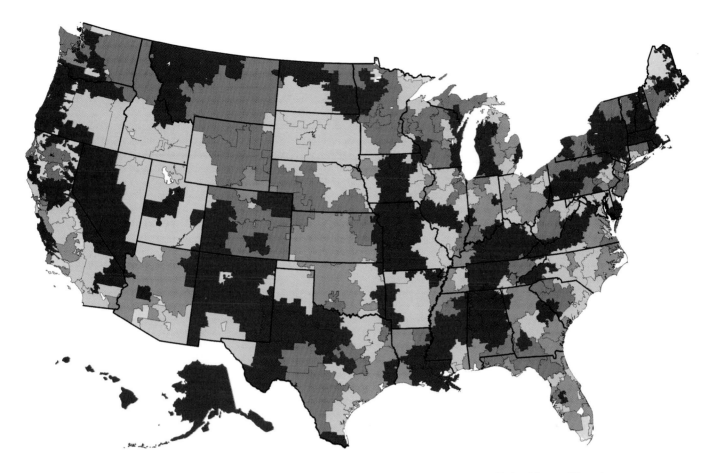

Map 5.4. Percutaneous Transluminal Coronary Angioplasty (1995-96)

The likelihood of undergoing balloon angioplasty was nearly random, depending on the enrollee's hospital referral region of residence; there were few regional patterns or logical distributions of the rates at which the procedure was performed. In some regions, enrollees were more than two and one-half times as likely as the national average to have the procedure; elsewhere, rates were more than 60% lower than the national average.

Ratio of Rates of Percutaneous Transluminal Coronary Angioplasty Procedures to the U.S. Average

by Hospital Referral Region (1995-96)

- 1.30 to   2.57   (54)
- 1.10 to < 1.30   (42)
- 0.90 to < 1.10   (89)
- 0.75 to < 0.90   (60)
- 0.37 to < 0.75   (61)
- Not Populated

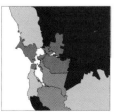

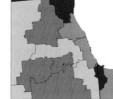

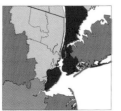

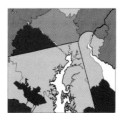

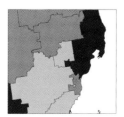

| San Francisco | Chicago | New York | Washington-Baltimore | Detroit |

Diagnostic Intensity As Source of Variation in Invasive Treatment

Coronary angiography is the primary diagnostic test for determining the severity of coronary artery disease. It is also a prerequisite to invasive treatment — neither bypass surgery nor angioplasty can be performed without the "road map" provided by angiography.

Physicians disagree about how severe patients' symptoms must be to warrant coronary angiography. This disagreement results in substantial variability in rates of angiography among hospital referral regions. In 1995-96, rates of coronary angiography among Medicare enrollees varied by a factor of 5.5, from 9.6 per 1,000 enrollees in the Grand Junction, Colorado hospital referral region to 53.1 per 1,000 among residents of the Houma, Louisiana hospital referral region.

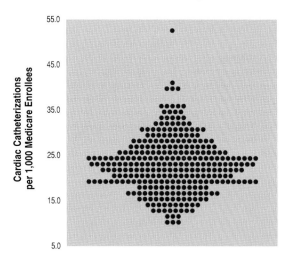

Figure 5.11. Rates of Cardiac Catheterization Among Hospital Referral Regions (1995-96)

Rates of cardiac catheterization ranged from fewer than 10 to more than 50 per 1,000 Medicare enrollees, after adjustment for differences in the age, sex, race, and illness levels of local populations. Each point represents one of the 306 hospital referral regions in the United States.

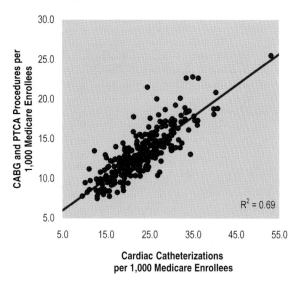

Figure 5.12. The Relationship Between Rates of Cardiac Catheterization and Rates of Invasive Coronary Procedures (Coronary Artery Bypass Grafting and Percutaneous Transluminal Coronary Angioplasty) (1995-96)

Rates of coronary angiography were strongly linked to rates of bypass surgery and coronary angioplasty, accounting for about 70% of the observed variation in surgery rates. The more physicians look for surgically treatable coronary artery disease, the more they find, and the more invasive treatment is provided ($R^2 = .69$).

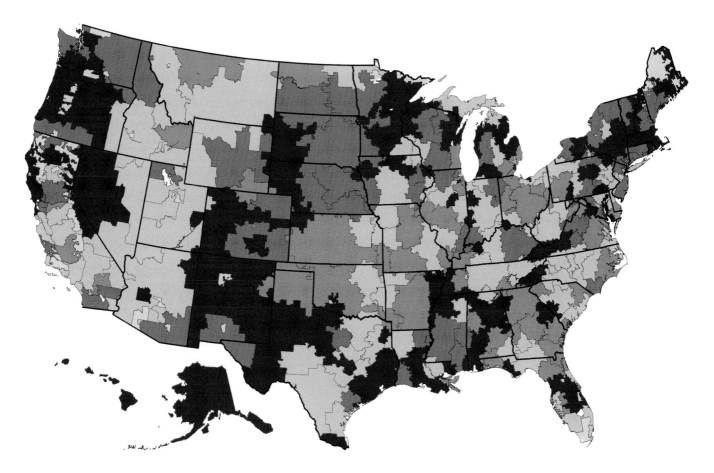

Map 5.5. Rates of Cardiac Catheterization Among Hospital Referral Regions (1995-96)

Variation in the use of invasive treatment for coronary artery disease is partly attributable to regional differences in diagnostic intensity. In 44 areas, rates were at least 30% higher than the national average; in 49 regions, rates were at least 25% lower than the national average.

Ratio of Rates of Cardiac Catheterization to the U.S. Average

by Hospital Referral Region (1995-96)

- 1.30 to 2.35 (44)
- 1.10 to < 1.30 (54)
- 0.90 to < 1.10 (97)
- 0.75 to < 0.90 (62)
- 0.42 to < 0.75 (49)
- Not Populated

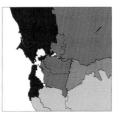

San Francisco

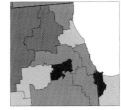

Chicago

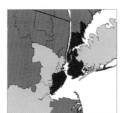

New York

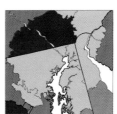

Washington-Baltimore

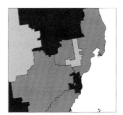

Detroit

The Quality of Medical Science and Importance of Patient Preferences

Several well-known clinical trials, all initiated in the 1970s, have described the effectiveness of bypass surgery. Compared to medical treatment, surgery was found in these studies to significantly improve angina symptoms and, in a few specific patient subgroups, to increase survival in patients with chronic stable angina. More recent trials have compared the relative effectiveness of bypass surgery and angioplasty. These studies have suggested lower short term morbidity and mortality with angioplasty, but longer lasting relief of symptoms with bypass surgery. Long term survival after the two procedures was found to be approximately equivalent.

However, our understanding of the risks and benefits of invasive treatment for coronary artery disease is limited in several ways. Because both medical treatment and surgical techniques have changed significantly since the 1970s, the results from surgery trials are outdated. Patients enrolled in the trials begun in the 1970s differed substantially from patients undergoing surgery in the 1990s. In the 1970s, patients were almost exclusively male; today approximately 30% of patients undergoing bypass surgery are women. The trials were based on elective bypass surgery in patients with stable coronary artery disease. Today, approximately one-half of all bypass surgery is done on an urgent basis, after heart attacks or for other acute conditions.

Finally, while the average age of patients in the trials was under 60, most patients undergoing surgery in the 1990s are over age 65, and bypass surgery rates are rising most dramatically in the very elderly. In 1996, almost 68,000 coronary artery bypass procedures were performed on Medicare enrollees age 74 and older.

The Quality of Surgical Performance: Coronary Artery Bypass Surgery

Optimal decision making about coronary artery bypass surgery depends on the risks of complications and mortality. The average 30-day mortality rate among Medicare enrollees undergoing bypass surgery between 1993 and 1996 was 5.2 deaths per 100 procedures (5.2%).

The quality of surgical performance varied widely among geographic regions. After adjusting for differences in population age, sex, and race, 30-day mortality rates varied by a factor of five, from 2.1% to 10.1%. In 46 hospital referral regions, mortality rates were less than 4%; 31 hospital referral regions had mortality rates in excess of 7%.

Claims data lack the clinical precision to account fully for differences in the severity of illness of patients undergoing surgery. Some hospital referral regions might have higher mortality rates because their patients are, on average, sicker than patients at hospitals with lower mortality rates. But case mix alone is unlikely to account for the five-fold variation in age, sex, and race adjusted mortality rates; some part of the variation must be attributable to variations in quality of care.

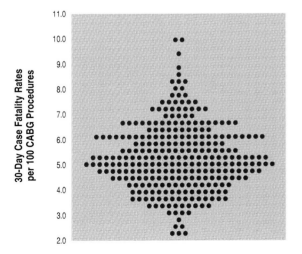

Figure 5.13. Thirty-Day Case Fatality Rates Following CABG Procedures Among Hospital Referral Regions (1993-96)
The likelihood of dying within 30 days of having bypass surgery ranged from 2% to 10%, after adjustments for differences in population age, sex and race. Each point represents one of the 306 hospital referral regions in the United States.

Improving Performance Quality: The Experience of the Northern New England Cardiovascular Disease Study Group

Founded in 1987, the Northern New England Cardiovascular Disease Study Group (NNECVDSG) is a voluntary research consortium involving clinicians, administrators, and epidemiologists from the five hospitals in Maine, New Hampshire, and Vermont that perform open heart surgery. The group collects detailed information on all patients undergoing coronary artery bypass surgery, heart valve surgery, and angioplasty in the region — approximately 85,000 patients since 1987. Data captured in the registry include patient characteristics (e.g., symptom and heart disease severity, co-existing conditions), variables describing the operation (e.g., how urgent the need for surgery was judged to be, technical details about how the surgery was performed), and patient outcomes after surgery (e.g., stroke and bleeding which made re-operation necessary, and death).

The NNECVDSG first focused on variation in mortality rates among providers. Among the five hospitals, rates of in-hospital mortality varied approximately three-fold, from 2% to 6%. Variation in surgical performance was even more dramatic among the 18 surgeons in the region, ranging from under 2% to almost 10%. These differences could not be explained by chance or because some surgeons operated on older, sicker patients and consequently had higher mortality rates.

Motivated by wide variation in surgical performance, the NNECVDSG then focused on differences in processes of care and quality improvement. To identify "best practices," the group organized round robin site visits among the five hospitals. Site visit teams from each hospital, consisting of cardiac surgeons, perfusionists, nurses, and administrators, reviewed how care was delivered at other centers. Teams focused on how patients were evaluated and treated before surgery, technical details of the operative procedure and anesthesia, and how patients were cared for in the intensive care unit and hospital ward after surgery. This review prompted changes in many areas of care at each hospital.

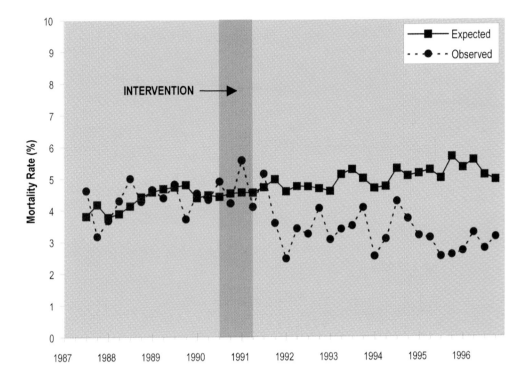

Figure 5.14. In-Hospital Mortality Rates Before and After Implementation of Quality Improvement Intervention (1987-1996)

A quality improvement effort implemented at five hospitals in northern New England reduced mortality rates by almost one-quarter, from 4.3% to 3.3% of patients undergoing bypass surgery. The initiative focused on patient evaluation and treatment prior to surgery, technical details of surgery and anesthesia, and postoperative care.

Source: The Journal of the American Medical Association (see Endnote).

Combining such quality improvement efforts with ongoing feedback to providers about performance paid substantial dividends. Overall, rates of in-hospital mortality in patients who had had coronary artery bypass grafting declined 24% (from 4.3% to 3.3%) among the five hospitals, and marked improvement in mortality rates was noted at each of the five surgery centers.

Chapter Five Table

All rates are age, sex, race and illness adjusted, and are expressed as rates per 1,000 Medicare enrollees. Surgical rates are for 1995-96, using a two year "person-year" denominator as given in the column labeled "Medicare Enrollees (1995 plus 1996)." Rates of radical prostatectomy are sex-specific. Data exclude Medicare enrollees who were members of risk bearing health maintenance organizations.

Where there were fewer than 25 expected cases of specific surgical procedures, the rate for the hospital referral region is bracketed in parentheses. Rates for hospital referral regions with 10 or fewer procedures are omitted from the table.

CABG = coronary artery bypass grafting
PTCA = percutaneous transluminal coronary angioplasty

Specific codes used to define the numerator for rates, and methods of age, sex, race and illness adjustment are included in the Appendix on Methods.

CHAPTER FIVE TABLE

Rates of Common Surgical Procedures Among Non-HMO Medicare Enrollees by Hospital Referral Region (1995-96)

Hospital Referral Region	Medicare Population (1995 plus 1996)	Hip Fracture Repair per 1,000 Medicare Enrollees (1995-96)	Colectomy for Colorectal Cancer per 1,000 Medicare Enrollees (1995-96)	Cholecystectomy per 1,000 Medicare Enrollees (1995-96)	CABG per 1,000 Medicare Enrollees (1995-96)	Hip Replacement per 1,000 Medicare Enrollees (1995-96)	Back Surgery per 1,000 Medicare Enrollees (1995-96)	Carotid Endarterectomy per 1,000 Medicare Enrollees (1995-96)	PTCA per 1,000 Medicare Enrollees (1995-96)	Lower Extremity Bypass per 1,000 Medicare Enrollees (1995-96)	Radical Prostatectomy per 1,000 Male Medicare Enrollees (1995-96)	Carotid Duplex Diagnostic Procedures per 1,000 Medicare Enrollees (1995-96)	Cardiac Catheterization per 1,000 Medicare Enrollees (1995-96)
Alabama													
Birmingham	531,198	9.2	2.3	6.6	8.5	2.0	4.6	4.6	9.4	2.0	1.6	60.9	32.3
Dothan	91,261	8.9	1.9	5.4	6.8	1.9	4.0	4.5	5.8	1.4	2.0	58.9	22.5
Huntsville	110,797	9.0	2.3	5.4	6.7	2.1	4.5	4.9	8.6	3.2	2.4	59.9	21.9
Mobile	164,496	8.6	2.5	7.0	9.3	2.0	3.1	4.4	7.9	4.1	2.2	42.9	32.2
Montgomery	98,631	9.2	2.4	6.1	5.8	2.0	6.1	4.4	12.1	2.2	1.7	58.8	27.1
Tuscaloosa	57,021	8.9	2.2	5.3	6.5	1.8	5.0	4.2	12.1	1.4	0.5	77.2	28.6
Alaska													
Anchorage	56,265	7.2	2.1	4.8	4.5	2.5	3.2	2.4	3.8	1.1	2.1	35.6	15.3
Arizona													
Mesa	107,378	7.8	2.3	4.5	5.8	3.2	3.7	2.7	6.8	2.1	2.0	47.8	24.1
Phoenix	372,696	8.5	2.1	5.1	5.0	2.5	3.3	2.8	7.8	2.0	1.8	45.9	22.5
Sun City	94,285	7.5	2.4	5.7	5.9	2.5	3.6	2.9	11.4	1.2	2.3	55.3	30.8
Tucson	148,037	8.7	1.9	4.9	4.0	2.5	4.5	1.8	6.7	1.5	1.7	21.0	19.8
Arkansas													
Fort Smith	88,931	9.5	2.2	4.7	6.3	1.7	2.5	2.4	4.6	1.5	1.3	53.1	22.8
Jonesboro	62,053	8.5	2.2	6.5	7.6	1.8	3.8	4.1	15.0	1.6	0.9	54.4	33.5
Little Rock	388,744	9.0	2.4	5.7	8.6	2.1	3.2	3.7	6.3	2.4	2.1	56.5	29.5
Springdale	95,202	8.6	2.0	5.8	5.5	2.2	2.5	2.8	7.0	1.0	1.9	39.1	21.1
Texarkana	69,646	9.2	2.6	6.2	6.1	2.0	4.7	4.5	4.6	1.7	1.5	50.9	27.3
California													
Orange Co.	270,153	7.8	2.2	3.6	5.1	2.6	3.1	2.5	7.2	1.6	2.2	55.4	22.0
Bakersfield	117,982	8.4	2.0	5.3	6.8	1.9	3.1	4.7	8.3	1.8	2.2	63.2	28.9
Chico	71,355	8.7	2.8	6.0	6.3	3.1	4.5	4.0	5.5	1.6	2.0	43.6	21.5
Contra Costa Co.	114,631	7.4	2.1	3.9	6.3	2.8	2.4	3.4	5.5	1.6	2.4	42.0	19.3
Fresno	153,777	7.3	2.2	4.7	5.3	2.2	3.0	2.8	6.9	1.9	2.4	39.2	22.5
Los Angeles	945,004	7.5	2.3	4.5	5.5	2.3	3.3	2.8	7.0	2.6	2.2	58.8	22.8
Modesto	112,858	8.1	2.4	4.4	5.3	2.3	3.2	3.6	6.0	2.4	1.3	55.2	21.2
Napa	68,998	8.2	2.2	4.6	6.7	3.4	3.9	5.3	13.4	2.2	2.1	61.9	32.1
Alameda Co.	187,366	7.2	2.1	4.3	4.9	2.3	3.0	2.7	8.4	1.9	1.4	41.6	19.6
Palm Spr/Rancho Mir	59,194	8.4	1.8	4.8	5.6	3.3	5.3	4.1	9.9	2.4	2.7	89.2	25.1
Redding	85,742	7.5	2.7	5.5	11.5	2.5	4.4	4.8	5.7	2.0	2.6	58.5	29.9
Sacramento	330,362	8.1	2.1	4.8	6.7	2.3	3.0	2.9	4.9	1.7	1.8	46.1	17.9
Salinas	63,756	7.4	1.8	4.8	7.0	2.7	4.1	3.8	14.4	1.8	1.5	42.4	24.6
San Bernardino	174,341	8.5	2.2	4.8	5.8	2.2	4.2	3.3	6.8	2.4	1.6	57.4	22.8
San Diego	325,134	7.7	1.9	4.8	4.6	2.5	4.1	2.6	6.1	2.1	2.1	45.2	20.2
San Francisco	216,897	6.7	2.1	3.1	4.5	2.5	2.9	2.1	5.0	1.8	1.6	25.3	13.2
San Jose	173,605	6.9	2.2	3.9	4.9	2.0	2.4	2.4	7.5	2.1	1.8	41.5	20.8
San Luis Obispo	42,298	7.6	2.2	4.8	4.9	3.0	5.6	2.7	4.6	1.8	2.4	34.0	18.3
San Mateo Co.	109,067	7.7	2.4	3.5	4.7	2.6	2.4	3.0	6.0	2.4	1.7	33.5	16.4
Santa Barbara	62,804	6.9	2.1	4.7	4.9	3.4	6.5	3.3	5.9	1.5	3.2	47.8	22.8

Hospital Referral Region	Medicare Population (1995 plus 1996)	Hip Fracture Repair per 1,000 Medicare Enrollees (1995-96)	Colectomy for Colorectal Cancer per 1,000 Medicare Enrollees (1995-96)	Cholecystectomy per 1,000 Medicare Enrollees (1995-96)	CABG per 1,000 Medicare Enrollees (1995-96)	Hip Replacement per 1,000 Medicare Enrollees (1995-96)	Back Surgery per 1,000 Medicare Enrollees (1995-96)	Carotid Endarterectomy per 1,000 Medicare Enrollees (1995-96)	PTCA per 1,000 Medicare Enrollees (1995-96)	Lower Extremity Bypass per 1,000 Medicare Enrollees (1995-96)	Radical Prostatectomy per 1,000 Male Medicare Enrollees (1995-96)	Carotid Duplex Diagnostic Procedures per 1,000 Medicare Enrollees (1995-96)	Cardiac Catheterization per 1,000 Medicare Enrollees (1995-96)
Santa Cruz	43,356	7.5	2.7	5.4	4.9	2.9	3.4	3.0	8.8	1.8	2.2	57.5	22.3
Santa Rosa	75,196	6.5	2.3	4.0	3.6	2.7	3.1	3.4	6.7	1.3	1.2	35.2	15.1
Stockton	73,773	7.9	2.5	4.4	6.4	1.8	3.7	3.6	13.6	2.8	1.5	57.6	26.7
Ventura	84,070	7.8	2.4	5.6	5.8	2.7	5.0	3.1	7.7	2.2	2.9	43.4	20.9
Colorado													
Boulder	29,397	9.1	2.3	5.4	4.9	3.2	4.3	3.0	6.8	1.0	(3.8)	30.2	19.8
Colorado Springs	117,647	9.0	2.2	4.5	5.8	2.7	3.1	2.6	5.8	1.6	1.4	34.9	19.0
Denver	291,391	8.8	2.0	3.9	3.8	3.1	3.7	2.1	5.9	1.5	2.0	38.9	16.1
Fort Collins	49,776	8.7	1.9	4.4	4.7	3.5	6.8	2.3	8.0	1.2	2.5	35.7	25.3
Grand Junction	61,540	6.5	1.8	7.4	3.5	3.3	2.8	1.8	4.2	0.9	2.4	18.9	9.6
Greeley	59,056	8.6	2.5	5.2	5.7	3.5	5.5	2.2	4.8	1.3	2.2	28.3	17.2
Pueblo	34,804	9.0	2.2	5.9	5.2	2.3	3.9	2.7	4.3	2.9	0.9	31.7	10.2
Connecticut													
Bridgeport	176,155	7.5	2.5	4.7	4.2	2.5	3.4	2.7	6.6	2.4	1.6	37.0	17.2
Hartford	379,442	7.1	2.5	4.4	6.8	2.4	2.5	2.3	5.0	2.9	1.5	32.4	18.4
New Haven	354,500	7.5	2.8	4.6	6.7	2.4	2.2	2.9	7.1	2.8	1.2	45.3	19.3
Delaware													
Wilmington	148,958	8.0	2.7	4.3	5.2	2.4	2.6	4.3	6.3	2.3	1.8	56.9	22.4
District of Columbia													
Washington	432,068	7.9	2.3	4.5	5.6	2.3	3.4	3.4	6.5	2.3	1.6	53.5	18.1
Florida													
Bradenton	95,601	7.9	3.1	4.0	6.6	2.7	4.6	4.7	6.0	2.2	1.8	63.7	21.4
Clearwater	179,366	8.4	2.7	4.7	6.1	2.8	4.4	4.4	8.6	2.3	2.5	84.0	26.5
Fort Lauderdale	626,104	8.5	2.6	3.9	7.3	2.6	3.4	3.9	7.6	2.1	1.8	76.6	25.0
Fort Myers	337,451	8.2	2.6	4.7	6.8	3.1	5.8	5.0	7.6	2.1	2.1	79.5	24.0
Gainesville	101,489	8.6	2.3	4.6	5.4	2.0	3.2	3.6	5.0	1.8	1.7	59.2	26.8
Hudson	160,882	7.7	2.8	6.0	9.4	2.4	4.5	5.0	7.9	2.3	1.1	84.9	36.1
Jacksonville	230,794	8.4	2.5	4.8	7.1	2.0	3.0	5.2	7.3	2.5	2.0	74.8	28.4
Lakeland	86,654	8.4	2.5	3.5	6.6	2.7	3.3	5.0	10.0	2.4	1.1	57.1	28.7
Miami	428,445	8.4	2.5	4.3	5.4	1.6	1.8	2.1	6.2	1.9	1.5	109.6	24.2
Ocala	165,671	7.5	2.7	4.8	7.0	2.7	4.4	4.9	6.5	2.4	2.5	74.8	30.0
Orlando	717,162	8.2	2.6	4.4	6.4	2.4	3.3	4.5	8.2	2.1	2.5	72.3	28.9
Ormond Beach	92,249	8.3	2.8	5.1	5.3	2.5	3.1	3.6	6.8	2.2	3.4	44.4	22.3
Panama City	45,564	8.3	2.4	4.8	7.0	2.0	3.7	4.4	7.4	2.0	1.5	71.7	32.4
Pensacola	155,000	8.7	2.2	4.5	7.6	2.1	4.4	3.5	5.8	2.1	2.7	59.5	26.0
Sarasota	192,292	8.3	2.6	4.1	7.9	3.1	3.8	4.1	6.5	3.0	2.8	70.7	29.3
St Petersburg	132,217	9.4	2.9	5.1	5.6	2.6	3.9	6.1	5.3	3.2	3.4	90.6	19.4
Tallahassee	146,930	8.6	2.0	5.6	6.5	2.1	3.6	3.9	5.0	1.3	1.8	64.1	22.8
Tampa	181,305	8.8	2.7	4.2	6.6	2.4	3.4	3.6	5.9	2.2	1.0	58.4	23.9
Georgia													
Albany	44,327	9.5	2.1	5.0	5.8	2.5	3.7	6.2	4.6	4.0	1.9	51.6	20.7
Atlanta	724,634	9.3	2.2	4.8	5.9	2.1	2.9	3.8	7.4	2.2	2.0	51.5	25.5
Augusta	126,511	8.2	1.9	5.0	7.0	2.0	3.8	3.8	11.8	1.5	1.2	55.0	33.2
Columbus	68,275	9.2	2.2	4.2	7.3	2.0	4.0	4.9	8.1	2.4	1.7	58.3	28.3
Macon	146,073	8.8	2.2	5.0	7.8	2.1	3.6	4.7	6.4	2.0	1.3	67.7	27.6
Rome	61,522	9.8	2.1	4.0	7.9	1.8	2.9	5.2	10.2	3.0	1.5	70.5	39.8

Hospital Referral Region	Medicare Population (1995 plus 1996)	Hip Fracture Repair per 1,000 Medicare Enrollees (1995-96)	Colectomy for Colorectal Cancer per 1,000 Medicare Enrollees (1995-96)	Cholecystectomy per 1,000 Medicare Enrollees (1995-96)	CABG per 1,000 Medicare Enrollees (1995-96)	Hip Replacement per 1,000 Medicare Enrollees (1995-96)	Back Surgery per 1,000 Medicare Enrollees (1995-96)	Carotid Endarterectomy per 1,000 Medicare Enrollees (1995-96)	PTCA per 1,000 Medicare Enrollees (1995-96)	Lower Extremity Bypass per 1,000 Medicare Enrollees (1995-96)	Radical Prostatectomy per 1,000 Male Medicare Enrollees (1995-96)	Carotid Duplex Diagnostic Procedures per 1,000 Medicare Enrollees (1995-96)	Cardiac Catheterization per 1,000 Medicare Enrollees (1995-96)
Savannah	144,045	8.4	2.1	4.7	7.0	2.6	4.9	4.4	7.5	2.1	2.0	52.8	27.6
Hawaii													
Honolulu	187,844	5.3	1.9	4.4	4.0	0.9	1.7	1.1	3.7	1.3	1.0	28.8	15.8
Idaho													
Boise	141,914	7.4	2.0	5.2	5.9	3.7	6.0	2.8	7.1	1.6	2.1	38.1	22.4
Idaho Falls	34,038	6.6	1.9	6.1	5.6	3.8	4.4	1.1	6.6	1.3	1.3	29.0	27.6
Illinois													
Aurora	33,873	8.8	2.6	5.6	8.5	2.8	3.1	3.9	5.4	1.0	2.0	48.7	22.7
Bloomington	38,683	8.1	2.8	5.3	9.8	3.5	4.4	3.7	5.6	1.7	1.3	54.4	30.1
Blue Island	187,921	7.1	2.6	4.7	7.6	2.4	2.7	3.8	6.5	2.5	2.0	51.9	25.2
Chicago	462,058	7.0	2.6	4.4	6.3	2.0	1.8	2.2	8.0	2.0	1.2	42.8	26.5
Elgin	85,637	7.5	2.5	4.1	6.9	2.7	3.1	3.2	5.8	1.8	1.2	47.1	20.3
Evanston	223,326	7.5	2.6	4.4	6.2	3.0	2.7	2.6	8.4	1.2	1.9	42.3	24.1
Hinsdale	63,880	8.0	2.7	3.9	8.0	2.8	3.1	2.9	5.9	1.5	1.8	41.2	31.0
Joliet	99,391	7.7	2.8	5.3	8.3	2.9	2.9	4.5	5.8	1.4	2.1	62.5	26.5
Melrose Park	262,951	7.3	2.6	5.0	7.8	2.6	2.5	2.8	7.0	1.8	1.5	41.4	26.1
Peoria	190,047	8.1	2.8	4.7	6.2	2.7	2.3	3.9	6.3	2.3	2.0	51.2	20.7
Rockford	173,322	7.7	2.8	5.0	6.8	2.9	2.1	3.7	6.9	2.1	1.7	40.7	20.2
Springfield	257,715	8.9	2.7	4.6	8.3	2.5	3.7	3.8	8.8	2.5	1.6	43.9	28.0
Urbana	113,172	7.4	2.6	4.6	7.1	2.6	2.7	3.3	6.8	2.5	1.6	44.9	23.9
Indiana													
Evansville	197,504	8.6	2.7	5.2	6.3	2.2	3.0	3.2	5.7	1.9	1.4	49.0	18.5
Fort Wayne	198,790	8.3	2.5	3.6	5.1	3.1	4.0	3.1	6.5	2.1	1.4	44.2	20.1
Gary	115,440	7.6	3.0	5.2	7.7	2.6	3.0	4.7	7.8	2.4	1.8	55.5	22.9
Indianapolis	581,059	8.4	2.5	4.3	5.7	2.5	2.4	3.7	8.1	2.3	1.4	48.4	23.8
Lafayette	46,183	8.3	2.5	3.4	6.4	2.3	3.1	2.1	7.0	1.6	1.7	26.5	12.4
Muncie	46,075	8.6	2.6	4.4	4.7	2.5	3.2	2.9	9.2	2.1	1.0	48.3	17.3
Munster	81,110	7.0	3.0	5.2	7.9	2.4	2.3	4.7	10.4	2.4	2.2	58.5	33.7
South Bend	167,946	7.6	2.6	3.8	7.1	2.8	2.8	3.5	5.1	2.2	1.3	39.4	24.7
Terre Haute	53,927	9.6	2.6	5.7	6.6	2.4	2.6	4.0	12.6	2.3	1.8	43.9	31.0
Iowa													
Cedar Rapids	71,240	7.8	2.8	4.0	6.6	3.5	3.3	3.1	6.0	2.7	2.3	43.4	18.1
Davenport	139,617	8.2	3.0	5.1	5.2	2.8	2.7	3.9	8.3	2.2	1.7	46.2	20.8
Des Moines	280,952	8.1	2.7	4.8	5.8	3.0	2.5	3.0	9.4	1.6	2.0	48.3	23.3
Dubuque	43,877	8.2	2.7	4.7	4.8	3.2	3.5	4.7	6.3	1.5	2.5	32.3	11.2
Iowa City	84,691	8.0	2.5	5.6	6.7	3.2	2.3	2.6	6.1	1.9	1.2	46.9	19.3
Mason City	53,653	7.6	2.6	4.0	8.0	3.8	4.0	3.8	9.3	1.1	1.7	54.9	35.4
Sioux City	80,240	8.0	3.2	5.7	4.7	3.9	3.2	4.4	7.5	1.4	1.8	51.5	16.1
Waterloo	63,821	8.1	2.7	4.8	5.0	3.7	3.0	3.0	4.9	1.9	2.7	49.9	12.8
Kansas													
Topeka	111,600	9.3	2.5	4.6	5.1	3.0	2.1	3.8	5.9	1.5	2.6	56.6	20.7
Wichita	353,253	9.2	2.4	5.3	7.3	2.7	3.4	4.6	7.5	1.5	2.4	58.3	28.1
Kentucky													
Covington	74,350	8.8	2.8	3.2	9.1	1.9	2.8	4.3	6.9	2.3	1.1	52.6	34.0
Lexington	306,484	8.3	2.3	5.3	6.8	1.9	2.0	2.8	4.3	1.5	1.0	49.0	19.4
Louisville	373,678	8.9	2.4	5.5	7.4	2.2	3.0	3.8	4.8	2.3	1.2	55.7	22.5

Hospital Referral Region	Medicare Population (1995 plus 1996)	Hip Fracture Repair per 1,000 Medicare Enrollees (1995-96)	Colectomy for Colorectal Cancer per 1,000 Medicare Enrollees (1995-96)	Cholecystectomy per 1,000 Medicare Enrollees (1995-96)	CABG per 1,000 Medicare Enrollees (1995-96)	Hip Replacement per 1,000 Medicare Enrollees (1995-96)	Back Surgery per 1,000 Medicare Enrollees (1995-96)	Carotid Endarterectomy per 1,000 Medicare Enrollees (1995-96)	PTCA per 1,000 Medicare Enrollees (1995-96)	Lower Extremity Bypass per 1,000 Medicare Enrollees (1995-96)	Radical Prostatectomy per 1,000 Male Medicare Enrollees (1995-96)	Carotid Duplex Diagnostic Procedures per 1,000 Medicare Enrollees (1995-96)	Cardiac Catheterization per 1,000 Medicare Enrollees (1995-96)
Owensboro	36,335	8.1	2.5	5.4	7.8	1.6	4.1	5.5	10.0	2.5	1.2	86.5	35.2
Paducah	113,236	8.7	2.9	8.0	6.7	2.1	3.5	5.5	8.5	3.0	1.3	90.7	25.7
Louisiana													
Alexandria	68,645	7.9	2.4	7.2	6.6	1.2	3.4	4.6	15.9	2.0	1.0	70.3	36.3
Baton Rouge	125,996	8.5	2.8	5.6	6.4	1.4	2.2	3.6	9.0	2.9	4.7	70.9	24.7
Houma	46,172	7.5	3.0	5.7	10.6	1.3	3.5	7.6	14.9	1.3	2.4	104.9	53.1
Lafayette	119,008	7.2	2.2	6.2	8.4	1.3	2.4	6.5	12.4	2.1	0.8	71.0	40.3
Lake Charles	53,138	7.9	2.2	5.6	6.5	1.6	3.0	5.2	8.0	1.5	2.5	62.8	18.9
Metairie	84,026	8.7	2.5	4.5	8.0	1.5	2.5	5.2	10.5	3.7	2.1	73.4	34.1
Monroe	68,197	8.7	2.1	6.4	6.3	2.1	3.2	2.2	5.0	1.2	1.4	39.4	19.7
New Orleans	157,397	8.1	2.7	5.0	6.9	1.6	2.4	5.4	8.8	2.3	1.7	76.1	25.4
Shreveport	169,234	8.5	2.3	5.5	6.5	1.5	3.9	4.6	7.8	1.8	2.1	51.4	23.4
Slidell	31,604	7.9	2.6	5.6	9.7	1.6	4.2	6.6	6.6	2.7	1.8	92.5	31.5
Maine													
Bangor	111,529	7.5	2.7	5.6	5.6	2.4	2.2	3.2	4.6	2.3	1.8	47.4	14.9
Portland	261,069	7.5	2.7	4.8	5.4	2.5	3.0	2.5	5.0	2.2	1.1	36.6	18.5
Maryland													
Baltimore	545,455	7.8	2.8	5.4	6.4	2.1	3.5	4.3	6.5	3.5	1.9	51.8	22.9
Salisbury	106,147	7.1	2.9	5.0	4.8	2.1	2.5	4.9	9.2	2.3	0.8	68.3	27.9
Takoma Park	131,825	7.4	2.3	4.3	4.7	2.1	3.2	3.3	9.9	2.2	1.8	67.7	22.1
Massachusetts													
Boston	1,090,114	7.8	2.8	4.1	5.3	2.3	2.3	3.2	4.5	2.8	1.8	44.9	16.0
Springfield	197,790	7.8	2.8	4.2	4.8	2.0	2.6	2.7	3.8	2.9	1.1	35.8	11.2
Worcester	136,618	8.5	2.8	4.4	4.8	2.4	2.5	3.4	4.6	3.0	2.1	47.4	13.2
Michigan													
Ann Arbor	267,884	7.4	2.4	4.1	6.1	2.7	2.9	4.0	6.4	2.1	1.6	73.6	26.3
Dearborn	146,494	6.9	2.7	4.3	7.0	2.3	2.6	4.4	8.4	2.6	1.7	104.6	30.1
Detroit	461,527	7.1	2.7	4.1	7.0	2.2	3.0	4.5	9.4	2.3	1.5	98.1	26.7
Flint	117,933	7.9	2.4	7.0	8.3	3.2	4.5	4.9	8.2	2.1	2.8	118.6	30.5
Grand Rapids	228,224	7.8	2.3	4.3	5.6	3.0	4.5	3.3	4.9	1.7	3.0	44.5	20.2
Kalamazoo	156,012	7.5	2.5	5.9	6.0	2.9	3.7	5.0	11.4	2.7	2.7	67.4	33.2
Lansing	128,215	7.1	2.3	4.5	7.6	3.4	3.8	4.1	8.0	1.7	3.4	80.0	24.0
Marquette	65,828	7.7	2.1	7.0	7.3	2.9	2.9	5.1	5.7	1.6	2.3	50.2	24.9
Muskegon	69,589	8.0	2.5	4.9	4.5	3.5	3.6	5.0	4.7	1.8	3.6	59.0	16.7
Petoskey	50,748	7.1	2.6	5.7	6.4	2.8	3.4	3.5	6.2	1.8	3.3	58.9	21.8
Pontiac	74,704	7.7	2.5	4.9	7.0	2.4	4.3	4.0	6.2	1.7	1.5	106.9	27.1
Royal Oak	165,149	7.5	2.3	4.9	6.0	2.6	3.3	4.3	10.5	1.8	1.5	102.7	24.9
Saginaw	191,457	7.0	2.7	6.1	8.3	3.2	4.2	5.3	8.4	2.1	2.0	90.1	30.7
St Joseph	39,623	6.2	2.3	3.7	5.7	2.7	3.4	4.8	11.4	2.8	3.2	61.8	29.8
Traverse City	64,232	7.2	2.9	6.2	7.1	3.0	3.9	5.3	10.4	1.8	3.4	66.1	30.2
Minnesota													
Duluth	109,464	7.1	2.6	5.8	5.2	3.0	2.3	1.9	7.0	1.3	1.8	29.4	16.5
Minneapolis	571,687	7.6	2.3	4.6	5.6	3.4	3.0	2.0	5.8	1.7	2.5	27.0	15.4
Rochester	111,509	7.7	2.5	3.9	5.3	3.4	2.1	1.6	6.3	1.3	2.8	30.3	22.2
St Cloud	51,664	7.6	2.4	4.4	5.2	3.4	2.4	2.5	5.6	1.9	2.7	37.3	19.3
St Paul	151,452	7.8	2.4	4.5	4.7	3.2	3.4	2.0	5.3	2.1	2.7	28.3	15.0

Hospital Referral Region	Medicare Population (1995 plus 1996)	Hip Fracture Repair per 1,000 Medicare Enrollees (1995-96)	Colectomy for Colorectal Cancer per 1,000 Medicare Enrollees (1995-96)	Cholecystectomy per 1,000 Medicare Enrollees (1995-96)	CABG per 1,000 Medicare Enrollees (1995-96)	Hip Replacement per 1,000 Medicare Enrollees (1995-96)	Back Surgery per 1,000 Medicare Enrollees (1995-96)	Carotid Endarterectomy per 1,000 Medicare Enrollees (1995-96)	PTCA per 1,000 Medicare Enrollees (1995-96)	Lower Extremity Bypass per 1,000 Medicare Enrollees (1995-96)	Radical Prostatectomy per 1,000 Male Medicare Enrollees (1995-96)	Carotid Duplex Diagnostic Procedures per 1,000 Medicare Enrollees (1995-96)	Cardiac Catheterization per 1,000 Medicare Enrollees (1995-96)
Mississippi													
Gulfport	38,727	7.7	2.4	6.3	6.0	1.6	3.4	6.4	6.4	2.4	1.6	69.3	18.7
Hattiesburg	64,370	7.7	2.0	7.2	5.4	1.8	3.0	4.1	7.2	2.3	4.2	74.6	20.0
Jackson	239,395	8.7	2.3	6.5	5.0	1.6	3.1	3.8	3.3	1.5	2.5	55.7	17.6
Meridian	53,549	7.7	2.2	5.0	7.2	2.1	3.4	3.7	4.5	1.2	2.9	56.4	18.7
Oxford	34,480	9.3	2.5	5.8	7.6	1.9	4.1	5.6	5.5	2.6		66.1	34.4
Tupelo	90,693	8.9	2.0	5.6	6.6	2.0	2.6	3.7	3.7	1.8	1.7	59.8	22.8
Missouri													
Cape Girardeau	76,675	8.5	2.7	4.1	7.5	1.8	3.5	4.1	6.2	1.7	1.1	59.9	26.5
Columbia	178,244	8.6	2.7	5.2	7.7	2.7	3.5	3.6	8.8	1.8	1.6	45.3	27.8
Joplin	104,566	9.4	2.3	5.2	6.0	2.6	3.3	4.4	9.5	1.9	2.2	77.6	26.6
Kansas City	479,005	9.3	2.7	4.6	5.6	2.6	2.9	4.2	8.9	2.1	2.7	55.3	24.3
Springfield	218,568	9.6	2.5	5.3	7.0	2.0	2.9	3.1	10.2	1.2	2.3	47.0	27.4
St Louis	807,992	9.1	2.7	4.4	7.2	2.2	3.0	3.2	6.4	2.4	3.0	42.4	23.9
Montana													
Billings	126,063	7.5	2.2	4.9	5.9	3.5	4.4	2.7	5.5	1.6	4.0	37.4	24.1
Great Falls	40,725	7.7	2.7	5.9	5.7	3.2	3.6	2.3	9.0	1.7	2.7	39.4	27.4
Missoula	86,069	8.3	2.3	5.6	4.6	3.6	3.5	3.0	11.2	1.1	1.8	39.4	21.3
Nebraska													
Lincoln	158,162	8.1	2.5	4.2	6.5	3.3	3.2	4.1	5.8	2.4	2.5	42.3	19.0
Omaha	305,122	8.3	2.7	4.5	6.2	3.1	3.5	3.5	6.2	2.0	2.0	40.9	18.4
Nevada													
Las Vegas	167,674	8.5	2.4	4.2	5.6	2.2	3.0	4.5	8.6	2.5	1.7	73.3	22.0
Reno	122,528	8.4	2.1	5.1	4.1	2.5	3.4	3.0	4.4	1.8	1.7	26.8	13.8
New Hampshire													
Lebanon	109,382	7.8	2.5	4.1	4.2	2.7	2.1	2.7	3.2	1.8	1.4	32.0	13.0
Manchester	171,865	7.7	2.7	4.1	6.3	2.3	2.5	3.6	4.9	2.3	1.2	42.9	18.8
New Jersey													
Camden	697,067	7.3	2.9	5.1	5.6	1.9	2.1	3.6	5.8	2.3	1.3	64.2	18.9
Hackensack	310,809	7.2	2.8	5.2	5.2	1.7	1.9	2.3	6.4	2.8	1.2	57.1	19.1
Morristown	212,488	7.9	2.7	5.0	5.0	2.2	2.0	2.5	5.2	2.3	2.0	57.4	19.0
New Brunswick	195,466	6.7	2.7	4.9	5.4	1.9	2.0	3.7	7.4	3.0	1.7	70.9	22.9
Newark	344,765	6.7	2.7	5.2	5.1	1.6	1.4	2.1	7.1	2.8	1.0	59.9	22.2
Paterson	81,774	7.6	3.1	5.2	5.5	1.7	1.7	2.2	6.5	2.8	0.9	58.6	19.8
Ridgewood	87,608	7.2	2.6	5.3	6.0	2.3	1.9	2.0	6.5	1.9	1.6	40.4	19.1
New Mexico													
Albuquerque	224,888	9.0	1.7	6.2	3.1	2.2	3.2	1.9	4.6	1.3	1.7	27.7	13.0
New York													
Albany	482,105	7.3	2.7	4.5	6.1	2.4	2.1	3.6	3.4	2.9	1.3	46.5	15.3
Binghamton	111,256	7.6	2.6	4.6	5.1	2.3	2.5	3.1	4.8	1.7	0.5	48.3	14.8
Bronx	197,752	7.8	2.6	4.4	4.7	1.4	1.3	1.7	3.7	2.3	1.2	38.3	14.0
Buffalo	415,614	7.2	2.6	5.1	6.3	2.6	2.3	4.0	3.1	2.3	2.4	63.8	20.0
Elmira	109,738	7.4	2.4	5.7	6.1	2.2	1.8	3.7	4.9	1.7	1.5	47.7	22.4
East Long Island	950,618	7.4	2.8	4.5	6.2	1.9	1.5	2.4	5.6	2.3	0.9	56.1	21.2
New York	881,446	7.5	2.6	4.0	5.3	1.6	1.6	2.1	4.5	2.2	0.8	53.7	16.9
Rochester	291,953	7.6	2.5	4.8	6.3	2.7	2.7	4.0	5.2	2.7	2.0	40.0	15.6

172 THE DARTMOUTH ATLAS OF HEALTH CARE 1999

Hospital Referral Region	Medicare Population (1995 plus 1996)	Hip Fracture Repair per 1,000 Medicare Enrollees (1995-96)	Colectomy for Colorectal Cancer per 1,000 Medicare Enrollees (1995-96)	Cholecystectomy per 1,000 Medicare Enrollees (1995-96)	CABG per 1,000 Medicare Enrollees (1995-96)	Hip Replacement per 1,000 Medicare Enrollees (1995-96)	Back Surgery per 1,000 Medicare Enrollees (1995-96)	Carotid Endarterectomy per 1,000 Medicare Enrollees (1995-96)	PTCA per 1,000 Medicare Enrollees (1995-96)	Lower Extremity Bypass per 1,000 Medicare Enrollees (1995-96)	Radical Prostatectomy per 1,000 Male Medicare Enrollees (1995-96)	Carotid Duplex Diagnostic Procedures per 1,000 Medicare Enrollees (1995-96)	Cardiac Catheterization per 1,000 Medicare Enrollees (1995-96)
Syracuse	269,858	7.5	2.5	5.4	5.4	2.8	1.5	4.1	4.5	2.6	1.8	59.9	19.2
White Plains	251,488	7.6	2.9	5.0	5.5	2.1	2.2	2.7	3.9	2.0	1.7	49.7	17.1
North Carolina													
Asheville	185,632	9.5	2.2	4.9	5.4	2.6	2.5	3.6	2.6	1.5	2.2	44.3	14.4
Charlotte	390,429	9.3	2.5	4.7	6.1	2.1	3.2	3.3	7.1	1.9	2.2	47.1	24.6
Durham	292,501	9.1	2.3	4.4	6.2	2.2	3.1	2.8	5.9	1.5	2.6	38.0	23.1
Greensboro	128,316	9.3	2.3	5.0	8.1	2.0	4.0	3.9	7.4	2.3	2.0	41.3	22.7
Greenville	169,580	8.8	2.4	5.0	6.9	2.3	3.7	4.7	7.4	2.0	2.6	54.2	25.9
Hickory	62,741	9.5	2.1	6.5	8.3	2.6	3.5	4.1	4.9	2.2	1.9	44.4	23.4
Raleigh	271,479	8.6	2.1	4.7	6.4	2.3	4.0	3.8	6.9	2.1	3.0	48.5	23.6
Wilmington	84,158	8.9	1.9	4.5	7.5	2.0	3.0	6.0	6.0	2.8	2.2	59.8	19.3
Winston-Salem	249,303	9.5	2.3	5.7	6.4	2.0	3.1	3.2	6.4	2.2	1.8	49.6	21.6
North Dakota													
Bismarck	62,854	7.3	2.5	5.0	5.8	3.5	4.3	3.7	6.3	2.2	1.8	51.9	18.0
Fargo Moorhead -Mn	144,946	7.6	2.7	6.1	5.6	3.5	2.8	2.4	4.7	2.1	2.6	32.8	17.2
Grand Forks	49,134	7.6	3.1	5.0	5.8	2.9	3.1	3.1	5.3	1.0	1.6	34.9	24.5
Minot	39,390	8.0	2.5	5.4	7.5	2.7	3.3	2.4	10.0	2.0	3.2	50.1	25.1
Ohio													
Akron	179,066	8.0	2.5	5.1	6.6	2.6	3.0	3.8	6.9	2.2	1.3	58.6	22.9
Canton	174,748	7.6	2.4	4.5	6.6	2.5	3.1	3.2	6.4	2.4	1.1	50.8	26.1
Cincinnati	366,415	8.8	2.7	4.2	5.9	2.2	3.4	3.7	7.0	2.4	1.8	48.3	22.9
Cleveland	557,531	7.9	2.6	4.3	6.6	2.6	2.9	4.6	5.7	2.8	1.5	60.3	23.7
Columbus	606,997	8.6	2.7	4.8	5.6	2.3	2.6	3.7	7.4	2.7	1.6	46.8	26.8
Dayton	283,883	8.1	2.7	4.7	7.4	2.6	3.3	3.7	8.3	2.5	1.4	52.0	26.0
Elyria	59,452	6.5	2.7	5.2	5.9	2.5	3.6	5.6	16.9	4.0	0.6	80.9	35.0
Kettering	96,363	9.0	2.6	4.3	7.0	2.4	3.0	4.3	7.1	2.6	3.6	57.1	25.1
Toledo	248,200	8.1	2.7	5.5	6.6	3.0	3.4	4.0	6.1	2.7	1.8	73.9	25.6
Youngstown	232,986	7.3	2.5	5.2	6.0	2.3	2.4	4.6	6.3	1.9	1.6	64.8	21.1
Oklahoma													
Lawton	48,926	9.2	2.3	6.1	8.0	2.1	3.1	4.1	5.9	1.6	1.4	66.3	32.0
Oklahoma City	407,045	9.2	2.5	5.8	6.6	2.0	3.3	3.7	7.4	1.6	2.9	43.5	27.6
Tulsa	288,289	9.1	2.1	4.6	5.0	1.9	3.9	2.7	7.1	1.3	1.8	47.1	24.6
Oregon													
Bend	40,794	7.1	2.4	6.4	6.5	3.5	7.3	4.0	6.4	1.3	4.1	42.0	14.9
Eugene	164,058	7.5	1.9	5.1	5.1	2.8	5.2	3.1	4.2	1.7	2.2	33.2	14.0
Medford	119,321	7.3	2.1	4.1	5.1	2.9	5.0	4.5	3.8	1.8	2.1	36.0	18.9
Portland	310,624	7.9	2.3	3.7	4.4	2.9	4.7	3.3	4.3	2.3	2.1	38.4	14.6
Salem	54,536	7.3	2.5	4.1	4.6	3.0	4.1	3.0	3.6	1.3	1.3	34.9	10.7
Pennsylvania													
Allentown	301,246	7.4	2.8	6.1	6.7	2.4	2.4	4.1	7.1	2.9	1.3	77.7	24.1
Altoona	94,974	7.2	2.8	5.6	7.5	2.1	2.3	2.5	4.4	1.9	1.4	54.0	22.9
Danville	143,082	7.9	2.8	5.6	4.8	2.2	3.2	3.7	3.3	1.6	1.7	61.1	13.3
Erie	227,568	7.8	2.6	4.5	5.8	2.4	3.0	3.1	5.6	1.9	1.8	58.9	21.4
Harrisburg	251,207	7.9	2.9	5.0	6.4	2.2	3.2	3.6	5.4	1.9	2.1	60.3	20.1
Johnstown	88,969	7.1	2.5	6.5	7.5	2.1	3.0	3.1	9.4	1.6	2.7	64.4	30.5
Lancaster	139,571	7.5	2.3	4.9	6.5	2.3	4.3	2.9	8.3	1.9	2.4	49.0	31.7

Hospital Referral Region	Medicare Population (1995 plus 1996)	Hip Fracture Repair per 1,000 Medicare Enrollees (1995-96)	Colectomy for Colorectal Cancer per 1,000 Medicare Enrollees (1995-96)	Cholecystectomy per 1,000 Medicare Enrollees (1995-96)	CABG per 1,000 Medicare Enrollees (1995-96)	Hip Replacement per 1,000 Medicare Enrollees (1995-96)	Back Surgery per 1,000 Medicare Enrollees (1995-96)	Carotid Endarterectomy per 1,000 Medicare Enrollees (1995-96)	PTCA per 1,000 Medicare Enrollees (1995-96)	Lower Extremity Bypass per 1,000 Medicare Enrollees (1995-96)	Radical Prostatectomy per 1,000 Male Medicare Enrollees (1995-96)	Carotid Duplex Diagnostic Procedures per 1,000 Medicare Enrollees (1995-96)	Cardiac Catheterization per 1,000 Medicare Enrollees (1995-96)
Philadelphia	900,104	8.1	2.8	4.8	6.2	2.2	2.5	3.2	5.8	2.5	1.5	62.1	21.7
Pittsburgh	975,984	7.6	2.8	5.9	7.2	2.3	3.4	3.8	8.9	2.7	2.0	60.1	26.6
Reading	163,121	7.2	2.6	5.7	6.3	2.2	2.7	3.3	6.9	2.6	1.9	62.8	24.7
Sayre	56,091	7.6	2.6	5.7	5.1	2.7	2.6	2.6	5.4	1.3	1.4	44.2	20.2
Scranton	110,662	7.2	2.9	6.7	5.9	1.7	2.3	3.1	4.9	2.7	0.8	57.2	13.7
Wilkes-Barre	90,912	7.2	2.8	5.4	7.2	2.0	2.4	3.0	4.9	2.4	1.2	92.1	20.6
York	97,457	7.7	3.2	5.3	7.6	2.2	2.7	3.5	2.5	2.2	0.9	38.6	16.6
Rhode Island													
Providence	302,229	7.0	2.9	4.7	5.1	2.1	1.8	3.0	4.7	2.3	1.1	47.9	16.8
South Carolina													
Charleston	167,086	8.1	2.4	4.8	5.6	2.3	3.8	3.4	7.0	2.1	2.2	47.5	24.3
Columbia	225,786	8.5	2.2	4.5	5.4	2.1	2.6	4.4	5.5	1.8	1.3	57.4	23.6
Florence	79,509	8.3	2.0	5.2	6.1	1.9	2.7	2.5	7.2	1.6	0.8	55.0	25.8
Greenville	178,591	9.5	2.3	5.2	6.9	2.0	3.1	3.3	5.9	1.8	2.2	44.6	25.7
Spartanburg	85,807	9.6	2.1	5.4	5.1	2.1	2.2	2.9	5.2	1.6	2.7	45.1	21.8
South Dakota													
Rapid City	46,330	8.3	2.1	5.2	7.2	2.9	5.3	3.4	6.7	1.3	2.0	35.1	29.9
Sioux Falls	234,742	7.6	2.9	6.1	6.2	3.8	3.4	3.2	7.1	1.1	2.2	48.3	20.2
Tennessee													
Chattanooga	151,930	9.0	2.0	6.0	7.2	1.9	2.7	3.4	6.0	1.3	1.6	43.6	25.8
Jackson	92,775	9.0	2.5	5.2	6.6	1.9	2.7	2.5	6.7	0.9	1.6	54.4	27.7
Johnson City	62,541	8.6	2.0	5.3	6.4	1.6	1.8	3.8	6.7	1.5	1.8	51.9	24.3
Kingsport	134,555	9.4	2.0	5.7	5.1	1.8	1.8	2.9	4.1	1.4	0.8	46.4	14.2
Knoxville	308,599	9.2	2.2	5.5	6.8	1.8	2.2	3.9	5.7	1.9	1.9	55.1	23.6
Memphis	368,719	9.1	2.6	4.7	8.3	1.9	2.6	3.6	7.5	1.9	1.7	57.4	30.6
Nashville	493,251	9.0	2.3	5.2	6.9	2.1	3.8	3.2	4.8	2.4	2.1	57.4	21.5
Texas													
Abilene	88,733	9.5	2.2	5.1	6.8	2.1	2.6	3.8	9.9	1.7	1.7	62.8	30.0
Amarillo	105,473	9.3	2.1	6.2	7.3	2.5	4.6	3.6	6.4	1.4	1.9	48.5	26.1
Austin	158,656	9.3	2.2	5.1	5.9	1.8	3.0	2.5	6.4	1.2	2.4	39.5	21.2
Beaumont	118,418	7.7	2.6	5.9	7.8	1.7	3.1	4.6	8.9	2.0	1.9	68.9	36.0
Bryan	37,939	8.0	2.5	5.7	6.4	1.5	3.4	2.6	5.6	1.2	2.9	32.5	20.8
Corpus Christi	99,580	8.7	2.4	5.8	6.7	1.4	2.6	4.0	6.0	3.4	1.3	70.1	22.0
Dallas	571,236	9.2	2.4	5.1	5.7	1.8	2.9	3.8	7.2	2.1	1.9	49.1	22.4
El Paso	168,495	7.3	1.6	5.8	5.2	1.4	2.5	2.0	6.6	1.9	0.8	31.8	19.7
Fort Worth	249,518	9.5	2.3	4.6	4.9	1.7	3.1	3.3	4.5	1.6	2.8	42.3	19.1
Harlingen	84,587	6.6	1.5	7.7	7.4	1.4	1.5	3.2	8.6	3.3	0.5	48.7	30.0
Houston	661,844	8.4	2.2	5.4	5.6	1.7	3.1	3.7	7.9	2.0	1.5	50.7	30.1
Longview	47,342	8.9	2.4	5.1	5.7	2.4	4.1	4.8	5.4	1.2	2.7	42.9	14.7
Lubbock	154,500	10.3	2.1	7.2	7.0	2.7	2.5	3.2	11.7	1.8	3.1	48.9	40.7
McAllen	70,740	6.6	1.7	8.1	8.5	1.4	1.3	2.8	9.8	2.7	1.4	62.2	33.3
Odessa	66,030	9.6	2.1	5.9	8.4	1.8	2.5	5.9	10.3	3.5	1.0	49.8	39.8
San Angelo	42,868	9.3	2.0	6.1	6.1	2.0	5.1	4.8	5.3	1.9	1.5	34.6	24.8
San Antonio	343,711	7.8	2.0	5.9	6.1	1.4	2.6	2.8	5.0	2.9	1.5	50.1	23.9
Temple	65,578	8.6	2.2	5.0	6.0	1.7	1.8	2.5	3.8	0.7	2.0	34.6	11.4
Tyler	138,956	8.5	2.6	5.9	6.5	1.9	3.0	5.6	6.2	1.8	2.0	65.8	24.0

Hospital Referral Region	Medicare Population (1995 plus 1996)	Hip Fracture Repair per 1,000 Medicare Enrollees (1995-96)	Colectomy for Colorectal Cancer per 1,000 Medicare Enrollees (1995-96)	Cholecystectomy per 1,000 Medicare Enrollees (1995-96)	CABG per 1,000 Medicare Enrollees (1995-96)	Hip Replacement per 1,000 Medicare Enrollees (1995-96)	Back Surgery per 1,000 Medicare Enrollees (1995-96)	Carotid Endarterectomy per 1,000 Medicare Enrollees (1995-96)	PTCA per 1,000 Medicare Enrollees (1995-96)	Lower Extremity Bypass per 1,000 Medicare Enrollees (1995-96)	Radical Prostatectomy per 1,000 Male Medicare Enrollees (1995-96)	Carotid Duplex Diagnostic Procedures per 1,000 Medicare Enrollees (1995-96)	Cardiac Catheterization per 1,000 Medicare Enrollees (1995-96)
Victoria	39,186	7.2	2.7	6.7	4.6	1.7	3.4	4.6	6.3	1.0	2.0	43.0	19.6
Waco	85,123	9.0	2.3	5.3	6.3	1.7	4.3	3.1	5.0	1.2	1.3	46.5	21.9
Wichita Falls	57,700	9.8	2.0	4.4	5.7	2.0	3.3	3.8	4.2	1.5	3.7	55.9	13.8
Utah													
Ogden	58,586	8.0	1.8	4.9	6.1	2.8	3.2	2.2	6.3	1.4	2.0	24.5	17.1
Provo	54,192	7.7	1.9	6.1	6.3	3.8	5.5	2.2	11.4	0.5	2.4	29.9	21.3
Salt Lake City	276,853	7.4	1.9	5.0	4.9	3.5	4.2	1.5	6.4	0.9	2.8	20.0	21.2
Vermont													
Burlington	141,153	7.9	2.5	4.8	5.1	2.9	2.1	2.8	5.6	2.3	1.9	42.7	19.9
Virginia													
Arlington	217,532	8.7	2.0	3.4	4.4	2.5	2.8	3.1	4.9	1.8	1.6	47.9	16.4
Charlottesville	119,093	8.4	2.2	4.1	4.6	2.5	3.2	1.6	3.8	1.3	1.8	31.1	19.0
Lynchburg	63,252	9.2	2.4	5.1	6.9	1.9	3.3	2.5	4.0	1.3	1.8	23.5	17.7
Newport News	100,986	8.9	2.2	4.8	6.6	2.3	5.6	3.7	6.0	3.2	2.2	37.2	24.6
Norfolk	223,741	8.8	2.5	4.9	7.1	2.2	4.2	3.8	5.8	3.0	1.0	71.2	24.5
Richmond	314,554	8.7	2.5	4.7	6.9	2.4	4.2	3.3	8.0	2.8	2.1	48.3	25.2
Roanoke	192,456	8.6	2.3	6.5	6.0	2.0	2.9	3.2	4.0	2.5	1.7	43.5	15.8
Winchester	81,227	8.7	2.5	5.7	6.9	2.1	3.4	2.2	7.0	1.3	1.2	35.1	28.3
Washington													
Everett	81,205	8.2	2.3	3.3	4.9	3.3	4.0	3.8	3.8	2.1	2.0	42.9	14.1
Olympia	67,206	7.9	2.1	4.0	4.6	3.7	3.6	3.6	8.0	2.2	2.2	51.0	15.1
Seattle	405,155	7.8	2.2	3.6	5.7	3.2	3.9	2.9	5.9	2.2	1.9	40.6	18.6
Spokane	289,363	8.0	2.3	4.3	5.8	3.2	4.6	3.1	5.1	1.8	2.3	39.3	18.0
Tacoma	112,312	7.6	2.2	3.7	5.2	3.4	4.5	2.6	3.3	3.4	2.5	41.6	12.8
Yakima	57,239	7.5	2.2	3.7	4.8	2.7	3.4	2.2	4.3	1.7	1.8	30.2	16.3
West Virginia													
Charleston	254,827	8.5	2.3	5.2	8.8	1.9	1.8	4.4	5.1	2.2	1.4	48.0	22.2
Huntington	100,854	8.4	2.6	4.7	5.7	1.7	2.6	3.4	6.9	1.2	1.5	52.3	22.4
Morgantown	114,046	8.6	2.6	5.0	5.9	2.0	2.2	4.0	6.6	1.9	1.4	43.4	23.9
Wisconsin													
Appleton	77,833	7.0	2.8	4.1	4.9	3.1	3.0	2.5	6.6	2.2	2.7	29.3	16.9
Green Bay	132,406	7.0	2.7	5.0	4.9	3.3	4.0	3.3	3.5	2.4	2.3	35.2	15.8
La Crosse	96,697	7.1	2.6	5.0	7.5	2.7	1.5	1.5	3.7	1.2	2.4	24.6	24.4
Madison	228,077	7.2	2.8	4.6	5.8	3.0	2.4	2.7	5.1	1.3	1.9	30.7	19.4
Marshfield	108,937	7.0	2.3	4.9	6.3	3.3	2.6	2.8	5.2	1.5	2.8	36.5	18.0
Milwaukee	574,765	7.4	2.7	4.5	7.4	2.7	2.7	3.1	9.8	2.0	1.5	44.1	28.7
Neenah	60,821	7.5	2.6	5.9	6.7	2.6	2.4	3.1	7.4	2.1	2.9	38.4	30.1
Wausau	54,206	7.0	2.8	5.5	5.6	3.0	3.2	4.3	5.9	2.4	2.1	48.1	19.3
Wyoming													
Casper	44,566	8.5	1.8	5.3	6.0	2.9	6.1	3.4	5.8	1.9	1.7	40.4	19.8
United States													
	57,875,844	8.1	2.5	4.9	6.2	2.4	3.1	3.4	6.6	2.2	1.9	53.0	22.7

The Quality of Care in the Last Six Months of Life

The Quality of Care in the Last Six Months of Life

The quality of medical intervention is often more a matter of the quality of caring than the quality of curing, and never more so than when life nears its end. Yet medicine's focus is disproportionately on curing, or at least on the ability to keep patients alive with life-support systems and other medical interventions. This ability to intervene at the end of life has raised a host of medical and ethical issues for patients, physicians, and policy makers.

The Dartmouth Atlas demonstrates that, to the extent that end of life issues are addressed in practice, they are resolved in ways that depend on where the patient happens to live, not on the patient's preferences or the power of care to extend life. The American experience of death varied remarkably from one community to another in 1995-96:

■ The chance that the decedent was an inpatient in an acute care hospital at the time of death varied by a factor of 2.8, from less than 20% to almost 50%.

■ The chance of being admitted to an intensive care unit at the time of death varied by a factor of 4.6, from 6.3% to almost 30% of all deaths.

■ Time spent in intensive care varied substantially. In some regions, more than 20% of patients spent a week or more in intensive care units during their last six months of life; in other regions, less than 4% did.

The intensity of care in the last six months of life also varied remarkably in 1995-96:

■ The number of visits to physicians varied by a factor of 5.6, from an average of less than nine to almost 50.

■ The number of physicians involved in patients' care varied substantially. In some regions more than 30% of patients saw ten or more physicians during their last six months of life; in other regions fewer than 3% were treated by that many different physicians.

■ Price adjusted reimbursements by the Medicare program for inpatient care during the last six months of life varied by a factor of three, from about $6,200 to almost $18,000 per decedent.

Like other medical decisions, end of life decisions about the use of resources are influenced by the available supply of acute care hospital resources and by individual physicians' practice styles. But is more better? The intensity of care in the last six months of life is an indicator of the propensity to use life saving technology. The question of whether more medical intervention is better must be framed in terms of the potential gain in life expectancy for populations living in regions with greater intensity of intervention. Research conducted in conjunction with the Atlas project provided evidence that populations living in regions with lower intensity of care in the last six months of life did not have higher mortality rates

More than 80% of patients say that they wish to avoid hospitalization and intensive care during the terminal phase of illness, but those wishes are often overridden by other factors. If more intense intervention does not improve life expectancy, and if most patients prefer less care when more intensive care is likely to be futile, the fundamental question is whether the quality of care in regions with fewer resources and more conservative practice styles is better than in regions where more aggressive treatment is the norm.

The Likelihood That Death Will Occur in a Hospital, Rather Than Elsewhere

In 1995-96, the likelihood of a hospitalized death was closely linked to where the enrollee lived. In one hospital referral region, fewer than 18% of Medicare deaths occurred in hospitals; in other regions, the proportion was almost 50%.

In 24 hospital referral regions, the chance of dying in a hospital was at least 40%, including Newark, New Jersey (49.0%); Manhattan (48.4%); East Long Island, New York (47.6%); and the Bronx, New York (46.3%). In five hospital referral regions, fewer than 20% of deaths occurred in hospitals: Bend, Oregon (17.2%); Ogden, Utah (19.6%); Mason City, Iowa (19.7%); and Tucson, Arizona (19.7%).

About one-third of the variation in the chance of a hospitalized death could be attributed to the numbers of hospital beds per 1,000 residents of hospital referral regions (R^2 = .34).

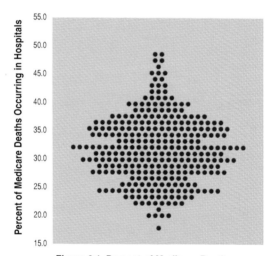

Figure 6.1. Percent of Medicare Deaths Occurring in Hospitals (1995-96)

The percent of Medicare deaths that occurred while the decedents were inpatients in hospitals ranged from less than 20% to almost 50%, after adjustment for differences in population age, sex, and race. Each point represents one of the 306 hospital referral regions in the United States.

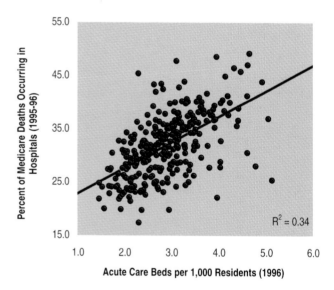

Acute Care Beds per 1,000 Residents (1996)

Figure 6.2. The Association between Hospital Beds per 1,000 Residents and the Likelihood that Death will Occur in Hospital (1995-96)

The numbers of hospital beds per 1,000 residents of hospital referral regions were correlated with the likelihood that when death occurred, it happened while the decedent was an inpatient in an acute care hospital (R^2 = .34).

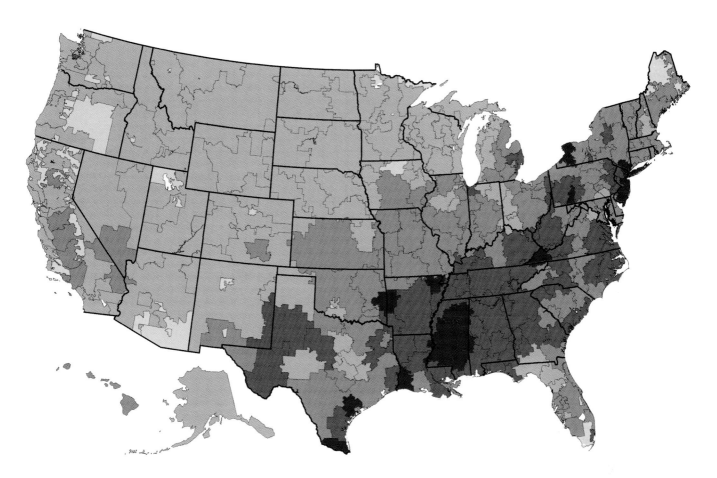

Map 6.1 Percent of Medicare Deaths Occurring in Hospitals (1995-96)

Medicare enrollees who lived in the Eastern and Southern United States were more likely to die as hospital inpatients than residents of the Western and Northwestern parts of the country. Rates were particularly high in the New York-New Jersey metropolitan area and in Mississippi, and much lower than average in Tucson, Arizona, Ogden, Utah, Bend, Oregon, and Mason City, Iowa.

Percent of Medicare Deaths Occurring in Hospitals
by Hospital Referral Region (1995-96)

- 40 or More   (24)
- 35 to < 40   (67)
- 30 to < 35   (102)
- 20 to < 30   (108)
- Less than 20   (5)
- Not Populated

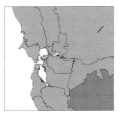

San Francisco

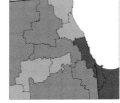

Chicago

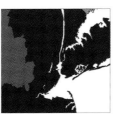

New York

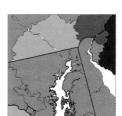

Washington-Baltimore

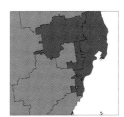

Detroit

The Likelihood of Being Admitted to an Intensive Care Unit During the Last Six Months of Life

The chances that the last six months of a Medicare enrollee's life included at least one stay in an intensive care unit varied by a factor of more than three. In one region, less than 15% of Medicare enrollees who died were admitted one or more times to intensive care units (including coronary intensive care) during their last six months of life; in other regions almost one-half of enrollees were admitted to intensive care at least once during their last six months of life.

In 18 hospital referral regions, the likelihood of one or more admissions to intensive care during the last six months of life was greater than 40%, including Miami (49.3%); Munster, Indiana (48.7%); Los Angeles (45.8%); St. Petersburg, Florida (44.2%); Beaumont, Texas (43.9%); and Newark, New Jersey (43.9%).

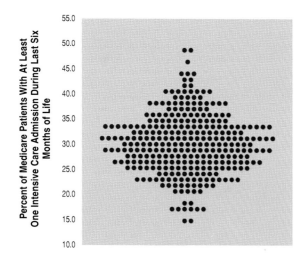

In ten hospital referral regions, the likelihood of admission to intensive care during the last six months of life was less than 20%, including Sun City, Arizona (14.2%); Bloomington, Illinois (15.2%); Bend, Oregon (16.6%); Wausau, Wisconsin (16.9%); Mason City, Iowa (16.9%); and Grand Junction, Colorado (17.4%).

Figure 6.3. Percent of Medicare Enrollees Admitted to Intensive Care During the Last Six Months of Life (1995-96)

The percent of all Medicare decedents who were admitted to intensive care units at least once during their final six months, after adjusting for differences in age, sex, and race, ranged from less than 15% to almost 50%. Each point represents one of the 306 hospital referral regions in the United States.

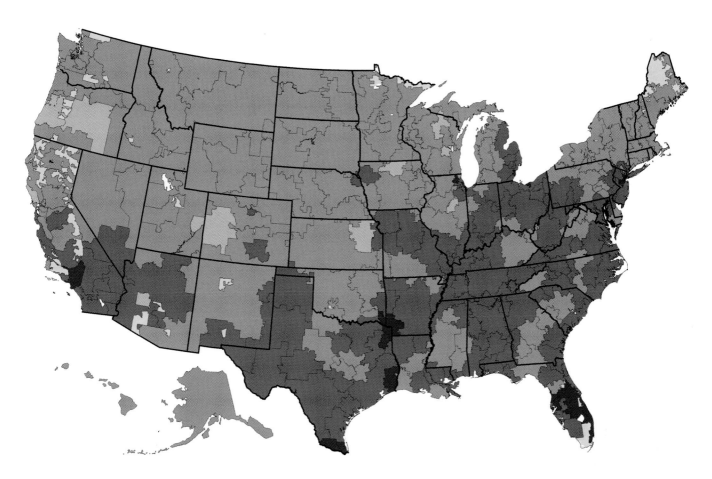

Map 6.2. Percent of Medicare Enrollees Admitted to Intensive Care During the Last Six Months of Life (1995-96)

The likelihood of at least one admission to intensive care during the last six months of life was generally higher in the Eastern and Southern United States than in the Western and Northwestern states.

Percent of Medicare Enrollees Admitted to Intensive Care During the Last Six Months of Life

by Hospital Referral Region (1995-96)

■ 40 or More	(18)
■ 30 to < 40	(137)
■ 20 to < 30	(141)
■ 10 to < 20	(10)
□ Less than 10	(0)
□ Not Populated	

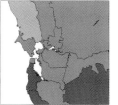

San Francisco

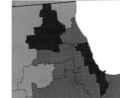

Chicago

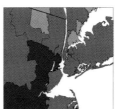

New York

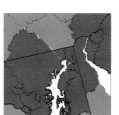

Washington-Baltimore

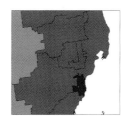

Detroit

The Likelihood of Spending Seven or More Days in an Intensive Care Unit During the Last Six Months of Life

The percent of Medicare enrollees who spent a week or more of their last six months in intensive care units is an indicator of aggressive end of life care. The likelihood of a week or more in intensive care ranged from less than 3% to more than 25%. The national average was 11.0%.

Among the hospital referral regions where decedents were had a better than 20% chance of spending a week or more in intensive care units during the last six months of their lives were Munster, Indiana (25.5%); Miami (23.5%); Beaumont, Texas (21.6%); and Los Angeles (20.4%).

Among the hospital referral regions where residents were less likely than average to spend seven or more days in intensive care at the end of life were Eugene, Oregon (2.9%); Grand Junction, Colorado (3.0%); Bend, Oregon (3.1%); Sun City, Arizona (3.2%); and Mason City, Iowa (3.4%).

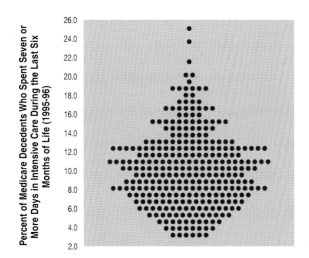

Figure 6.4. Percent of Medicare Enrollees Who Spent Seven or More Days in Intensive Care During Their Last Six Months of Life (1995-96)

The percent of Medicare enrollees who spent seven or more days of their last six months of life in an intensive care unit ranged from less than 5% to more than 25%, after adjustment for differences in population age, sex, and race. Each point represents one of the 306 hospital referral regions in the United States.

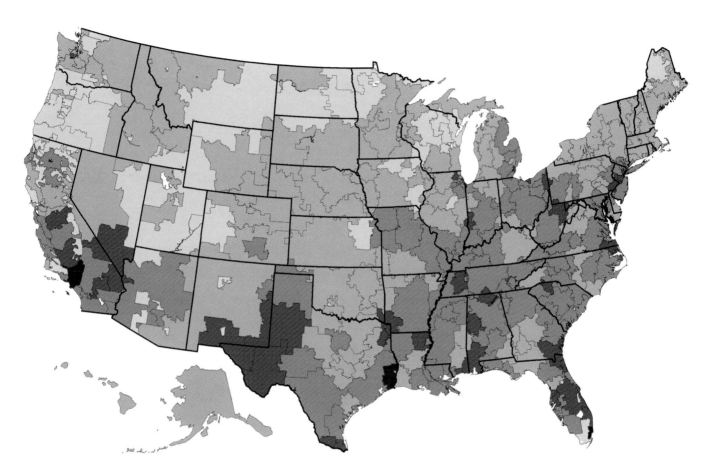

Map 6.3. Percent of Medicare Enrollees Who Spent Seven or More Days in Intensive Care During Their Last Six Months of Life (1995-96)

The likelihood of spending at least one week of the last six months of life in intensive care was higher among enrollees in the East, Midwest, Texas and southern California. Medicare residents of the Upper Midwest, Mountain states, and Oregon were on average less likely to spend seven or more days in intensive care at the end of life.

Percent of Medicare Enrollees Who Spent Seven or More Days in Intensive Care During the Last Six Months of Life

by Hospital Referral Region (1995-96)

- ■ 20 or More   (4)
- ■ 15 to < 20   (35)
- ■ 10 to < 15   (115)
- ■ 5 to < 10   (128)
- ■ Less than 5   (24)
- ■ Not Populated

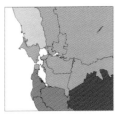

San Francisco

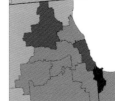

Chicago

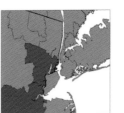

New York

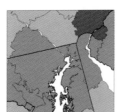

Washington-Baltimore

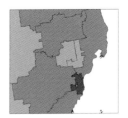

Detroit

The Likelihood of Being Admitted to an Intensive Care Unit During the Terminal Hospitalization

Another measure of the intensity of hospital care at the end of life is the likelihood that Medicare enrollees would be admitted to intensive care units during the hospitalization in which they died. The chance that an enrollee who died in a hospital had been admitted to an intensive care unit during that hospitalization varied by a factor of almost five, from less than 6.5% to almost 30%.

In six hospital referral regions, dying Medicare enrollees had a one-in-four or greater chance of being admitted to intensive care during their terminal hospitalization: Newark, New Jersey (29.0%); Munster, Indiana (26.3%); Harlingen, Texas (25.6%); McAllen, Texas (25.3%); New Brunswick, New Jersey (25.1%); and Miami (25.0%).

In eleven hospital referral regions, the chance of being admitted to intensive care at the time of death was less than one in ten, including Bend, Oregon (6.3%); Sun City, Arizona (7.1%); Bloomington, Illinois (8.4%); Mason City, Iowa (8.6%); Santa Rosa, California (8.6%); and Grand Junction, Colorado (9.3%).

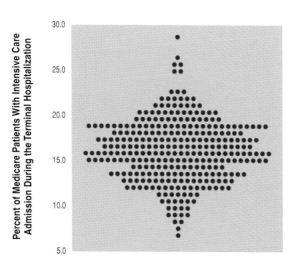

Figure 6.5. Percent of Medicare Enrollees Admitted to Intensive Care During the Terminal Hospitalization (1995-96)

The proportion of enrollees who were admitted to intensive care units during their terminal hospitalizations ranged from about 6% to almost 30%, after adjustment for differences in population age, sex, and race. Each point represents one of the 306 hospital referral regions in the United States.

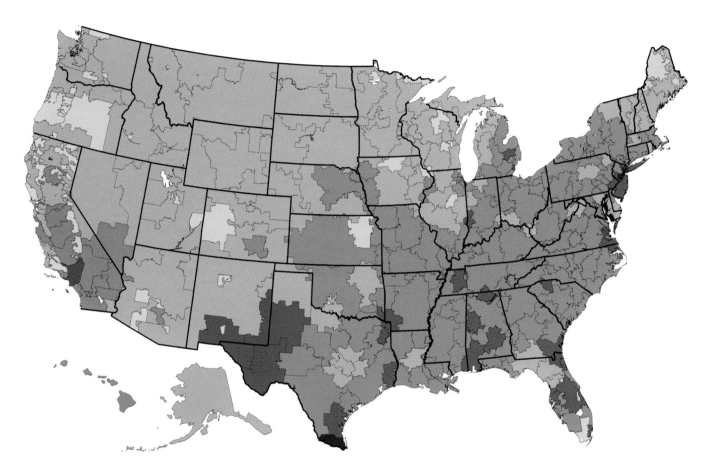

Map 6.4. Percent of Medicare Enrollees Admitted to Intensive Care During the Terminal Hospitalization (1995-96)

Admissions to intensive care during terminal hospitalizations were more likely among Medicare enrollees who lived in the East and South than among those in the West, with the exception of parts of California.

Percent of Medicare Enrollees Admitted to Intensive Care During the Terminal Hospitalization

by Hospital Referral Region (1995-96)

■	25 or More	(5)
■	20 to < 25	(31)
■	15 to < 20	(161)
■	10 to < 15	(98)
■	Less than 10	(11)
■	Not Populated	

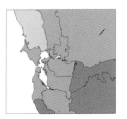

San Francisco

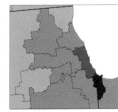

Chicago

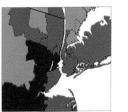

New York

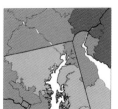

Washington-Baltimore

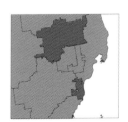

Detroit

Physician Visits During the Last Six Months of Life

Although people in the last six months of their lives are generally quite sick, the intensity of physician care that Medicare enrollees in their last six months of life were likely to receive, as measured by the average number of visits to physicians, varied from fewer than nine visits per decedent to almost 50. The national average was 24.4. About 90% of physician visits in the last six months of life were with either primary care physicians or medical specialists; surgeons were visited much less frequently.

The average number of physician visits during the last six months of life was almost double the national average among residents of the Miami hospital referral region (47.9). Rates of visits were also high in the New York-Northern New Jersey metropolitan area, including Newark, New Jersey (45.5); Ridgewood, New Jersey (43.0); New Brunswick, New Jersey (42.4); Paterson, New Jersey (42.2); East Long Island, New York (40.0); and Manhattan (39.4).

Dying residents of other hospital referral regions were much less likely to make multiple visits to doctors during the last six months of life. Hospital referral regions where rates of visits were low included Grand Junction, Colorado (8.5); Ogden, Utah (8.6); Salt Lake City (10.9); Mason City, Iowa (11.0); and Salem, Oregon (11.0).

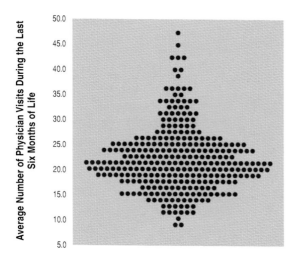

Figure 6.6. Average Number of Physician Visits per Decedent During the Last Six Months of Life (1995-96)

The number of physician visits during the last six months of life varied by a factor of about five, from fewer than 10 to almost 50, after adjustment for differences in population age, sex, and race. Each point represents one of the 306 hospital referral regions in the United States.

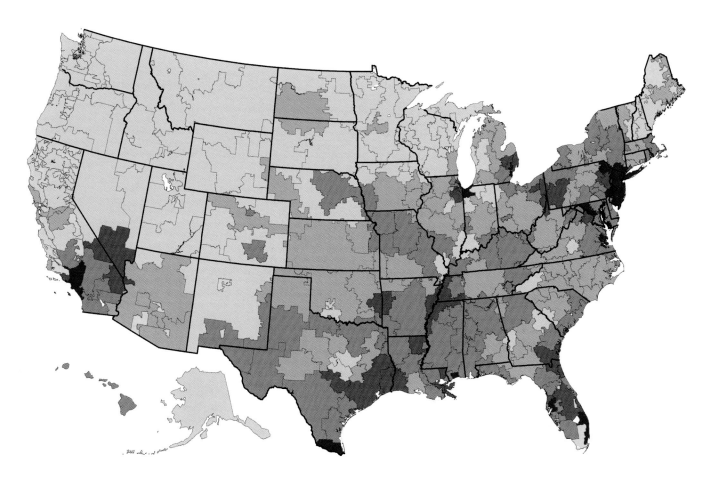

Map 6.5. Physician Visits During the Last Six Months of Life (1995-96)

Rates of physician visits during the last six months of life were higher than the national average in the Eastern United States, and lower in the West and Northwest. Rates were at least 30% higher than the national average in 27 hospital referral regions, most of which were in Florida, New York, New Jersey, Texas and California.

Ratio of Rates of Physician Visits During the Last Six Months of Life to the U.S. Average

by Hospital Referral Region (1995-96)

- 1.30 to 1.97 (27)
- 1.10 to < 1.30 (27)
- 0.90 to < 1.10 (85)
- 0.75 to < 0.90 (91)
- 0.34 to < 0.75 (76)
- Not Populated

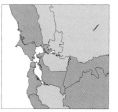

San Francisco

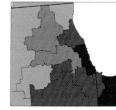

Chicago

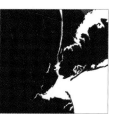

New York

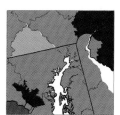

Washington-Baltimore

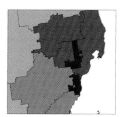

Detroit

Primary Care Physician Visits During the Last Six Months of Life

Almost one-half of all physician visits among Medicare enrollees in their last six months of life were with primary care physicians. As with total physician visits, treatment by primary care physicians was extremely variable, according to where the enrollee lived. Such visits varied by a factor of almost four, from fewer than five per decedent to almost 20.

In five hospital referral regions, enrollees in their last six months of life averaged more than 18 primary care physician visits, including Gulfport, Mississippi (19.0); Newark, New Jersey (18.5); Ridgewood, New Jersey (18.3); East Long Island, New York (18.1); and Dearborn, Michigan (18.1).

Residents of other hospital referral regions had many fewer visits with primary care physicians during the last six months of their lives than the national average of 11.5, including those in Ogden, Utah (4.5); Salem, Oregon (4.8); Grand Junction, Colorado (4.9); Bend, Oregon (5.9); Provo, Utah (6.0); and Salt Lake City (6.0).

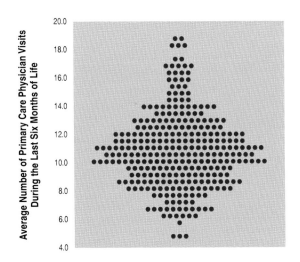

Figure 6.7. Average Number of Primary Care Physician Visits During the Last Six Months of Life (1995-96)

Visits to primary care physicians by Medicare enrollees in their last six months of life varied by a factor of more than four, from fewer than five to almost 20, after adjustment for differences in population age, sex, and race. Each point represents one of the 306 hospital referral regions in the United States.

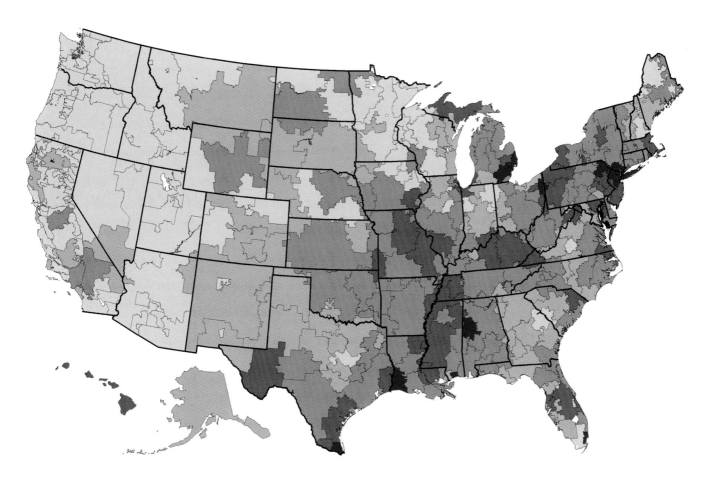

Map 6.6. Primary Care Physician Visits During the Last Six Months of Life (1995-96)

The intensity of primary care physician visits was higher, generally, in the East and Midwest, and lower in the Western states.

Ratio of Rates of Primary Care Physician Visits During the Last Six Months of Life to the U.S. Average

by Hospital Referral Region (1995-96)

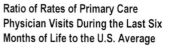

- 1.30 to 1.65   (23)
- 1.10 to < 1.30   (44)
- 0.90 to < 1.10 (101)
- 0.75 to < 0.90   (74)
- 0.39 to < 0.75   (64)
- Not Populated

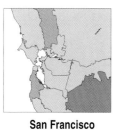

San Francisco

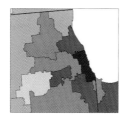

Chicago

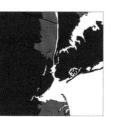

New York

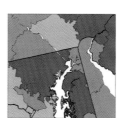

Washington-Baltimore

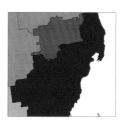

Detroit

Visits to Medical Specialists During the Last Six Months of Life

More than 40% of Medicare enrollees' visits with physicians during the last six months of the enrollees' lives were with medical (non-surgical) specialists. The number of such visits varied by a factor of more than ten, from 2.0 to 25.1. There was no evidence that Medicare enrollees in the last six months of life were seen by primary care doctors instead of visiting medical specialists (a substitution effect); indeed, regions with higher visit rates for primary care tended also to have higher visit rates for specialist care (R^2 = .22).

Among the hospital referral regions where medical specialist visits were higher than the national average of 10.3 were Miami (25.1); Newark, New Jersey (23.8); Los Angeles (22.9); and New Brunswick, New Jersey (22.5).

Among the hospital referral regions where Medicare enrollees had fewer than average visits to medical specialists were Mason City, Iowa (2.0); Grand Junction, Colorado (2.6); Ogden, Utah (2.6); and Lebanon, New Hampshire (2.6).

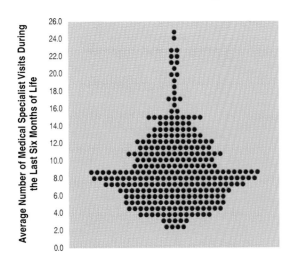

Figure 6.8. Average Number of Visits to Medical Specialists During the Last Six Months of Life (1995-96)

The average number of visits to medical specialists during the last six months of life varied by a factor of more than ten, from 2 to 25, after adjustment for differences in population age, sex, and race. Each point represents one of the 306 hospital referral regions in the United States.

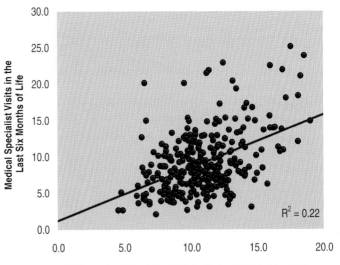

Figure 6.9. The Relationship Between Rates of Visits to Primary Care Doctors and Rates of Visits to Medical Specialists During the Last Six Months of Life (1995-96)

There was no evidence that Medicare enrollees who had higher rates of visits to primary care physicians during their last six months of life saw fewer medical specialists in the same period; there was, in fact, a positive correlation (R^2 = .22).

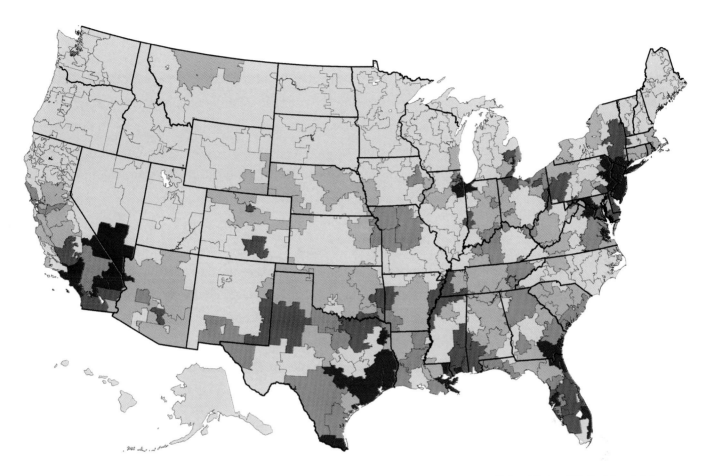

Map 6.7. Visits to Medical Specialists During the Last Six Months of Life (1995-96)

Visits to medical specialists by Medicare enrollees during the last six months of life were higher than the national average in the Eastern and Southern United States than in the West and Upper Midwest. Residents of 41 hospital referral regions had at least 30% more visits than the national average.

Ratio of Rates of Medical Specialist Visits During the Last Six Months of Life to the U.S. Average

by Hospital Referral Region (1995-96)

- 1.30 to 2.43 (41)
- 1.10 to < 1.30 (33)
- 0.90 to < 1.10 (48)
- 0.75 to < 0.90 (58)
- 0.19 to < 0.75 (126)
- Not Populated

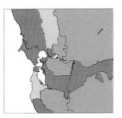
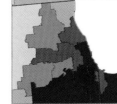
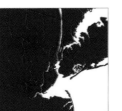
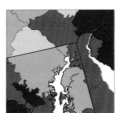
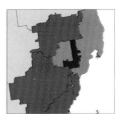

San Francisco   Chicago   New York   Washington-Baltimore   Detroit

The Likelihood of Seeing Ten or More Physicians in the Last Six Months of Life

Another way of measuring the intensity of the use of physician care in the last six months of life is to measure the number of different physicians involved in the treatment of individual enrollees in the last six months of their lives. To measure this "propensity to refer," an index was developed by counting the number of physicians who provided one or more patient visits within the last six months of life to each patient in the 5% sample of Part B Medicare claims. (The index is explained in more detail in the Appendix on Methods.)

According to this index, the propensity to refer varied by a factor of 27 among the 306 hospital referral regions in the United States. Only 1.3% of patients in the Bloomington, Illinois hospital referral region saw ten or more physicians during their last six months of life. In the Miami hospital referral region, more than a third of patients (34.7%) saw ten or more physicians. Propensity to refer was strongly correlated with visit rates in last six months of life (Figure 6.11).

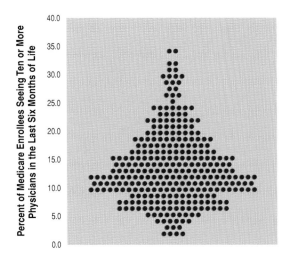

Figure 6.10. Percent of Medicare Enrollees Seeing Ten or More Physicians During the Last Six Months of Life (1995-96)

The proportion of Medicare enrollees who saw ten or more physicians during the last six months of the enrollees' lives ranged from less than 2% to almost 35%, after adjustment for differences in population age, sex, and race. Each point represents one of the 306 hospital referral regions in the United States.

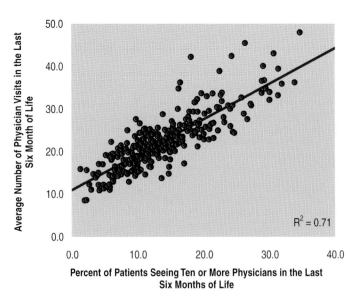

Figure 6.11. The Relationship Between the Propensity to Refer to Multiple Physicians and the Average Number of Physician Visits Among Enrollees in the Last Six Months of Life (1995-96)

The number of different physicians Medicare enrollees saw during the last six months of their lives was strongly correlated with the average number of total physician visits (R^2 = .71).

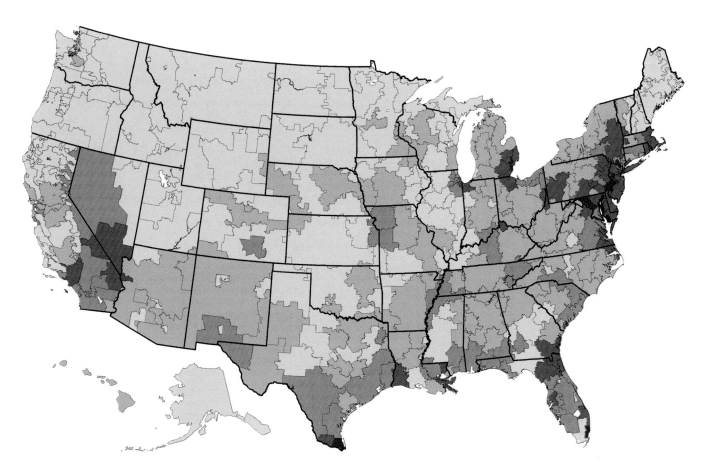

Map 6.8. Propensity to Refer to Multiple Physicians During the Last Six Months of Life (1995-96)

Medicare residents of the Eastern Seaboard and parts of Texas, Florida, California and Nevada were more likely to see ten or more physicians during their last six months of life. The propensity to refer dying patients to many different physicians was lower in the West, Upper Midwest, and Northwest.

Percent of Medicare Enrollees Seeing Ten or More Physicians During the Last Six Months of Life

by Hospital Referral Region (1995-96)

- 30 or More   (8)
- 20 to < 30   (41)
- 15 to < 20   (59)
- 10 to < 15   (105)
- Less than 10 (93)
- Not Populated

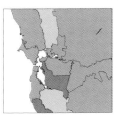

San Francisco

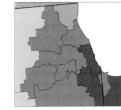

Chicago

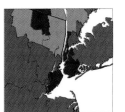

New York

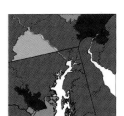

Washington-Baltimore

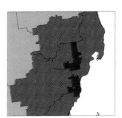

Detroit

Reimbursements for Inpatient Care During the Last Six Months of Life

Per-enrollee Medicare spending for inpatient care (Part A reimbursements) provides another measure of the intensity of care in the last six months of life. In 1995-96, the price adjusted amount of money spent by the Medicare program for inpatient care of enrollees during the last six months of their lives varied by a factor of three, from about $6,200 per enrollee to almost $18,000.

Four hospital referral regions had per-enrollee reimbursements for inpatient care of more than $15,000, including Manhattan ($17,797); Harlingen, Texas ($16,938); McAllen, Texas ($16,504); and the Bronx, New York ($16,499). Residents of the hospital referral regions in Miami ($14,986); Chicago ($13,580); and Los Angeles ($13,160) also had higher than average reimbursements for inpatient care.

Among the hospital referral regions with the lowest per enrollee reimbursements during the last six months of life were Bend, Oregon ($6,198); Appleton, Wisconsin ($6,346); Salem, Oregon ($6,602); Dubuque, Iowa ($6,648); and San Luis Obispo, California ($6,672).

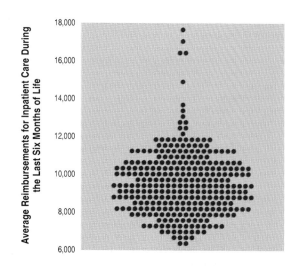

Figure 6.12. Average per Decedent Reimbursements for Inpatient Care During the Last Six Months of Life (1995-96)

Average reimbursements for inpatient hospital care during the last six months of life, after adjusting for price, age, sex and race, ranged from less about $6,200 to almost $18,000. Each point represents one of the 306 hospital referral regions in the United States.

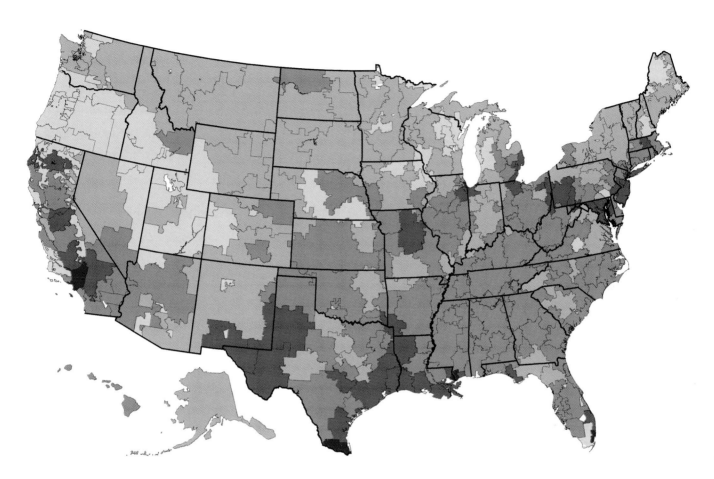

Map 6.9. Average Reimbursements for Inpatient Care During the Last Six Months of Life (1995-96)

Price adjusted per enrollee reimbursements for inpatient care during the last six months of life were highest along the Washington-to-Boston corridor, in Detroit, Chicago, and some hospital referral regions in California. Reimbursements were substantially below the national average in the majority of hospital referral regions.

Ratio of Rates of Price Adjusted Medicare Reimbursements for Inpatient Care During the Last Six Months of Life to U.S. Average
by Hospital Referral Region (1995-96)

- 1.30 to 1.79   (8)
- 1.10 to < 1.30   (45)
- 0.90 to < 1.10 (134)
- 0.75 to < 0.90   (90)
- 0.62 to < 0.75   (29)
- Not Populated

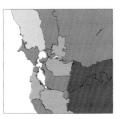

San Francisco

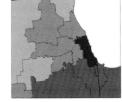

Chicago

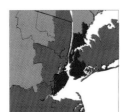

New York

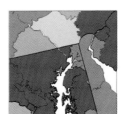

Washington-Baltimore

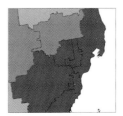

Detroit

How Effective is Medicare Spending in the Last Six Months of Life?

There were wide differences in the treatment provided to people who spent their last six months of life during 1995-96. Did the greater intensity provided in some hospital referral regions actually save lives, or increase the survival of the elderly sick? At the very heart of the question is the economics of the end of life, and the question, What are we getting for our investment in the very aggressive care provided to some members of the Medicare population?

Answering this question is complex, since sicker people might be expected to account for more health care spending, and also are more likely to die. But the treatment of people in their last six months of life is an excellent marker for the treatment being given to everyone in the Medicare population who is seriously ill. For example, there was a strong relationship between the intensity of inpatient health care spending in the last six months of life and average per capita Medicare reimbursements for all enrollees (Figure 6.13).

Despite the fact that this indicator of intensity of care is highly correlated with overall per capita spending among the Medicare population, it is not closely associated with standard measures of health status, such as population-based rates of acute myocardial infarction, stroke, and hip fracture. In other words, how people are treated in the last six months of their lives is a good indicator of the overall intensity of medical intervention in the population, but it does not reflect the underlying level of illness or sickness.

In turn, the intensity of care, while raising spending, does not appear to have had an impact on the overall mortality level of the community. Regions providing more intensive levels of medical interventions to the elderly sick yielded no discernible improvement in life expectancy, suggesting that the United States might be on the "flat of the curve" in terms of the relationship between spending (inputs) and survival (outputs).

Simply measuring mortality does not capture the entire spectrum of possible benefits of end of life spending. The quality of health care includes more than the ability to prevent or postpone death; it also includes the capacity to improve the quality of life. While the extra resources devoted to health care intensity in some regions might provide comfort, if not life extension, to the population of people who are near death, it is unclear by what measure or mechanism more intensive acute care per capita resulted in improved quality of care at the end of life.

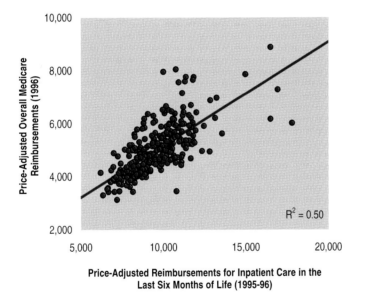

Figure 6.13. The Association Between Inpatient Medicare Spending in the Last Six Months of Life and Overall Per Capita Spending in the General Medicare Population (1995-96)

The intensity of care in the last six months of life, measured by Medicare Part A spending, is closely correlated with overall Medicare per capita spending (Part A and B) for the entire Medicare population.

Capacity, Patient Preferences and the Likelihood of a Hospitalized Death

Quality medical care includes respect for the patients' preferences about the end of life. There is growing concern in the United States about the quality of how we die. In two Gallup polls, one in 1992 and a second in 1996, nine out of ten Americans said they would prefer to be cared for at home if they were terminally ill. Of course, answers to this hypothetical question might not correspond to the preferences of those actually facing death. Another study, called SUPPORT (Study to Understand Preferences for Prognoses and Outcomes of Treatments) examined preferences about the place of death among patients who were facing death — those with very serious, life-threatening illnesses. The vast majority — 82% — reported that if a doctor told them they had "very little time to live," they would prefer death at home, rather than in a hospital. In most cases, however, those who die do not know with certainty that they will die within a certain time frame. Different people might place different degrees of importance on the (perhaps small) chance of surviving, versus the discomforts and risks of high-technology interventions. Some people die in intensive care units not because they prefer them to other settings, but because they were willing to take the risk of intense intervention in exchange for the chance of recovery.

The degree of regional variation in how many people die in hospitals, and how many have been admitted to intensive care units at least once during the last six months of their lives, however, is surprising, given the almost universal expression of a desire for death to happen elsewhere, and otherwise. Can this be explained by patient preferences — are people in some areas are more willing to take the risks associated with intensive medical interventions than similar people living elsewhere? Probably not. The SUPPORT study is unique among studies of terminal care and advance directives because it sought to "re-engineer" the clinical setting in order to respect and incorporate into the care plan the individual patient's own preferences at the time of death. The core of the intervention was specially trained and philosophically committed nurses who "spent all of their time counseling patients and families, convening meetings with physicians and others, eliciting preferences, making plans for future contingencies and ensuring that the best possible information about prognosis and preferences was available to the care team."

The intervention failed. The majority of patients who had expressed their preference for dying at home were actually in the hospital at the time of death, despite the best efforts of the SUPPORT group to redirect the clinical pathway.

Why did this happen? Probably the best explanation is that the local supply of hospital resources, and local physicians' practice styles, are far more dominant determinants of how care is given at the end of life than either patient preferences or the best clinical strategies to avoid unwelcome interventions. The SUPPORT study took place at five different hospitals in five different hospital referral regions. The percent of study patients who died in hospitals ranged from a low of 29% to a high of 66%. The variations were not explained by sociodemographic characteristics, clinical profiles, or patients' preferences.

Among the Medicare population, there was a strong, and apparently prevailing, association between acute care hospital capacity and the likelihood of a hospitalized death. Indeed, the supply of acute care hospital beds per 1,000 residents explained 71% of the variance among sites in place of death, and patient days per 1,000 Medicare enrollees explained 88% of the variance among sites in place of death. As with medical care and surgical interventions, in death geography is destiny. The place of death and the intensity of interventions provided depend much more on the region's patterns of use of acute care hospital resources than on what dying patients say that they want.

Population-based studies strongly suggest that greater intensity of medical care does not yield benefits, either in terms of longevity or in terms of providing patients with the kinds of deaths that they want. Clearly, below some critical level, less care is harmful because treatable illnesses go untreated or are under-treated; and we might be unable to identify such groups in population-based studies. Nevertheless, the evidence presented in this chapter characterizes a system in which large amounts of money are spent on medical intervention that provides no benefit, whether that benefit is measured in longevity or in honoring patients' preferences.

Chapter Six Table

All hospitalization and utilization rates are based on Medicare deaths occurring during the period July 1, 1995 — December 31, 1996, and are expressed as rates per person (per decedent). Rates are age, sex and race adjusted, and reimbursements are also adjusted for regional differences in prices. Data exclude Medicare enrollees who were members of risk bearing health maintenance organizations.

Specific codes used to define the numerator for rates, and methods of age, sex, race and illness adjustment are included in the Appendix on Methods.

CHAPTER SIX TABLE

Medical Care in the Last Six Months of Life by Hospital Referral Regions (1995-96)

Hospital Referral Region	Medicare Deaths (1995 plus 1996)	Percent of Medicare Deaths Occurring in Hospitals (1995-96)	Percent of Medicare Enrollees Admitted to Intensive Care During the Last Six Months of Life (1995-96)	Percent of Medicare Enrollees Spending Seven or More Days in Intensive Care During the Last Six Months of Life (1995-96)	Percent of Medicare Enrollees Admitted to Intensive Care During the Terminal Hospitalization (1995-96)	Physician Visits per Decedent During the Last Six Months of Life (1995-96)	Primary Care Physician Visits per Decedent During the Last Six Months of Life (1995-96)	Medical Specialist Visits per Decedent During the Last Six Months of Life (1995-96)	Percent of Medicare Enrollees Seeing Ten or More Physicians During the Last Six Months of Life (1995-96)	Price Adjusted Reimb. for Inpatient Care During the Last Six Months of Life per Decedent (1995-96)
Alabama										
Birmingham	22,119	39.8	34.4	12.6	19.9	22.9	12.1	8.5	12.0	10,441
Dothan	3,613	36.5	30.4	8.6	17.0	21.8	12.4	7.2	15.7	9,450
Huntsville	4,257	37.9	37.6	15.8	21.4	22.1	11.2	8.4	13.2	9,572
Mobile	6,569	38.4	38.7	15.3	21.2	25.2	10.6	11.5	17.9	10,306
Montgomery	4,236	38.0	33.4	10.7	20.3	20.5	10.5	7.9	10.8	9,768
Tuscaloosa	2,388	36.7	36.3	17.4	20.4	24.3	15.7	6.2	10.3	9,623
Alaska										
Anchorage	1,952	25.0	25.9	9.9	12.0	15.7	10.0	5.1	7.6	8,423
Arizona										
Mesa	3,784	23.9	33.3	12.2	15.6	20.5	6.3	12.6	13.5	8,170
Phoenix	13,896	24.0	30.9	10.2	14.2	18.5	8.0	8.7	14.2	9,029
Sun City	3,034	25.8	14.2	3.2	7.1	19.7	7.2	10.6	12.6	8,155
Tucson	5,959	19.7	28.5	8.8	11.9	18.9	8.1	8.6	11.6	8,095
Arkansas										
Fort Smith	3,794	40.0	32.4	7.1	18.8	27.6	12.5	12.5	9.8	9,059
Jonesboro	2,611	40.5	29.2	8.5	17.8	21.6	12.5	7.2	12.8	10,381
Little Rock	16,128	37.7	32.0	10.3	18.0	22.9	11.9	8.7	10.8	10,302
Springdale	3,541	30.6	30.9	6.4	16.1	18.8	11.5	5.5	5.8	8,098
Texarkana	3,002	38.7	41.5	17.5	21.5	24.4	11.7	10.9	10.5	12,020
California										
Orange Co.	10,550	29.7	39.3	13.4	18.7	32.3	9.5	20.1	19.0	10,650
Bakersfield	5,056	33.7	34.8	15.1	17.6	25.5	10.3	12.9	13.1	11,117
Chico	3,013	30.1	28.8	10.2	15.3	17.0	8.4	7.1	4.7	10,595
Contra Costa Co.	4,466	24.7	23.8	7.0	10.7	16.5	6.4	8.5	11.8	8,725
Fresno	5,943	30.9	29.4	10.2	15.1	18.0	7.7	8.7	8.4	8,957
Los Angeles	37,006	33.8	45.8	20.4	22.5	38.9	12.4	22.9	22.4	13,160
Modesto	4,483	31.6	36.9	15.0	19.3	21.5	10.5	9.2	12.6	11,823
Napa	2,906	24.6	23.6	7.1	11.9	17.1	8.8	5.8	8.8	9,792
Alameda Co.	7,591	27.3	26.7	7.8	13.3	20.6	8.4	9.9	15.4	10,494
Palm Spr/Rancho Mir	2,180	28.2	38.6	16.2	18.0	26.7	6.6	14.9	18.8	10,853
Redding	3,374	29.4	29.5	11.0	14.9	16.9	10.2	5.3	8.0	11,628
Sacramento	12,747	27.3	27.1	9.5	13.3	18.1	8.6	8.0	11.7	10,202
Salinas	2,323	23.4	36.7	13.1	16.3	17.9	7.0	8.9	9.8	10,877
San Bernardino	8,091	29.4	38.4	14.7	19.3	24.0	10.5	11.1	16.1	11,691
San Diego	12,946	25.5	31.0	10.9	15.1	23.8	8.6	13.2	15.2	10,208
San Francisco	8,702	25.9	28.3	8.7	13.0	20.1	8.5	9.4	10.9	9,824
San Jose	6,545	26.2	29.4	10.1	14.3	18.1	7.9	8.6	8.8	8,941
San Luis Obispo	1,636	23.3	33.2	11.6	14.9	16.3	7.8	6.9	9.6	6,672
San Mateo Co.	3,991	22.7	32.5	12.4	13.3	18.4	9.0	7.2	11.2	8,250
Santa Barbara	2,320	23.4	25.8	6.5	12.4	18.7	9.0	7.8	7.0	7,386

Hospital Referral Region	Medicare Deaths (1995 plus 1996)	Percent of Medicare Deaths Occurring in Hospitals (1995-96)	Percent of Medicare Enrollees Admitted to Intensive Care During the Last Six Months of Life (1995-96)	Percent of Medicare Enrollees Spending Seven or More Days in Intensive Care During the Last Six Months of Life (1995-96)	Percent of Medicare Enrollees Admitted to Intensive Care During the Terminal Hospitalization (1995-96)	Physician Visits per Decedent During the Last Six Months of Life (1995-96)	Primary Care Physician Visits per Decedent During the Last Six Months of Life (1995-96)	Medical Specialist Visits per Decedent During the Last Six Months of Life (1995-96)	Percent of Medicare Enrollees Seeing Ten or More Physicians During the Last Six Months of Life (1995-96)	Price Adjusted Reimb. for Inpatient Care During the Last Six Months of Life per Decedent (1995-96)
Santa Cruz	1,771	26.4	33.3	12.1	15.2	21.4	8.1	10.7	17.0	9,754
Santa Rosa	3,108	23.9	17.7	3.7	8.6	21.4	8.1	11.4	13.9	7,395
Stockton	2,936	29.3	28.8	9.8	15.6	20.5	8.2	10.0	13.3	11,822
Ventura	3,202	30.3	31.1	11.1	16.9	29.4	6.5	20.1	18.5	9,723
Colorado										
Boulder	1,212	19.9	30.6	8.4	13.7	22.6	7.8	11.7	14.0	6,993
Colorado Springs	4,287	25.6	23.2	5.6	13.4	15.3	8.7	5.1	9.0	7,930
Denver	11,795	23.0	26.7	7.5	13.0	18.9	8.7	8.3	10.6	8,544
Fort Collins	1,791	24.1	23.6	7.4	12.2	16.3	6.8	7.8	7.1	7,672
Grand Junction	2,142	21.3	17.4	3.0	9.3	8.5	4.9	2.6	1.9	7,054
Greeley	2,188	25.7	22.4	6.1	12.1	17.2	7.5	7.4	8.3	9,336
Pueblo	1,329	31.2	33.0	12.6	19.4	25.1	9.4	12.6	19.7	10,064
Connecticut										
Bridgeport	6,464	33.3	29.6	11.0	17.5	29.6	12.8	13.6	20.8	9,022
Hartford	14,457	30.7	27.3	8.5	15.3	21.9	10.6	8.4	16.2	9,212
New Haven	13,313	30.3	28.7	8.5	15.8	20.9	10.4	7.9	14.1	9,068
Delaware										
Wilmington	5,796	32.4	33.5	13.0	17.5	25.8	10.8	12.8	20.3	9,530
District of Columbia										
Washington	16,512	33.6	31.0	12.3	16.7	25.1	10.2	12.4	19.0	11,112
Florida										
Bradenton	3,392	30.2	38.1	14.7	17.4	23.5	9.9	10.6	16.8	9,293
Clearwater	6,925	29.0	34.5	12.0	17.5	26.6	9.7	13.9	17.9	9,878
Fort Lauderdale	22,059	31.1	40.2	17.0	19.4	36.7	11.3	21.8	29.2	11,268
Fort Myers	10,405	30.0	33.1	12.3	17.3	25.2	10.0	12.0	17.4	9,547
Gainesville	4,180	26.0	32.4	13.2	14.7	22.8	12.0	8.8	20.8	8,869
Hudson	5,580	32.4	41.2	15.6	20.2	27.3	13.0	10.8	19.4	10,901
Jacksonville	9,550	33.1	39.9	18.5	20.1	28.8	11.2	14.8	26.1	10,764
Lakeland	3,119	30.3	32.3	11.5	17.3	23.8	9.7	10.8	18.3	10,150
Miami	17,220	38.1	49.3	23.5	25.0	47.9	17.5	25.1	34.7	14,986
Ocala	5,395	28.5	28.2	8.9	14.1	22.6	9.4	9.9	16.8	8,987
Orlando	24,792	31.8	38.9	15.4	19.5	26.5	10.3	13.1	19.3	9,933
Ormond Beach	3,469	31.3	37.8	13.6	19.3	25.5	10.6	11.9	17.7	9,543
Panama City	1,774	35.9	31.2	13.1	18.8	24.4	9.8	9.6	16.1	11,563
Pensacola	5,639	36.4	33.9	12.2	18.9	24.3	10.7	10.6	18.7	10,680
Sarasota	6,266	27.7	34.5	12.9	17.1	25.2	9.6	12.9	16.3	9,444
St Petersburg	5,632	29.2	44.2	18.4	21.0	26.1	11.6	12.2	17.1	10,199
Tallahassee	6,184	24.9	26.2	7.9	10.8	20.3	10.0	7.8	7.7	8,461
Tampa	7,246	31.8	40.8	18.2	20.9	32.7	14.3	15.2	25.7	10,273
Georgia										
Albany	1,743	38.5	29.4	7.6	17.8	21.7	10.1	9.4	15.9	10,445
Atlanta	28,912	36.5	32.0	10.4	17.7	22.3	8.9	11.0	14.7	10,310
Augusta	5,360	34.8	26.9	10.2	15.6	18.0	8.4	7.9	6.0	9,612
Columbus	2,853	38.3	31.5	9.8	19.2	18.2	8.9	7.4	9.2	9,093
Macon	6,155	36.4	29.7	9.0	16.4	18.3	8.7	7.6	6.1	9,889
Rome	2,522	35.5	34.0	11.3	18.7	19.3	10.2	6.6	13.0	10,014

Hospital Referral Region	Medicare Deaths (1995 plus 1996)	Percent of Medicare Deaths Occurring in Hospitals (1995-96)	Percent of Medicare Enrollees Admitted to Intensive Care During the Last Six Months of Life (1995-96)	Percent of Medicare Enrollees Spending Seven or More Days in Intensive Care During the Last Six Months of Life (1995-96)	Percent of Medicare Enrollees Admitted to Intensive Care During the Terminal Hospitalization (1995-96)	Physician Visits per Decedent During the Last Six Months of Life (1995-96)	Primary Care Physician Visits per Decedent During the Last Six Months of Life (1995-96)	Medical Specialist Visits per Decedent During the Last Six Months of Life (1995-96)	Percent of Medicare Enrollees Seeing Ten or More Physicians During the Last Six Months of Life (1995-96)	Price-Adjusted Reimb. for Inpatient Care During the Last Six Months of Life per Decedent (1995-96)
Savannah	5,729	36.1	31.4	10.9	16.5	23.6	10.1	10.5	11.2	10,479
Hawaii										
Honolulu	5,471	34.2	23.5	6.8	15.7	24.3	14.9	7.7	11.5	10,804
Idaho										
Boise	5,190	23.3	23.4	5.0	11.5	12.9	6.6	4.9	6.3	6,848
Idaho Falls	1,211	23.5	24.9	9.1	12.7	12.2	6.4	4.7	4.1	9,262
Illinois										
Aurora	1,418	29.6	29.2	10.1	14.2	20.1	8.4	9.5	15.6	8,025
Bloomington	1,489	27.8	15.2	3.6	8.4	15.9	8.2	5.6	1.3	8,958
Blue Island	7,806	33.3	36.0	13.1	17.8	30.8	13.3	15.2	23.7	11,257
Chicago	20,273	35.4	40.5	16.9	21.7	33.0	16.2	13.9	20.5	13,580
Elgin	3,534	30.7	40.9	15.2	19.3	24.8	10.9	10.5	18.6	10,255
Evanston	7,678	29.1	34.7	10.9	16.6	28.1	13.8	11.6	17.7	10,437
Hinsdale	2,484	27.1	33.6	12.0	15.3	27.6	14.1	11.2	17.3	9,871
Joliet	4,003	34.0	34.6	11.1	17.1	31.6	12.6	15.3	18.7	10,991
Melrose Park	10,372	30.4	34.8	13.1	17.7	26.2	12.1	11.6	16.4	10,650
Peoria	7,522	29.7	24.9	6.1	14.5	20.8	10.2	7.9	7.0	9,417
Rockford	6,544	30.2	29.2	9.5	14.7	19.2	10.0	6.6	9.3	8,788
Springfield	10,387	31.3	26.9	8.5	13.9	18.9	11.2	5.3	5.7	9,375
Urbana	4,580	31.6	27.1	8.9	14.8	20.1	11.2	6.6	7.3	9,148
Indiana										
Evansville	8,098	30.9	31.9	10.1	15.6	18.1	10.9	5.7	7.9	8,390
Fort Wayne	7,542	27.5	32.0	9.9	16.6	18.1	8.5	7.8	14.9	7,458
Gary	4,627	37.4	34.2	15.0	18.9	33.6	14.6	16.7	21.4	11,574
Indianapolis	23,865	30.3	30.3	10.2	15.9	19.8	9.1	9.2	14.9	8,943
Lafayette	1,874	30.1	25.3	9.2	13.3	15.9	7.1	7.0	9.8	8,162
Muncie	1,845	33.8	35.1	13.2	18.3	19.3	8.0	10.1	6.0	9,917
Munster	3,202	39.2	48.7	25.5	26.3	27.1	12.5	12.4	15.2	11,708
South Bend	6,505	27.6	27.1	7.8	13.6	17.2	9.3	6.3	10.0	7,659
Terre Haute	2,388	34.6	39.4	18.5	20.3	22.8	9.1	12.1	12.0	10,020
Iowa										
Cedar Rapids	2,566	27.2	22.5	7.6	13.1	19.2	7.6	10.1	5.2	7,083
Davenport	5,452	31.8	29.1	8.3	16.1	21.3	10.5	8.6	9.4	8,786
Des Moines	10,987	30.3	27.5	8.1	14.7	20.0	10.5	7.6	14.8	8,686
Dubuque	1,651	24.3	21.7	5.8	9.9	12.2	6.4	4.1	2.7	6,648
Iowa City	3,308	32.8	23.2	4.6	13.6	18.8	12.9	4.1	6.3	9,050
Mason City	2,005	19.7	16.9	3.4	8.6	11.0	7.4	2.0	5.8	7,343
Sioux City	3,138	28.2	30.3	9.5	15.3	15.0	9.6	3.7	4.1	7,969
Waterloo	2,391	26.2	24.8	3.9	13.3	13.8	8.4	3.8	6.4	7,638
Kansas										
Topeka	4,548	26.5	17.6	3.8	9.9	19.2	9.4	7.8	6.3	7,931
Wichita	13,694	31.7	25.7	6.7	15.0	21.1	11.4	6.9	9.9	9,790
Kentucky										
Covington	3,120	29.0	33.7	11.5	15.6	24.6	12.2	10.2	24.4	8,756
Lexington	12,855	36.6	29.1	9.2	16.2	22.6	12.8	7.7	10.0	10,151
Louisville	15,409	33.2	31.5	12.1	16.8	25.8	12.9	10.6	15.3	9,879

Hospital Referral Region	Medicare Deaths (1995 plus 1996)	Percent of Medicare Deaths Occurring in Hospitals (1995-96)	Percent of Medicare Enrollees Admitted to Intensive Care During the Last Six Months of Life (1995-96)	Percent of Medicare Enrollees Spending Seven or More Days in Intensive Care During the Last Six Months of Life (1995-96)	Percent of Medicare Enrollees Admitted to Intensive Care During the Terminal Hospitalization (1995-96)	Physician Visits per Decedent During the Last Six Months of Life (1995-96)	Primary Care Physician Visits per Decedent During the Last Six Months of Life (1995-96)	Medical Specialist Visits per Decedent During the Last Six Months of Life (1995-96)	Percent of Medicare Enrollees Seeing Ten or More Physicians During the Last Six Months of Life (1995-96)	Price Adjusted Reimb. for Inpatient Care During the Last Six Months of Life per Decedent (1995-96)
Owensboro	1,454	35.1	33.2	11.3	18.8	21.4	9.2	10.3	7.5	9,396
Paducah	4,536	36.0	33.4	11.3	17.8	22.0	12.0	7.2	8.4	9,960
Louisiana										
Alexandria	2,911	36.5	27.5	7.8	14.5	24.7	11.7	9.8	12.1	10,711
Baton Rouge	5,396	37.2	36.1	14.8	18.5	24.6	13.0	9.0	18.7	10,009
Houma	1,756	37.5	29.1	10.8	16.4	23.2	10.7	9.8	13.3	11,324
Lafayette	4,673	32.6	32.1	11.2	15.4	20.2	10.4	7.2	7.4	11,184
Lake Charles	2,104	41.1	27.0	8.1	16.5	30.1	16.8	10.9	22.2	11,793
Metairie	3,288	35.1	31.6	11.9	16.9	30.3	11.8	14.5	22.3	11,857
Monroe	3,071	36.8	37.8	16.4	17.2	28.7	14.9	10.1	13.8	10,773
New Orleans	6,950	30.4	32.8	12.6	16.4	30.8	11.9	15.1	24.4	10,942
Shreveport	7,046	38.0	31.3	10.3	17.9	23.0	11.6	8.5	11.0	11,222
Slidell	1,276	35.7	33.6	11.4	17.7	24.3	9.5	12.4	11.3	13,252
Maine										
Bangor	4,383	33.0	26.7	8.9	13.8	19.5	11.9	5.8	6.3	8,844
Portland	10,039	30.3	23.1	5.4	12.6	17.6	9.6	6.2	9.7	8,110
Maryland										
Baltimore	21,938	33.9	30.1	10.4	14.9	24.9	13.3	8.7	22.1	11,768
Salisbury	4,073	31.9	25.4	8.3	14.0	26.5	11.0	12.9	21.1	9,473
Takoma Park	4,787	32.2	33.2	14.4	16.3	35.9	11.2	21.5	31.9	12,364
Massachusetts										
Boston	42,841	32.6	28.1	8.4	15.9	25.3	12.9	9.0	20.8	10,369
Springfield	7,853	30.9	22.5	5.9	12.9	20.3	11.3	5.7	13.9	9,053
Worcester	6,023	32.9	26.9	6.9	16.1	21.2	12.3	6.3	19.0	11,128
Michigan										
Ann Arbor	10,526	32.0	37.1	13.3	19.4	25.9	15.4	8.4	24.1	10,214
Dearborn	5,508	36.5	42.6	17.3	22.1	33.2	18.1	12.0	31.3	11,568
Detroit	19,016	35.4	34.1	14.5	19.0	30.8	16.5	11.3	27.2	11,842
Flint	4,771	37.3	36.0	13.9	21.8	28.0	13.9	12.0	23.0	10,692
Grand Rapids	8,721	23.9	28.4	8.0	13.7	17.8	11.2	4.4	11.1	7,451
Kalamazoo	6,176	30.3	27.7	8.2	16.1	18.5	10.0	6.3	13.2	8,866
Lansing	5,241	31.3	27.7	7.6	16.0	20.6	11.2	6.8	13.4	9,078
Marquette	2,575	27.1	24.8	5.0	13.3	17.6	12.8	3.4	9.8	8,312
Muskegon	2,665	26.9	24.0	5.3	12.5	16.4	11.3	3.1	14.8	7,332
Petoskey	1,765	27.7	28.3	8.6	14.4	20.0	12.7	5.4	12.2	8,116
Pontiac	3,035	32.1	30.3	9.7	16.0	30.4	16.9	10.9	22.0	11,106
Royal Oak	6,054	35.1	30.1	10.0	17.3	33.9	16.2	13.9	30.0	11,385
Saginaw	7,066	31.5	33.0	11.9	18.1	21.5	12.2	7.2	14.2	8,618
St Joseph	1,529	29.8	27.7	7.4	15.6	19.9	14.5	3.0	8.7	8,579
Traverse City	2,299	26.0	26.9	8.6	13.3	18.9	11.2	5.8	10.4	8,630
Minnesota										
Duluth	4,292	28.4	26.3	7.5	13.4	11.6	6.5	4.0	5.8	7,477
Minneapolis	21,628	24.2	22.8	5.3	11.3	12.9	7.7	3.8	8.7	7,775
Rochester	4,164	24.7	25.8	6.2	12.3	13.7	8.6	3.7	13.6	8,410
St Cloud	1,882	23.0	25.3	6.0	12.0	19.3	10.3	7.3	12.9	7,333
St Paul	5,973	23.2	28.7	7.9	13.4	14.8	8.0	5.5	14.7	8,106

Hospital Referral Region	Medicare Deaths (1995 plus 1996)	Percent of Medicare Deaths Occurring in Hospitals (1995-96)	Percent of Medicare Enrollees Admitted to Intensive Care During the Last Six Months of Life (1995-96)	Percent of Medicare Enrollees Spending Seven or More Days in Intensive Care During the Last Six Months of Life (1995-96)	Percent of Medicare Enrollees Admitted to Intensive Care During the Terminal Hospitalization (1995-96)	Physician Visits per Decedent During the Last Six Months of Life (1995-96)	Primary Care Physician Visits per Decedent During the Last Six Months of Life (1995-96)	Medical Specialist Visits per Decedent During the Last Six Months of Life (1995-96)	Percent of Medicare Enrollees Seeing Ten or More Physicians During the Last Six Months of Life (1995-96)	Price Adjusted Reimb. for Inpatient Care During the Last Six Months of Life per Decedent (1995-96)
Mississippi										
Gulfport	1,616	39.3	37.9	16.3	19.2	36.2	19.0	14.9	16.5	12,868
Hattiesburg	2,665	46.9	27.2	8.1	17.7	26.3	11.5	12.8	19.1	10,676
Jackson	10,283	41.1	27.1	10.4	15.5	23.6	14.0	7.5	9.6	9,522
Meridian	2,120	43.7	26.9	7.4	16.3	26.6	11.9	12.9	10.3	10,342
Oxford	1,477	45.6	26.7	10.6	16.9	25.0	11.9	8.3	8.5	10,081
Tupelo	3,691	44.7	31.5	12.2	17.8	24.1	14.0	7.3	13.0	9,522
Missouri										
Cape Girardeau	3,349	31.3	33.6	12.3	16.7	17.1	10.4	4.7	4.1	8,796
Columbia	7,188	32.2	31.7	10.4	16.4	24.6	12.9	9.3	12.3	11,150
Joplin	4,501	34.1	28.4	6.4	15.9	19.8	13.1	4.6	7.0	9,681
Kansas City	19,734	31.0	34.0	12.0	17.4	23.6	12.2	9.3	15.6	9,461
Springfield	8,545	30.1	27.6	6.5	15.8	19.0	10.6	6.2	9.9	8,616
St Louis	33,647	31.7	33.4	11.9	17.3	22.0	12.8	6.7	11.1	10,025
Montana										
Billings	4,652	24.8	21.0	4.3	10.7	14.7	8.8	4.8	7.5	7,671
Great Falls	1,556	28.6	26.8	8.5	14.0	16.2	6.5	7.8	7.1	8,885
Missoula	3,181	24.8	22.5	6.0	11.2	15.2	8.0	6.0	6.7	7,873
Nebraska										
Lincoln	6,123	24.0	20.6	5.4	10.6	14.5	8.3	4.9	5.7	7,293
Omaha	12,055	28.7	29.1	9.2	15.3	22.4	11.5	8.8	12.4	9,485
Nevada										
Las Vegas	6,415	32.6	34.7	16.7	18.7	27.6	9.7	15.3	26.6	10,152
Reno	4,587	28.6	24.4	7.4	13.4	17.2	7.5	7.7	17.0	8,285
New Hampshire										
Lebanon	4,198	30.2	21.9	5.1	12.9	14.3	9.7	2.6	9.6	8,547
Manchester	6,713	29.2	22.7	5.8	13.3	15.4	8.0	5.2	7.9	7,294
New Jersey										
Camden	27,881	42.3	35.9	14.9	20.7	33.8	14.0	16.7	28.8	11,177
Hackensack	11,080	43.8	32.6	12.3	20.9	34.8	14.2	17.3	16.2	11,091
Morristown	7,879	37.5	31.6	11.3	19.2	33.8	15.9	15.6	22.8	9,021
New Brunswick	7,015	43.3	40.3	18.9	25.1	42.4	15.9	22.5	24.2	11,116
Newark	13,648	49.0	43.9	19.9	29.0	45.5	18.5	23.8	26.3	11,674
Paterson	3,469	42.7	32.9	11.8	20.9	42.2	16.9	21.9	18.1	9,866
Ridgewood	3,298	41.8	29.6	10.5	18.2	43.0	18.3	21.0	30.7	10,698
New Mexico										
Albuquerque	8,076	26.5	26.6	8.1	13.2	16.2	9.1	5.0	10.1	7,987
New York										
Albany	19,044	33.8	26.4	8.1	15.5	26.2	12.0	11.5	21.0	8,266
Binghamton	4,173	33.9	25.1	5.6	15.3	20.8	11.4	7.5	15.2	7,466
Bronx	8,609	46.3	26.9	11.3	17.1	34.7	16.3	14.0	29.5	16,499
Buffalo	16,478	40.0	28.8	9.5	18.9	24.1	13.7	7.8	13.1	9,226
Elmira	4,322	37.9	28.9	8.7	17.2	23.4	13.8	7.7	14.4	8,262
East Long Island	36,238	47.6	30.6	12.1	20.4	40.0	18.1	18.3	29.1	12,835
New York	35,164	48.4	30.5	13.6	20.8	39.4	17.1	18.0	31.4	17,797
Rochester	11,435	32.3	25.7	7.3	15.4	18.5	12.5	4.6	10.7	8,723

Hospital Referral Region	Medicare Deaths (1995 plus 1996)	Percent of Medicare Deaths Occurring in Hospitals (1995-96)	Percent of Medicare Enrollees Admitted to Intensive Care During the Last Six Months of Life (1995-96)	Percent of Medicare Enrollees Spending Seven or More Days in Intensive Care During the Last Six Months of Life (1995-96)	Percent of Medicare Enrollees Admitted to Intensive Care During the Terminal Hospitalization (1995-96)	Physician Visits per Decedent During the Last Six Months of Life (1995-96)	Primary Care Physician Visits per Decedent During the Last Six Months of Life (1995-96)	Medical Specialist Visits per Decedent During the Last Six Months of Life (1995-96)	Percent of Medicare Enrollees Seeing Ten or More Physicians During the Last Six Months of Life (1995-96)	Price Adjusted Reimb. for Inpatient Care During the Last Six Months of Life per Decedent (1995-96)
Syracuse	10,446	33.7	26.2	8.0	15.8	22.1	11.2	8.3	14.8	7,708
White Plains	9,484	40.1	30.0	11.3	17.3	33.7	16.8	13.8	19.6	10,754
North Carolina										
Asheville	6,971	30.4	28.0	8.3	15.4	17.6	10.9	4.9	12.1	8,180
Charlotte	15,483	35.9	33.9	13.2	19.9	20.7	12.6	6.1	15.1	9,415
Durham	11,496	34.3	29.7	9.7	17.4	18.9	9.3	7.2	11.6	9,778
Greensboro	4,861	34.2	31.5	12.8	18.7	18.4	10.0	6.0	9.1	8,338
Greenville	6,876	36.1	33.0	12.0	17.7	19.5	11.7	5.9	12.3	9,953
Hickory	2,389	33.0	33.8	12.2	19.0	19.6	12.2	6.0	9.2	9,893
Raleigh	10,802	39.1	32.1	11.5	18.4	20.6	11.3	7.2	11.5	9,751
Wilmington	3,231	34.9	30.1	8.7	17.5	20.0	10.3	7.0	14.9	9,419
Winston-Salem	9,742	35.7	32.2	11.2	18.8	21.1	11.0	7.9	12.2	9,916
North Dakota										
Bismarck	2,198	27.9	21.7	4.1	11.4	18.8	10.5	6.1	6.0	8,936
Fargo Moorhead -Mn	5,626	25.6	22.1	4.9	12.0	14.7	8.4	4.8	9.8	8,231
Grand Forks	2,006	28.7	21.0	4.2	11.9	16.6	11.1	4.0	7.6	8,764
Minot	1,519	25.2	23.5	6.1	12.7	16.5	8.4	4.4	6.6	9,225
Ohio										
Akron	7,034	33.8	35.3	13.1	18.5	27.3	13.1	11.9	17.8	11,432
Canton	6,769	32.5	36.0	14.9	19.9	22.0	11.7	8.5	13.3	8,906
Cincinnati	15,311	27.5	26.4	7.4	14.0	20.9	9.8	8.4	14.2	8,955
Cleveland	22,387	31.9	37.2	13.7	18.9	24.1	10.0	11.2	20.0	10,493
Columbus	25,503	30.6	32.9	11.6	16.8	20.2	11.0	7.0	13.9	9,589
Dayton	11,487	27.3	30.1	12.0	16.1	20.5	9.9	8.7	12.6	9,211
Elyria	2,292	28.0	40.6	17.9	18.4	23.5	9.6	12.5	13.0	7,878
Kettering	3,604	28.8	31.0	11.2	17.1	24.9	11.9	11.3	14.7	9,500
Toledo	10,143	31.0	36.2	13.6	18.6	26.7	12.4	11.4	21.5	10,979
Youngstown	8,846	35.3	38.3	15.1	19.9	29.3	15.3	10.9	19.1	11,384
Oklahoma										
Lawton	2,064	28.2	26.9	6.8	12.9	18.2	9.2	6.4	10.3	9,356
Oklahoma City	17,119	34.8	27.7	7.7	15.8	20.9	10.7	8.1	9.3	9,407
Tulsa	11,986	31.6	25.9	7.0	14.7	21.8	11.1	8.9	12.0	8,733
Oregon										
Bend	1,414	17.2	16.6	3.1	6.3	12.2	5.9	4.6	4.8	6,198
Eugene	6,131	21.7	18.4	2.9	9.4	11.3	6.9	3.4	4.9	7,040
Medford	4,558	22.0	20.8	4.6	10.4	11.9	6.6	3.9	5.4	7,002
Portland	12,979	22.1	21.9	4.3	11.3	12.3	6.9	3.7	5.7	7,285
Salem	2,206	24.1	29.0	9.2	14.4	11.0	4.8	5.1	3.0	6,602
Pennsylvania										
Allentown	11,701	36.2	32.1	11.0	18.1	31.2	13.9	13.9	27.1	10,185
Altoona	3,655	37.7	33.3	10.6	19.4	21.4	11.7	7.1	10.2	10,086
Danville	5,718	30.4	25.6	6.7	13.4	21.6	11.8	7.6	12.2	8,199
Erie	8,890	32.5	28.9	8.5	15.9	25.2	14.0	8.1	11.9	8,829
Harrisburg	9,939	31.8	29.3	8.7	16.3	22.8	12.0	7.8	20.0	9,100
Johnstown	3,302	41.5	32.5	9.5	18.9	21.1	12.5	6.9	13.9	11,912
Lancaster	5,343	25.6	29.9	9.5	15.3	24.4	9.8	12.2	24.6	7,417

Hospital Referral Region	Medicare Deaths (1995 plus 1996)	Percent of Medicare Deaths Occurring in Hospitals (1995-96)	Percent of Medicare Enrollees Admitted to Intensive Care During the Last Six Months of Life (1995-96)	Percent of Medicare Enrollees Spending Seven or More Days in Intensive Care During the Last Six Months of Life (1995-96)	Percent of Medicare Enrollees Admitted to Intensive Care During the Terminal Hospitalization (1995-96)	Physician Visits per Decedent During the Last Six Months of Life (1995-96)	Primary Care Physician Visits per Decedent During the Last Six Months of Life	Medical Specialist Visits per Decedent During the Last Six Months of Life (1995-96)	Percent of Medicare Enrollees Seeing Ten or More Physicians During the Last Six Months of Life (1995-96)	Price Adjusted Reimb. for Inpatient Care During the Last Six Months of Life per Decedent (1995-96)
Philadelphia	37,907	35.8	38.1	15.3	20.5	36.2	13.4	19.3	33.9	12,478
Pittsburgh	39,652	36.2	35.3	12.1	19.0	30.0	13.4	13.3	24.0	11,576
Reading	6,510	34.0	28.0	7.5	15.9	23.3	12.7	7.7	19.4	8,478
Sayre	2,235	34.7	25.4	5.6	15.1	18.8	11.4	5.7	10.1	8,634
Scranton	4,510	36.1	25.6	6.9	14.9	33.3	15.9	13.9	22.6	9,661
Wilkes-Barre	3,827	31.7	29.7	8.4	15.4	28.9	16.7	10.7	20.1	8,246
York	3,843	27.5	31.8	10.5	16.3	19.6	11.4	6.1	11.6	8,365
Rhode Island										
Providence	11,731	32.4	24.7	7.5	14.5	23.1	10.9	9.3	21.5	9,789
South Carolina										
Charleston	6,088	35.2	31.7	13.2	18.5	22.6	11.1	9.4	15.1	10,526
Columbia	8,890	34.9	29.1	11.1	17.4	20.8	9.9	8.4	10.7	8,739
Florence	3,381	34.0	32.0	12.1	16.0	23.6	13.5	7.9	15.7	10,577
Greenville	6,993	36.2	30.5	11.2	18.4	20.5	10.2	8.0	13.0	9,542
Spartanburg	3,537	39.7	37.2	16.3	21.7	21.9	11.2	8.6	10.6	8,599
South Dakota										
Rapid City	1,675	26.1	23.2	7.2	11.7	17.3	9.3	6.2	9.6	8,079
Sioux Falls	8,614	27.6	24.2	6.1	13.0	15.1	9.3	4.2	7.2	8,347
Tennessee										
Chattanooga	6,097	36.5	35.2	12.2	18.9	21.0	10.1	8.7	12.3	10,282
Jackson	3,953	39.7	36.0	16.7	20.2	25.4	14.3	8.5	11.1	10,227
Johnson City	2,526	34.9	31.0	10.8	17.7	21.4	11.8	6.7	13.9	10,434
Kingsport	5,565	40.8	36.1	14.5	19.2	19.4	13.0	4.8	11.3	10,370
Knoxville	12,509	39.9	33.3	12.1	18.9	24.8	12.1	9.8	17.5	10,198
Memphis	16,383	39.9	30.9	12.6	18.7	30.0	13.7	13.4	16.1	10,696
Nashville	20,165	35.4	33.6	12.1	18.0	21.2	11.0	7.8	11.1	10,504
Texas										
Abilene	3,646	35.1	30.0	8.1	15.8	19.5	9.3	7.9	7.7	10,045
Amarillo	4,300	22.0	30.8	10.4	12.2	20.7	10.3	8.4	8.3	9,312
Austin	5,841	30.3	25.3	6.5	13.7	21.3	9.0	10.2	12.7	8,277
Beaumont	4,814	39.8	43.9	21.6	22.3	31.6	14.8	14.9	18.6	11,814
Bryan	1,528	28.5	26.0	8.6	12.3	18.4	11.1	4.7	11.3	8,800
Corpus Christi	3,952	37.8	35.5	11.4	20.5	25.2	13.3	9.7	15.4	11,382
Dallas	23,471	31.1	30.7	9.8	16.4	24.3	10.3	11.9	14.5	9,401
El Paso	5,485	32.6	38.1	17.0	20.2	23.4	10.0	11.3	16.7	11,971
Fort Worth	10,671	28.3	32.9	10.9	16.0	20.4	9.3	9.4	11.6	8,852
Harlingen	2,742	43.2	42.6	19.5	25.6	32.1	15.4	13.6	30.0	16,938
Houston	27,223	31.5	37.8	14.4	18.9	29.4	12.1	14.8	17.8	11,682
Longview	1,898	35.0	40.8	17.3	21.8	26.5	10.3	13.6	15.4	10,440
Lubbock	5,977	37.5	37.9	16.5	20.7	25.1	9.9	12.9	14.1	11,241
McAllen	2,114	45.3	40.7	19.0	25.3	36.6	13.1	20.4	28.9	16,504
Odessa	2,540	37.4	39.8	18.4	22.3	23.7	14.8	6.8	11.7	11,154
San Angelo	1,805	29.5	30.6	11.2	15.2	21.3	12.2	6.4	9.8	8,408
San Antonio	13,237	31.8	34.7	13.8	18.6	24.5	11.4	11.1	16.0	10,176
Temple	2,591	29.2	25.1	5.1	12.8	15.7	8.8	5.4	10.5	9,748
Tyler	5,826	35.2	30.8	9.6	16.9	19.8	10.8	6.8	8.6	9,969

Hospital Referral Region	Medicare Deaths (1995 plus 1996)	Percent of Medicare Deaths Occurring in Hospitals (1995-96)	Percent of Medicare Enrollees Admitted to Intensive Care During the Last Six Months of Life (1995-96)	Percent of Medicare Enrollees Spending Seven or More Days in Intensive Care During the Last Six Months of Life (1995-96)	Percent of Medicare Enrollees Admitted to Intensive Care During the Terminal Hospitalization (1995-96)	Physician Visits per Decedent During the Last Six Months of Life (1995-96)	Primary Care Physician Visits per Decedent During the Last Six Months of Life (1995-96)	Medical Specialist Visits per Decedent During the Last Six Months of Life (1995-96)	Percent of Medicare Enrollees Seeing Ten or More Physicians During the Last Six Months of Life (1995-96)	Price Adjusted Reimb. for Inpatient Care During the Last Six Months of Life per Decedent (1995-96)
Victoria	1,523	40.3	30.1	7.0	18.1	25.2	13.7	9.2	11.0	10,579
Waco	3,548	27.1	23.4	5.4	12.4	13.8	8.2	4.0	6.2	7,916
Wichita Falls	2,431	34.1	27.5	9.0	14.7	22.3	9.7	10.1	6.0	8,276
Utah										
Ogden	1,944	19.6	22.6	5.1	11.8	8.6	4.5	2.6	2.2	6,806
Provo	1,891	25.6	23.2	6.9	13.7	13.1	6.0	6.0	6.3	7,967
Salt Lake City	9,500	22.5	20.6	4.1	10.8	10.9	6.0	3.6	4.2	6,970
Vermont										
Burlington	5,402	32.2	26.5	7.1	14.8	18.4	11.7	4.5	10.6	8,167
Virginia										
Arlington	7,581	27.4	27.9	9.0	15.1	26.9	9.8	14.9	23.1	7,864
Charlottesville	4,603	31.4	29.1	9.8	15.0	19.4	10.2	7.0	11.5	9,154
Lynchburg	2,530	32.1	34.8	12.7	17.4	15.7	8.1	6.3	6.5	7,194
Newport News	3,819	35.3	36.6	14.8	20.9	31.8	12.1	17.2	22.8	8,294
Norfolk	8,905	38.1	35.5	15.3	20.1	25.0	13.4	8.9	22.1	8,968
Richmond	12,625	36.5	30.1	11.7	16.6	23.3	10.7	10.2	16.0	8,877
Roanoke	7,879	36.0	30.8	10.1	17.0	20.5	10.1	8.6	10.3	9,126
Winchester	3,140	33.8	24.3	6.6	13.0	22.3	12.8	7.8	12.3	8,194
Washington										
Everett	3,093	21.7	21.3	4.7	10.0	14.3	7.7	5.1	6.2	7,249
Olympia	2,619	22.5	27.3	5.8	11.8	14.7	7.1	5.4	3.3	7,844
Seattle	15,477	24.0	25.9	6.5	13.2	15.6	6.7	7.4	9.2	7,909
Spokane	10,944	24.5	22.9	6.1	11.7	14.7	8.3	5.1	8.5	7,792
Tacoma	4,617	23.9	29.2	7.3	14.4	14.6	6.8	6.4	11.2	7,768
Yakima	2,188	24.9	25.4	6.3	12.8	14.4	7.9	4.7	3.9	7,773
West Virginia										
Charleston	10,666	39.0	31.0	11.2	17.3	21.6	11.0	7.9	14.3	10,904
Huntington	4,285	36.7	24.8	7.3	14.7	24.0	11.7	10.5	12.3	10,548
Morgantown	4,692	34.3	37.5	15.5	19.1	20.4	11.3	6.8	13.0	10,858
Wisconsin										
Appleton	2,975	23.7	21.3	4.5	11.4	15.0	9.0	4.5	8.3	6,346
Green Bay	5,034	28.7	24.1	4.8	13.0	15.5	9.3	4.9	9.2	6,976
La Crosse	3,809	23.0	22.3	4.4	11.1	15.3	10.4	3.0	10.2	7,309
Madison	8,639	25.8	23.9	5.7	12.5	14.3	8.6	4.2	7.1	7,813
Marshfield	3,966	28.7	22.0	4.4	12.7	16.4	8.3	6.5	12.0	7,997
Milwaukee	22,632	29.9	27.6	8.6	14.7	21.0	10.2	8.6	14.3	8,776
Neenah	2,344	23.9	18.5	4.1	9.6	15.7	9.9	4.3	7.3	7,345
Wausau	1,986	22.9	16.9	3.7	9.3	13.9	8.7	3.6	3.7	7,117
Wyoming										
Casper	1,650	27.7	24.9	6.0	12.3	15.7	10.5	3.7	2.3	8,815
United States										
	2,278,277	33.0	31.4	11.0	16.9	24.4	11.5	10.3	16.1	9,943

The Quality of Medical Care in the United States

Overuse, Underuse, and Misuse of Care

There is extensive evidence in support of the National Roundtable on Health Care Quality's conclusions about the quality of care in the United States: "Serious and widespread quality problems exist throughout American medicine." In this chapter, "best practices" benchmarks are used to measure the extent of underuse, overuse and misuse of medical care.

■ The patterns of practice of preventive services, including care known to prevent heart attacks and complications of diabetes are evaluated using guidelines drawn from evidence-based assessments of optimal practice and benchmarks from managed care plans.

■ Overuse of discretionary surgery is evaluated by using benchmarks from health plans where the rates of surgery reflect the demand of patients who were fully informed about their treatment options and encouraged to choose according their own preferences.

■ Overuse of hospitals in the treatment of patients with medical conditions and in the intensity of care provided in the last six months of life is evaluated using benchmark regions selected because of the apparent efficiency of their patterns of practice.

The Roundtable defined misuse of care as the occurrence of a preventable complication. Although egregious medical error speaks for itself — and demands immediate rectification — variations in treatment outcomes such as mortality following surgery often occur for unknown reasons. Fixing "errors" related to variations in surgical mortality requires a concerted effort to understand and improve the processes of care. This can only be accomplished if the necessary infrastructure is in place and a proper learning environment is established. Chapter Five reports on one such project to improve the outcomes of cardiac surgery in northern New England.

The Atlas extends the definition of misuse to include inefficiency in the allocation of medical resources. Benchmarks for efficient allocation of medical resources, selected from among the 306 hospital referral regions, are used to estimate the possible costs of poor quality in the allocation resources. When value is considered in terms of benefit gained per dollar spent, it is hard to find evidence that more resources are required to improve the quality of care in fee-for-service Medicare. We find, instead, evidence of large scale waste and inefficiency in the delivery system; scarcity, where it exists, is most likely to result from the misallocation of resources. Improving the overall quality of care in the Medicare program cannot be achieved by spending more; the task is to improve the quality of clinical science, the quality of clinical decision making, and the quality of resource allocation.

Underuse of Effective Medical Care

Underuse represents a failure to provide diagnostic tests, preventive services and treatments that are proven effective in improving health status. The 1999 edition of the Atlas and related studies confirm several of the findings of underuse cited in the Roundtable's report. Among hospital referral regions, there are striking variations in Medicare enrollees' use of:

■ Immunizations of demonstrated efficacy in preventing pneumonia (Chapter Four);
■ Tests and drugs widely believed to reduce complications in patients with diabetes (Chapter Four);
■ Treatments proven effective in lowering mortality rates of patients with heart attacks (below).

For services such as these, there can be little debate over the question, Which rate is right? The interventions are known to be effective, and the benefits far exceed associated risks. Moreover, Medicare enrollees want these benefits. The right rate — the "best practices" benchmark — is the rate when all eligible patients are provided with appropriate care. In actual practice, there is evidence of extensive waste of the opportunity to prevent serious illness (Figures 7.1 and 7.2).

Why is there underuse of services that work — and that patients want — in a nation so amply endowed with medical resources? Underuse cannot be explained by an inadequate supply of either primary care physicians or specialists, because underservice is prevalent in hospital referral regions with both high and low supplies of all these resources. Nor is underuse related to access to physicians or the continuity of ambulatory care (Chapter Four). If undersupply is not the cause of underuse, then spending more is not the cure for the problem (Figure 7.4). There is little consistency in the quality of performance; regions that approach the standard for "best practice" for one preventive service commonly do notably poorly in other measures. Performance seems to vary in an idiosyncratic way, reflecting local physicians' opinions and practice styles (Figure 4.9). The extent of underuse, and the haphazard nature of compliance with recommended guidelines, indicate there is substantial opportunity to improve the quality of care by improving the process by which preventive and therapeutic services are delivered.

Measuring the Underuse of Preventive Care

Screening for Breast Cancer. The United States Task Force on Preventive Disease guidelines recommend mammograms at least once every two years for Medicare women age 65-69. In 1995-96, only 28.3% of women in this age group received at least one mammogram; compliance with the guideline for women between 65 and 69 varied from a low of 12% to a high of 50% (Figure 4.2). No hospital referral regions came close to the "best practice" benchmark provided by Kaiser-Permanente South, a California health maintenance organization, in which 82% of Medicare seniors received breast cancer screening (Figure 7.1). If 82% is the benchmark of achievable quality, there is extensive underuse of mammography in the rest of the United States: in 1995-96, 2.25 million, or 65% of eligible Medicare enrollees, did not have the mammograms they would have received had the quality of their care equaled that provided by the Kaiser Permanente Health Plan.

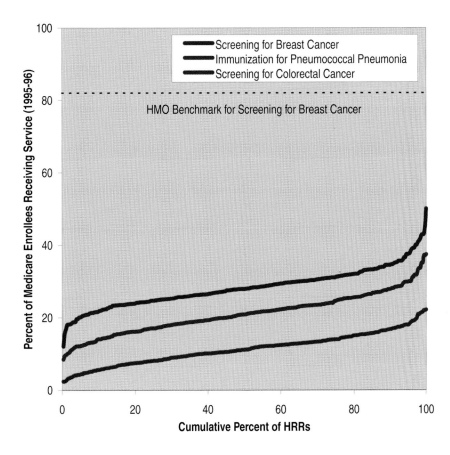

Figure 7.1. The Use of Selected Preventive Services by Medicare Enrollees by Hospital Referral Regions (1995-96)

The vertical axis shows the percent of Medicare enrollees receiving one or more of the selected preventive services in 1995-96. The horizontal axis is the cumulative percent of hospital referral regions, ranked from lowest (left) to highest in percent compliance with guideline. The figure also indicates the "best practice" benchmark for screening for breast cancer. All hospital referral regions fell well below the benchmark.

Immunization against Pneumococcal Pneumonia. To meet the minimal expectation for protection, the United States Task Force guidelines call for vaccination at least once every ten years, meaning that over the two year period 1995-96 at least 20%, or 5.8 million Medicare enrollees in fee-for-service Medicare, should have been vaccinated. Using this standard implies massive underservice: in 1995-96, only 21% of the 5.8 million Americans enrolled in fee-for-service Medicare received one or more vaccinations. Compliance with the guideline for vaccination varied from 9% of those who were eligible to 38% (Figure 4.1). We found no audited reports from health maintenance organizations to use as a "best practice" benchmark.

Screening for Colorectal Cancer. The United States Task Force calls for annual colorectal cancer screening by either fecal occult blood test or colonoscopy, or both. During 1995-96, years when Medicare did not pay for screening for colorectal cancer, only 12% of the 29.4 million Americans enrolled in fee-for-service Medicare had one or more colonoscopy or occult blood test. The percent of enrollees receiving screening ranged from 2% to 22% (Figure 4.3). We found no audited reports from health maintenance organizations to use as a "best practice" benchmark.

Measuring the Underuse of Care for Diabetic Patients

Eye Examinations. The Diabetes Quality Improvement Project recommends annual retinal eye examinations for diabetics. In 1995-96, 45.3% of the 3.1 million Medicare enrollees who were diagnosed diabetics received one or more eye examinations. According to this recommendation, 1.7 million Medicare patients with diabetes were underserved: compliance with the guideline ranged from 25% to 66%. No hospital referral region came close to the "best practice" benchmark provided by Kaiser-Permanente North, a California health maintenance organization (Figure 7.2), in which 69% of Medicare diabetics received at least one eye examination. Using 69% as the benchmark of achievable quality, there is evidence of extensive underservice among other Medicare populations. Although a few hospital referral regions came close (notably Fort Lauderdale, Florida), most were well below the quality benchmark. in 1995-96, 731,000 Medicare diabetics did not receive the services they would have received had the quality of their care equaled that provided by the Kaiser Permanente Health Plan.

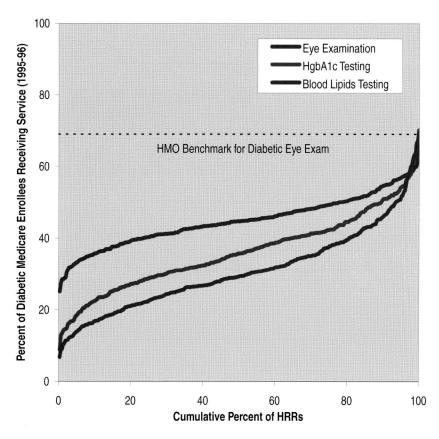

Figure 7.2. The Use of Selected Services by Medicare Diabetics by Hospital Referral Regions (1995-96)

The vertical axis shows the percent of Medicare enrollees receiving one or more of the selected services in 1995-96. The horizontal axis is the cumulative percent of hospital referral regions, ranked from lowest (left) to highest in percent compliance with guideline. The guideline calls for 100% of diabetic patients to have the service at least once annually. The "best practice" benchmark for diabetic eye examination is indicated. Compliance was well below the guidelines and the Kaiser-Permanente "achievable best practice" benchmark for eye examinations in all hospital referral regions.

Monitoring Glucose Control. The Diabetes Quality Improvement Project recommends routine monitoring of HgbAlc protein, a marker for glucose. Compliance with the guideline, however, fell far short of the recommendation. Two million diabetics went without the test during 1995-96; only 35.6% of diabetic patients had one or more tests. The proportion receiving the service ranged from 9% to 70%. We found no audited reports from health maintenance organizations to use as a "best practice" benchmark.

Blood Lipid Examinations. The Diabetes Quality Improvement Project recommends annual blood lipid examinations for diabetics. Compliance with this guideline was poor. Over the two year period 1995-96, only 33% of diabetic patients had one or more blood lipid examinations. In fee-for-service Medicare, 2.1 million diabetics went without the test. We found no audited reports from health maintenance organizations to use as a "best practice" benchmark.

The Underuse of Care for Medicare Enrollees Who Have Had Heart Attacks

Each year about one and a half million people in the United States have heart attacks. The toll in lives is heavy; about one-third of these patients die in the acute phase. The annual economic burden is more than $60 billion.

Because acute myocardial infarction is both common and serious, it has been the topic of intense scientific and clinical interest. One effort to incorporate evidence-based practice guidelines into the care of heart attack patients, begun in 1992, is the Health Care Financing Administration's Health Care Quality Improvement Initiative Cooperative Cardiovascular Project.

The Cooperative Cardiovascular Project developed quality indicators which were based heavily on clinical practice guidelines developed by the American College of Cardiology and the American Heart Association. Information about more than 200,000 patients admitted to hospitals for treatment of heart attacks was obtained from clinical records. Patients were classified as "eligible" or "ideal" for the specific therapies described by the quality indicators.

A study published in the Journal of the American Medical Association in February of 1999 found wide variations among hospital referral regions in the proportion of heart attack patients judged "ideal" for various treatments who actually received the recommended therapies (see the Endnote). The study documented substantial underuse of four potentially life saving treatments:

Beta-blockers at discharge. The American Heart Association and the American College of Cardiology recommend the use of beta blockers for all eligible patients at the time of discharge from the hospital following acute myocardial infarction. According to the Health Care Financing Administration's Cooperative Cardiovascular Project, compliance with this guideline varied substantially among hospital referral regions. Overall, only 49.5% of Medicare enrollees judged "ideal" candidates for beta-blockers actually got the medication. The proportion receiving the service ranged from 5.0% to 93.2%. In 25.7% of regions, less than 40% of "ideal" candi-

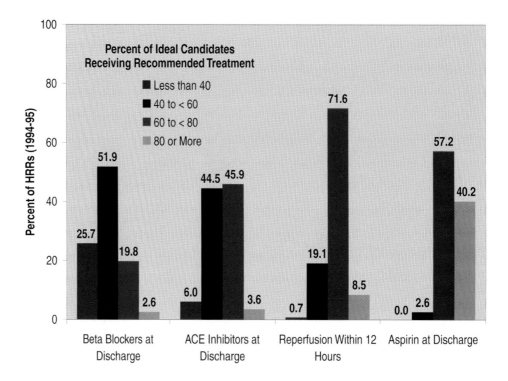

Figure 7.3. Percent of Medicare Residents with Heart Attacks Receiving Recommended Treatments by Hospital Referral Regions (1994-95)
The vertical axis shows the percent of regions, and the horizontal axis is the recommended treatment. For example, the light blue bar represents regions in which 80% or more of "ideal" patients actually received the treatment. Only 2.6% of regions achieved a level of at least 80% compliance with the guideline for beta-blockers at discharge. In 25.7% of hospital referral regions less than 40% of "ideal" patients were adequately treated (red bar). Only three regions had compliance with the guideline greater than the Kaiser-Permanente South "best practice" benchmark. (The guideline recommends that 100% of eligible heart attack patients receive beta-blockers.) In most hospital referral regions there was substantial underuse for each of these effective treatments.

dates received prescriptions for beta blockers; only a few regions exceeded the best practice benchmark of Kaiser-Permanente South, where 89% of "ideal" candidates received beta-blockers at discharge (Figure 7.3).

Angiotensin converting enzyme (ACE) inhibitors at discharge. The standards of care call for the use of ACE inhibitors at the time of discharge from the hospital for all eligible patients. Compliance with the this guideline varied substantially; overall, only 59.3% of Medicare enrollees who were judged as ideal candidates for ACE inhibitors following heart attacks actually got the medication. The proportion receiving the service ranged from 6.7% to 100%. In 6.0% of regions, less than 40% of ideal candidates received a prescription for ACE inhibitors. In 3.6%, 80% or more received the recommended care. We found no audited reports from health maintenance organizations to use as a "best practice" benchmark (Figure 7.3).

Reperfusion with thrombolytic agents or percutaneous transluminal coronary angioplasty. The Cooperative Cardiovascular Project found that compliance with the guideline recommending reperfusion varied substantially. The proportion of "ideal" candidates who received the recommended reperfusion following heart attacks ranged from 33% to 93%. Overall, 62% of ideal candidates received the recommended treatment. In 0.7% of regions, less than 40% of ideal candidates were reperfused according to the guideline; in 8.5%, 80% or more received the recommended care. We found no audited reports from health maintenance organizations to use as a "best practice" benchmark (Figure 7.3).

Aspirin prescribed at discharge. Aspirin has been shown in randomized clinical trials to reduce mortality in patients who have had heart attacks. Compared to the other three guidelines, fee for service Medicare performed best when it came to prescribing aspirin at the time of discharge. Only about 22.2% of "ideal" candidates failed to get the recommended treatment. Compliance with the guideline ranged from 96% to 52%; no hospital referral regions had less than 40% compliance with the guideline, and 40.2% had better than 80% compliance. We found no audited reports from health maintenance organizations to use as a "best practice" benchmark (Figure 7.3).

More Medicare Spending Does Not Cure Underservice

The Dartmouth Atlas series has focused on the wide geographic variations in both underservice and variations in overall Medicare resources and utilization. But do areas that have larger per capita expenditures also provide better quality care? This is obviously a complicated and multidimensional question, and we cannot entirely resolve it. However, we can ask whether there is a relationship between areas with higher per capita Medicare expenditures and the rates at which enrollees receive appropriate and recommended screening tests. Figure 7.4 shows per capita Medicare spending by hospital referral regions, adjusted for age, sex, race, regional price levels, and illness burden (on the horizontal axis). The vertical axis is an index of underservice: the average proportion, by hospital referral region, of Medicare enrollees who (1) received immunizations for pneumococcal pneumonia; (2) had at least one mammogram (women age 65-69); (3) were screened for colorectal cancer; and (4)the proportion of diabetics receiving annual eye examinations; (5) the proportion of diabetics receiving glucose (Hgba1c) screening; and (6) the proportion of diabetics receiving LDL blood lipids testing. A score of 100 would mean that each eligible person had received the appropriate screen or tests; a score of zero would mean that no eligible person received the recommended preventive care. A higher index is indicative of better compliance with the guidelines for preventive and screening services.

Figure 7.4 demonstrates that there was no correlation between overall Medicare spending in hospital referral regions and the index of the quality of preventive services (R^2 = .01). It appears that, even in areas that spent up to $3,000 per capita more than other regions, the quality of preventive care was no better (and very slightly worse) than in regions with lower per capita lower spending.

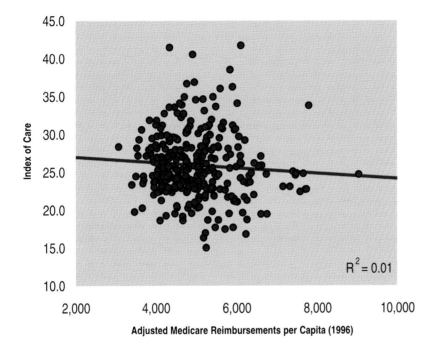

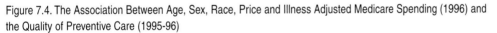

Figure 7.4. The Association Between Age, Sex, Race, Price and Illness Adjusted Medicare Spending (1996) and the Quality of Preventive Care (1995-96)

The vertical axis gives the values for the quality of care index (see text); the horizontal axis gives the fully adjusted Medicare per capita spending. There was little association between spending level and the quality of preventive care (R^2 = .01).

Underuse and Overuse of Surgery and The Quality of Clinical Science

Which surgical rate is "right?" Do patients in high rate areas suffer from overtreatment, while those in low rate areas receive less than adequate care? According to the Roundtable report, underuse represents the failure to provide effective treatments, and overuse means that patients are subjected to treatments for which the associated harms exceed the expected benefits. How do we know when treatments are effective, and when harms exceed benefits? Answering this question depends fundamentally on outcomes research — clinical trials and cohort studies which study the outcomes of care according to the treatment used. In many situations, however, judgments about overuse or underuse are impossible because medical science is so poor that we cannot make accurate prognoses for the use of given treatments. The research required to arrive at conclusions about harms and benefits has never been done.

The ten-fold variation in the incidence of surgery for prostate cancer is one example of how poor medical science inhibits the valid interpretation of outcomes. Rates of prostate cancer vary much less than rates of treatment, from which it can be inferred that in regions with low rates of surgery for prostate cancer, the condition is being treated in other ways (or not diagnosed at all). From the perspective of the outcome that matters most — life expectancy — the value of care has not been determined.

It cannot be said, on the basis of science, that active treatment of prostate cancer helps; nor can it be said that it does not. Under a strict interpretation of the Roundtable criteria, such as one the Food and Drug Administration uses in determining the value of drugs, any use of an unproven intervention in everyday practice is "overuse." Indeed, if prostate cancer surgery were a drug, rather than a procedure, its use would be forbidden by law until proof of efficacy had been established. Under the rules of everyday medical practice, however, most non-drug innovations escape rigorous evaluation. For such innovations, it is impossible to say, on the basis of evidence concerning outcomes, whether the observed rates constitute either underuse or overuse. Failure to evaluate the outcomes of care is, moreover, an incredible waste of the opportunity to learn what works and what patients want.

The Overuse of Discretionary Surgery

In the absence of good scientific evidence of efficacy, outcomes researchers have sometimes relied on medical opinion to define overuse and underuse of care. Panels of experts are asked to make group judgments about whether the benefits of a particular intervention exceed its risks. Over the past 15 years, the RAND corporation has used a group judgment process (The Delphi Approach) to develop detailed judgments about which groups of patients will benefit from surgery and which will not. RAND then applied the judgments to actual patients to classify surgery according to "appropriateness." Surgery in cases in which the panel felt the benefits exceeded the risks was judged "appropriate;" for those patients for whom the risks exceed the benefits, surgery was classified as "inappropriate," or unnecessary. The Roundtable report used these studies to estimate the extent of overuse of specific surgical procedures. For surgical procedures common in the Medicare population, the Roundtable's estimates of overuse ranged from 17% of all cases (coronary angiography) to 32% (carotid endarterectomy).

Several studies have attempted to understand the relationship between inappropriate use of care, as defined by panels of experts, and geographic variations in surgical rates. While many researchers had assumed that areas with high rates of surgery would have a greater percentage of unnecessary care, the studies failed to confirm that hypothesis. Overuse as defined by experts accounts for very little of the variation (see the Endnote).

Discretionary Surgery and the Question of Which Rate is Right

Sparing patients from surgery that experts believe is actually harmful obviously improves the quality of care; and on purely ethical grounds, such care should not even be offered. However, the overuse of harmful care or care that patients do not want does not explain geographic variations, and the elimination of overuse would not be sufficient to define what care patients actually want.

Increasingly, outcomes researchers are documenting the importance of patients' preferences in deciding which treatment best meets the individual patient's needs and wishes. A treatment is discretionary precisely because medical practice offers patients at least one other option. A woman with breast cancer, for example, has a choice between breast sparing surgery and mastectomy. Extensive clinical trials have shown that improvement in survival (the main goal of either treatment) is about the same for both options. However, other outcomes of the two interventions are not the same, and the choice between them involves trade-offs. The patient who undergoes lumpectomy will need radiation therapy, and faces a risk of local recurrence of her breast cancer. The patient who undergoes mastectomy avoids radiation and local recurrence, but must deal with the loss of her breast. Individual women differ substantially in how they evaluate the risks and benefits of these two treatment options. Breast sparing surgery is appropriate for some patients, and mastectomy is the right choice for others. Since the trade-offs must be made according to the preferences and values of individuals, the decision rightfully belongs to the patient — and not to panels of experts, managed care companies, surgeons, or patient advocates. The definition of unnecessary care must be expanded to include care that does not reflect what individual patients actually want.

Benign prostatic hyperplasia is a common disease in men over the age of 50, and there is considerable debate about how — and whether — the condition should be treated. Traditionally, men with benign prostatic hyperplasia have relied on their physicians to decide on the course of treatment for them, assuming that "the doctor knows best." Outcomes research has clarified the theoretical reasons for treatment, which is primarily to improve the quality of life by reducing the intensity of symptoms. For most men, surgery does not increase the length of life and, in fact, might shorten life expectancy slightly because of the risk of operative mortality. The importance — the necessity — of the patient's active involvement in the choice of treatment is illuminated by these outcomes studies, because they have shown that the most important consideration for the patient is the tradeoff between risks and outcomes. Surgery is superior in improving urinary tract symptoms; foregoing surgery is superior to surgery in avoiding surgical complications, including impotence, incontinence, and retrograde ejaculation. Individual patients differ substantially in how they assess their own situations, including their feelings about sexual activity. There is nothing in a given patient's physical examination, clinical history, or laboratory test results that would allow a physician to prescribe the treatment that a patient who was informed and involved in the decision making process would prefer. The patient must be actively involved in the decision process.

An observational study of treatment choice for benign prostatic hyperplasia conducted in two health maintenance organizations showed that in a program of shared decision making, treatment choice was determined by the individual patient's own assessment of two subjective factors: how much his symptoms bothered him (not the severity of symptoms, but the extent to which symptoms at any level of severity were considered bothersome) and his concern about side effects, particularly the impact of surgery on sexuality.

Shared Decision Making and the Right Rate for Discretionary Surgery

If patients were informed about the risks and benefits of available treatments, and were actively involved in the decision making process, surgical rates would be based on patient choice among the "appropriate" options, rather than the preferences of individual physicians or the recommendations of panels of experts. The rates of surgery that would result from the incorporation of informed patients' choices into the decision making process would then be available as measures of how much surgery is necessary according to patients. We would also know whether the amount that informed patients want is less or more than the amount now being prescribed by physicians and experts.

Several studies have found that the level of demand for surgery that results from shared decision making is different and sometimes substantially less than in circumstances in which patients are not involved in decisions about surgical options. When informed about the risks and benefits of the alternative treatments, and invited to make decisions according to their own preferences, patients with benign prostatic hyperplasia and coronary artery disease demanded more conservative treatments and less surgery than was being performed before shared decision making was implemented (Figure 7.5).

Rates of prostate surgery in the two health maintenance organizations were already substantially lower than the national average when the study began. Among men who participated in the study, rates dropped even lower — more than 40% below the health maintenance organization's baseline. There was no reduction in demand among men in the control groups. (A subsequent randomized clinical trial showed a similar result, but the trial was underpowered and the result was not statistically significant.)

Current rates of other kinds of surgery might, by the same token, be lower than the rates that would be demanded by patients who were informed and actively engaged in decision making. The point is that learning which rate is right (and how much underuse or overuse of surgery there is in the United States) depends on improving the quality of clinical decision making. The extreme variations in the rates of most surgical treatments (Chapter Five) is evidence of the extent of the decision quality aspect of the problem of overuse, underuse, and misuse of care.

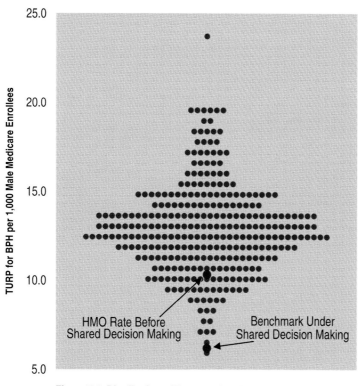

Figure 7.5. Distribution of Transurethral Prostatectomies for Benign Prostatic Hyperplasia Among Hospital Referral Regions (1992-93) Compared to Shared Decision Making Benchmark in Two Staff Model HMOs

The rate of surgery fell about 40% after implementation of shared decision making, although the rate prior to the intervention was lower than the national average. Rates in the control region did not change.

The Shared Decision Making Benchmark:
Patient Demand for Surgery for Benign Prostatic Hyperplasia

The experience of the health maintenance organization in implementing shared decision making provides a benchmark for addressing the question, Which rate is right? In 1992-93, the last years of the shared decision making observational study, the rates of surgery for benign prostatic hyperplasia among men participating in shared decision making were comparable to the rates in the hospital referral regions with the lowest rates in the United States (Figure 7.5). If the preferences about surgical treatment of the men who participated in the shared decision making study reflect the preferences of most men, then the amount of surgery for benign prostate disease being performed in the United States in those years substantially exceeded the amount that informed men would actually have wanted. In 1992-93, 309,000 operations for benign prostatic hyperplasia were performed among men enrolled in fee-for-service Medicare. The health maintenance organization benchmark predicts that patient demand was less than half the amount supplied — that about 160,000 more procedures were performed on Medicare men than would have been wanted, had shared decision making been the standard of care in those years.

The quality problem of surgery that patients don't really want has another dimension: the misapplication of resources. For example, in 1992-93, Medicare reimbursements for hospital care alone related to surgery for benign prostatic hyperplasia exceeded $1.08 billion. The level of spending predicted by the health maintenance organization benchmark — the amount of surgery patients actually wanted — was $511 million, less than half that amount. More than 1.6 million days of hospitalization were allocated to the care of patients having surgery for benign prostatic hyperplasia; had the health maintenance organization benchmark prevailed throughout the United States, such patients would have used almost 800,000 fewer hospital days.

The health maintenance organization benchmark can be used to estimate the extent of excess use of surgery for benign prostatic hyperplasia by hospital referral regions (Figure 7.6).

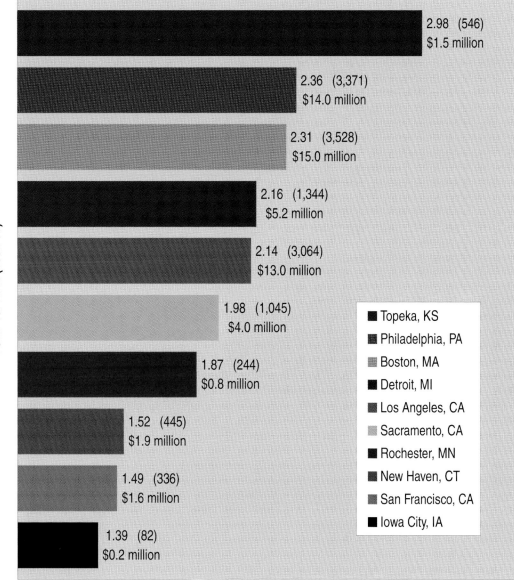

Figure 7.6. Predicted Overuse of Surgery for Benign Prostatic Hyperplasia in Selected Hospital Referral Regions According to a Shared Decision Making Benchmark (1992-93)

The figure gives the ratio of the rate of surgery in the selected hospital referral regions to the rate in two health maintenance organizations after the implementation of shared decision making. It also indicates the numbers of surgical procedures (in parentheses) and the reimbursements for hospitalization in excess of that predicted by the health maintenance organization benchmark. For example, in the Boston hospital referral region, the rate of prostate surgery in 1992-93 exceeded the benchmark rate by a factor of 2.3. If the rate of surgery had been the same as in the benchmark health maintenance organization, 3,371 fewer procedures would have been performed and Medicare reimbursements for inpatient care would have been $15.0 million less.

Overuse and Underuse of Hospitals for Medical Conditions

Variations in rates of discretionary surgery reflect differences in choices among alternative ways of treating specific conditions. Variations in rates of use of hospitals for medical conditions raise a different set of issues of overuse and underuse (Chapter Three). There are at least four important issues raised by variations in the rates at which acute care hospital inpatient resources are used to treat patients with medical conditions:

■ First, for most medical conditions, the supply of hospital beds is closely associated with the incidence of hospitalization, and this relationship cannot be explained on the basis of differences in illness rates among hospital referral regions.

■ Second, the effect of increasing hospital capacity is to decrease the threshold for admitting patients for virtually all acute and chronic medical conditions which can be treated on an inpatient basis.

■ Third, physicians are not aware of the propensity to hospitalize in their own hospital referral regions, or in the particular hospitals in which they practice; nor, when asked, do physicians practicing in regions with low rates of hospitalizations for medical conditions feel they are rationing hospital care.

■ Fourth, on an illness adjusted basis, the outcomes of treatment reflected in mortality rates are not better in regions with greater propensity to hospitalize. In other words, there is no apparent marginal gain in terms of improved life expectancy.

Given that these things are true, the "best practices" benchmarks come from hospital referral regions with low acute care hospital capacity and correspondingly low rates of utilization, because these regions are more efficient: that is, spending is lower and there is no apparent loss of benefit. The benchmark hospital referral regions selected for purposes of illustration in Map 7.1 and Table 7.1 are Salt Lake City, San Francisco, and Hartford, Connecticut.

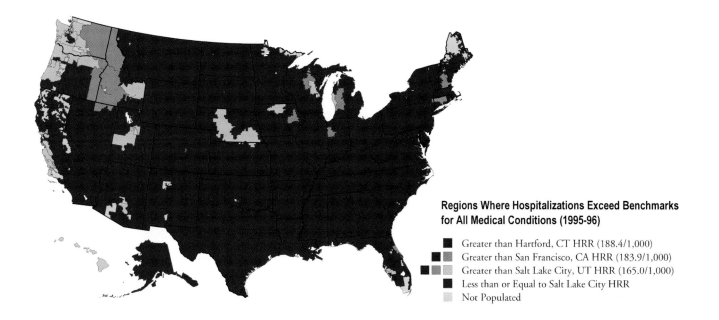

Regions Where Hospitalizations Exceed Benchmarks
for All Medical Conditions (1995-96)

- Greater than Hartford, CT HRR (188.4/1,000)
- Greater than San Francisco, CA HRR (183.9/1,000)
- Greater than Salt Lake City, UT HRR (165.0/1,000)
- Less than or Equal to Salt Lake City HRR
- Not Populated

Map 7.1. Regions Where Age Sex, Race and Illness Adjusted Rates for Discharges for Medical Conditions Exceed the Benchmark Regions (1995-96)

The hospitalization rates for medical conditions exceed the Salt Lake City benchmark in almost all regions. If, in 1995-96, the benchmark rate had prevailed in all regions with higher rates, hospitalization rates in the Medicare population would have been 27% lower; there would have been 3.5 million fewer hospitalizations; and allocations for inpatient care of patients with medical (non-surgical) conditions would have been $15.2 billion less. The rates in most hospital referral regions exceeded the San Francisco and Hartford benchmarks; Table 7.1 estimates the excess numbers of hospitalizations and the excess Medicare spending according to these benchmarks.

Benchmark	# Regions Higher	% U.S. Population	Excess Hospitalizations (millions)	Excess Dollars Spent (billions)
Hartford, CT	266	91.1	2.2	9.6
San Francisco, CA	276	93.7	2.5	10.6
Salt Lake City, UT	298	98.5	3.5	15.2

Table 7.1. Overuse of Hospitalizations Predicted by Selected Benchmark Hospital Referral Regions

Compared to rates in the hospital referral regions in Hartford, Connecticut, San Francisco, and Salt Lake City, there was substantial overuse of hospitalizations for medical conditions in other regions of the United States. The estimated excess number of hospitalizations ranged from 2.2 million to 3.5 million; the excess spending for such hospitalizations is estimated at between $9.6 billion and $15.2 billion.

Overuse and Underuse of End of Life Care

Variations in the intensity of care provided at the end of life (Chapter Six) raise a similar set of issues. The intensity of care (measured, for example, by the number of physician visits to medical specialists, the frequency of use of intensive care, and total spending in the last six months of life) varies substantially. The relative supply of medical resources and the intensity of care delivered in the last six months of life are directly correlated; but what about the value gained from spending more on the acute care of the very sick? Do the populations living in regions with more aggressive patterns of care live longer because more is spent on saving lives?

In research conducted in conjunction with the 1999 edition of the Atlas, we sought answers to these questions. We examined the association between intensity of care and mortality rates among Medicare enrollees, taking as the measures of intensity of care Medicare spending for inpatient care and the number of days spent in intensive care units during the last six months of life. The goal was to evaluate the marginal productivity of increased spending: Is more better? Are we on the flat of the curve? Or, is it conceivable that more is actually worse — that in regions with greater intensity of care the risks might actually exceed the benefits? (See Endnote)

Our investigation yielded no evidence that more intervention results in better outcomes. The associations between Medicare spending in last six months of life and mortality, even after correcting for a number of illness-related variables, were consistent with the flat-of-the-curve hypothesis that there is no marginal benefit from incremental increases in spending or intensity of care. In other words, populations living in regions with relatively low supplies of resources and intensity of medical intervention do not appear to be losing life expectancy as a result of any "underuse" of care. Indeed, greater intensity of care, measured by use of intensive care units, was actually associated with a slight increase in mortality, a finding compatible with the hypothesis that more intervention is actually associated with worse outcomes. Moreover, most patients appear to prefer less intensive care at the end of life, and those who live in regions with lower intensity of care are more likely to receive the care

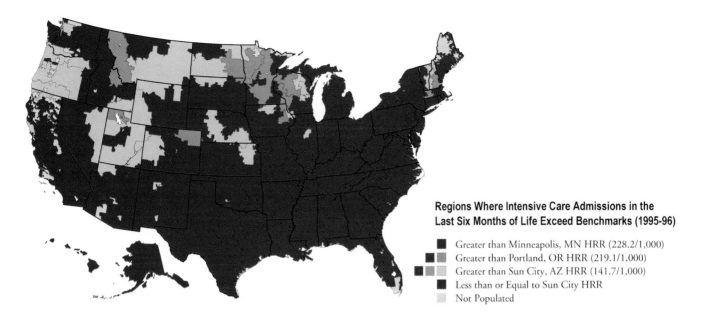

Regions Where Intensive Care Admissions in the
Last Six Months of Life Exceed Benchmarks (1995-96)

■ Greater than Minneapolis, MN HRR (228.2/1,000)
■ Greater than Portland, OR HRR (219.1/1,000)
■ Greater than Sun City, AZ HRR (141.7/1,000)
■ Less than or Equal to Sun City HRR
■ Not Populated

Map 7.2. Regions Where The Percent of Medicare Patients Admitted to Intensive Care in Last Six Months of Life Exceeds the Benchmark Regions (1995-96)

The proportion of enrollees admitted one or more times to an intensive care unit in the last six months of life exceeded the Sun City, Arizona benchmark in all other hospital referral regions. If, in 1995-96, the benchmark rate had prevailed in all other regions, there would have been 391,000 fewer admissions to intensive care units among Medicare enrollees in the last six months of their lives. Enrollees would have spent 3.7 million fewer days in intensive care units, and the Medicare program would have reimbursed $3 billion less for care in intensive care units. The rates in most regions exceeded the Minneapolis and Portland, Oregon benchmarks.

Benchmark	# Regions Higher	% U.S. Population	Excess ICU Admissions (thousands)	Excess Dollars Spent (billions)
Minneapolis, MN	275	93.8	196.5	1.4
Portland, OR	285	96.4	216.3	1.5
Sun City, AZ	305	99.9	391.0	3.0

Table 7.2. Overuse of Intensive Care Units in Last Six Months of Life as Predicted by Selected Benchmark Hospital Referral Regions

Table 7.2 estimates the excess numbers of enrollees admitted to intensive care units one or more times in the last six months of life, the excess number of days of care in an intensive care unit and the excess dollars spent, compared to the benchmarks. Estimated excess admissions ranged from 197,000 to 391,000; excess spending for such admissions from $1.4 billion to $3.0 billion.

they say they want (which is generally less than most people now receive). It is reasonable to use those regions in which the intensity of end of life care is low as "best practice" benchmarks of efficiency, because in those areas, lower spending results in no known loss of benefit, and appears to reflect actual patient preferences for end of life care. Three hospital referral regions provide such benchmarks for the use of intensive care in the last six months of life: Sun City, Arizona, Portland, Oregon, and Minneapolis.

Benchmark	# Regions Higher	% U.S. Population	Excess Visits to Medical Specialists (thousands)	Excess Dollars Spent (millions)
Rochester, NY	273	93.0	643.7	40.9
Rochester, MN	293	98.0	749.8	47.4
Lebanon, NH	302	99.6	867.5	54.6

Table 7.3. Overuse of Visits to Medical Specialists in Last Six Months of Life as Predicted by Selected Benchmark Hospital Referral Regions (1995-96)
Estimated excess number of visits to medical specialists during the last six months Medicare enrollees' lives, according to the selected benchmarks, ranged from 643,700 to 868,500; excess spending on such visits was estimated to be from $40.9 million to $54.6 million.

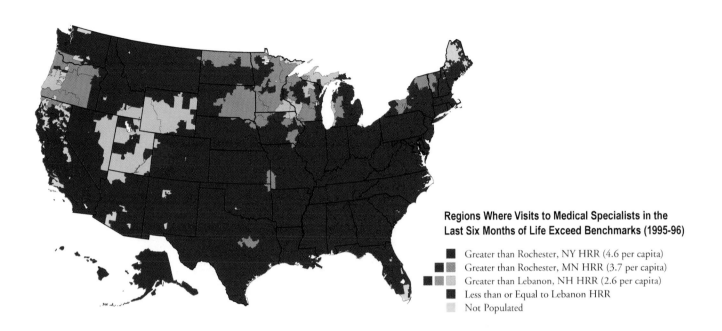

Regions Where Visits to Medical Specialists in the
Last Six Months of Life Exceed Benchmarks (1995-96)

- Greater than Rochester, NY HRR (4.6 per capita)
- Greater than Rochester, MN HRR (3.7 per capita)
- Greater than Lebanon, NH HRR (2.6 per capita)
- Less than or Equal to Lebanon HRR
- Not Populated

Map 7.3. Regions Where Average Visits Per Person to Medical Specialists During the Last Six Months of Life Exceeds the Benchmark Regions (1995-96)

The number of visits to medical specialists in the last six months of life exceeded the benchmark of the Lebanon, New Hampshire hospital referral region in all but three other regions. If the benchmark rate had prevailed in all regions with higher rates, Medicare enrollees in the last six months of life would have made 867,500 fewer visits to medical specialists and the Medicare program would have reimbursed $54.6 million less for such services. The rates in most regions exceeded that of the Rochester, Minnesota hospital referral region, home of the Mayo Clinic, as well as the Rochester, New York, hospital referral region, home of the University of Rochester Medical School. Table 7.3 estimates the excess numbers of Medicare enrollees' visits to medical specialists in the last six months of enrollees' lives.

Misuse of Resources: Inefficiency in the Allocation of the Physician Workforce

The numbers of clinically active physicians, both specialists and generalists, vary substantially among hospital referral regions (Chapter Two). How many physicians constitute an adequate workforce? Traditional approaches to workforce planning have depended on either need-based or demand-based planning to identify the appropriate supply of physicians. Both approaches have flaws (see Endnote). Benchmarking provides an alternative approach, by comparing physician resources with health plans or regions which have relatively low supplies of physicians but are able to provide care without discernible loss of benefit.

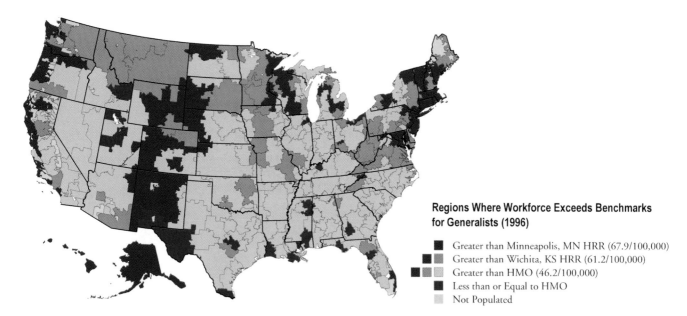

Regions Where Workforce Exceeds Benchmarks for Generalists (1996)

- Greater than Minneapolis, MN HRR (67.9/100,000)
- Greater than Wichita, KS HRR (61.2/100,000)
- Greater than HMO (46.2/100,000)
- Less than or Equal to HMO
- Not Populated

Map 7.4 Regions Where Workforce Exceeds Benchmark for Generalists (1996)

Benchmark	# Regions Higher	% U.S. Population	Excess Generalists
Minneapolis, MN	75	32.1	9,951
Wichita, KS	137	54.7	17,704
HMO	288	97.8	49,600

Table 7.4. Excess Supply of Generalist Physicians as Predicted by Selected Benchmark Hospital Referral Regions (1996)

The supply of generalists in the United States exceeds the prepaid group practice benchmark by 49,600 full time equivalents; the Wichita benchmark by 17,700 full time equivalents, and the Minneapolis benchmark by 9,950 full time equivalents.

Three benchmarks have been used in Atlas analyses: a large prepaid group practice; the clinically active workforce serving the Minneapolis hospital referral region, and the workforce in the Wichita, Kansas hospital referral region. The Minneapolis hospital referral region has high managed care penetration (39.4% of the Medicare population in 1995) and the Wichita hospital referral market is a predominantly fee-for-service market with low managed care penetration (4.5% of the Medicare population in 1995). In contrast to populations served by health maintenance organizations, populations of hospital referral regions are not biased by selection against the disabled, the uninsured and the very elderly.

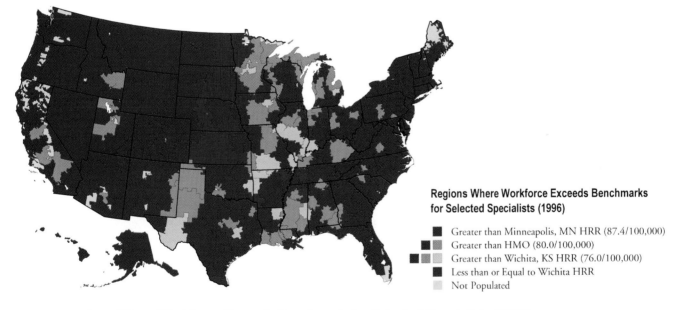

Regions Where Workforce Exceeds Benchmarks for Selected Specialists (1996)

■ Greater than Minneapolis, MN HRR (87.4/100,000)
■ Greater than HMO (80.0/100,000)
■ Greater than Wichita, KS HRR (76.0/100,000)
■ Less than or Equal to Wichita HRR
  Not Populated

Map 7.5 Regions Where Workforce Exceeds Benchmark for Selected Specialists (1996)

Benchmark	# Regions Higher	% U.S. Population	Excess Specialists
Minneapolis, MN	225	84.7	55,395
HMO	275	95.2	72,898
Wichita, KS	288	97.1	83,066

Table 7.5. Excess Supply of Specialist Physicians as Predicted by Selected Benchmark Hospital Referral Regions (1996)
The supply of selected specialists in the United States exceeded the Wichita benchmark by 27.5% (83,000 full time equivalents); the prepaid group practice benchmark by 24.1% (72,900 full time equivalents); and the Minneapolis benchmark by 18.3% (55,400 full time equivalents).

Summing Up: Inefficiency in the Allocation of Medicare Spending

Per capita Medicare spending varies substantially among the nation's hospital referral regions, even after adjustments for differences in regional prices and illness rates, but there is little evidence that greater spending brings better health. In the example of the underuse of services known to be effective (Figure 7.4), more spending does not result in less underservice. In other words, the "cure" for underservice, as demonstrated by the best practice health maintenance organization benchmark, appears to be better management of resources, not more spending. In the case of spending for discretionary surgery, more does not appear to be better: in the case of surgery for benign prostate disease, the amount provided by fee-for-service Medicare exceeds the amount demanded by informed patients (Figure 7.5). In the case of use of hospitals for medical conditions and for treatment of the seriously ill, greater use and greater spending does not appear to improve life expectancy. While populations living in regions with greater supplies of physicians have more visits per capita and greater spending per capita for physician services, more physicians do not assure less underservice (Chapter Four) or the participation of patients in shared decision making.

Improving Quality and Achieving Efficiency

The evidence in this edition of the Dartmouth Atlas confirms the conclusion of the National Roundtable that "serious and widespread quality problems exist throughout American medicine." Some of these problems can be addressed by improving the management of care. This is particularly the case for errors of omission, such as the failure to provide effective care that patients want, including immunizations, mammograms, eye care for diabetics and the timely use of effective drugs for patients who have had heart attacks. Managed care, to the extent that it can bring discipline to the workplace, offers a important opportunity to improve the quality of this aspect of care.

Managed care might also provide important solutions to the problem of medical error, particularly when it arises from failure to conform to reasonable standards of the prudent practice of medicine. But many quality problems require a different focus. Those that derive from poor science require improvement in the quality of clinical science. Those that emerge from inefficiency in medical spending and resource use require improvement in the quality of resource allocation.

The Quality of Clinical Science

The evaluative sciences need to be applied in a systematic way to medical innovation, whether it arises from biomedical research or from the efforts of practicing physicians to adopt existing technologies to new purposes. We must assure that medical theory is tested in an orderly way in order to make accurate prognoses and to improve the process of care.

The Quality of Clinical Decision Making

Quality problems that emerge from failure to base the choice of discretionary care on the preferences of the patient require improvement in the quality of clinical decision making. The subtle, often unrecognized influences that physicians have on choices among available treatments is the major cause of variations in the rates of surgery and of many other common interventions. Discretionary interventions involve trade-offs that only patients can make, and to make good decisions patients must have access to up to date, evidence-based assessments of the outcomes that matter to them. Moreover, patients must be encouraged to choose according to their own preferences, particularly in situations where individuals have very different attitudes and preferences.

The Quality of Resource Allocation Decisions

For decades, the health care debate has taken place against the background assumption that more is better; but from the perspective of patients and the welfare of populations, the Atlas provides ample evidence that this assumption is not necessarily true. It will not be possible to come to terms with the problem of increasing medical costs without dealing with the quality of resource allocation decisions. This raises a number of questions. Why does the nation continue to subsidize growth in the physician workforce? Will managed care and competition — as it is now structured — clear the medical market of excess capacity? How can the nation promote population-based strategies for resource allocation? Can the private sector accomplish strategies to implement "best practice" benchmarks for the efficient allocation of health care resources — for example, can the successes in achieving an efficient physician workforce of population based health plans such as Kaiser Permanente be replicated in different practice settings, medical cultures and forms of organizing the delivery system? Can such systems achieve similar efficiency in acute care resources? Can purchasers, including insurers and employers, influence private sector health planning? Is it time to reconsider the possibilities for public sector health planning?

The Economics of Quality

Improving the quality of clinical science, decision making, and resource allocation is linked to the problem of growth in Medicare spending. A recent study by the Congressional Budget Office projects a rapid increase in the proportion of the gross domestic product invested in medical care, if Medicare's current defined benefit (fee-for-service) program is left unchanged. An increase of this magnitude in total costs of care is widely regarded as politically unsustainable. One proposal for reducing this increase is to move the age of eligibility for the Medicare program to 67 by 2025 and to 70 by 2032. A second proposal is to change the benefit package from the present fee-for-service plan to a defined contribution plan. Under this option, spending per capita would increase 4% per year after the baseline year, 2000.

The Congressional Budget Office has examined the effect of these options on projected increases in the proportion of the gross domestic product allocated to Medicare. Delaying retirement helps a little, reducing spending by 11% in years 2030 and beyond. But the best strategy for reducing the rate of growth is the defined contribution approach, which results in a 38% reduction in the projected increase in proportion of gross domestic product.

The projections are based on average per capita spending —which assumes that average spending is somehow the efficient amount to spend. But the national average has no inherent validity; it is simply the weighted average of all hospital referral regions (Figure 7.7). In 1995, price adjusted Medicare spending for residents of the Miami hospital referral region was $7,955 per enrollee, a rate which if nationalized would be equivalent to about 4.2% of gross domestic product. Spending in the Minneapolis hospital referral region for the fee-for-service defined benefit plan was $3,528, or about 1.9%.

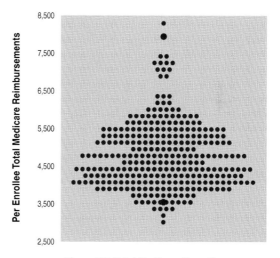

Figure 7.7. Total Medicare Spending per Enrollee (1995)

Per enrollee spending varied from less than $3,000 to more than $8,000. Levels of the Minneapolis and Miami hospital referral regions are indicated in red. Other hospital referral regions are represented by the blue points.

Spending projections are clearly sensitive to the health care market used as a benchmark. When Minneapolis, rather than the national average, is used as a benchmark, projections of the percent of gross domestic product allocated to the defined benefit fee-for-service program are very different. Indeed, if all regions in the United States were to spend at the level of Minneapolis, spending would be lower than the Congressional Budget Office's projection for the defined contribution plan until late in the 2020s (Figure 7.8).

It is important to link the problem of Medicare spending with the issues of improving the quality of care. Much of medical care is not governed by well-articulated medical theory, much less by empirical evidence about the outcomes of care. Although our medical culture is dominated by the assumption that more is better, greater total per capita spending does not buy better outcomes. There is no apparent advantage in terms of life expectancy of spending more on acute hospital care or intensive care, and no relationship between spending and the quality of ambulatory and preventive care.

The implications for the quality debate seem straightforward. We must pay attention to the quality of medical science, making sure that common treatments that now escape systematic evaluation are brought under protocol. Likewise, the quality of clinical decision making should focus on the empowerment of patients to participate in the choice of their own treatments. Finally, we must review the quality of resource allocation decisions.

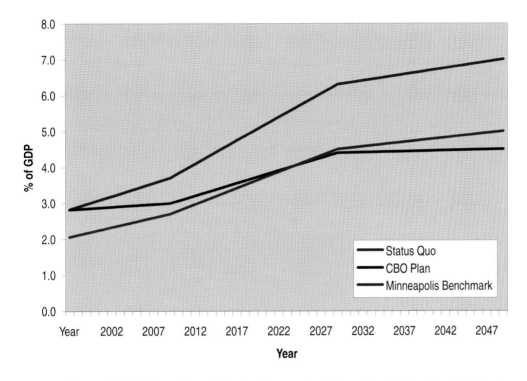

Figure 7.8. Projections of Spending Using Congressional Budget Office Projections for Defined Contribution Plan Spending, and Projections Based on Current per Enrollee Spending in the Minneapolis Hospital Referral Region (1998-2050)

Chapter Seven Table

The data in the table provide benchmarks for each hospital referral region. The benchmarks are used to answer the question: If all regions with higher rates were brought down to the rate of the benchmark region, and all regions with rates below the benchmark remained the same, how many excess admissions to ICUs, hospitalizations, specialist visits, etc, would there have been in the United States during the designated year(s)? For example, if in 1996 the suppply of generalists in all regions with more generalists per 100,000 residents than were allocated to the Birmingham, Alabama hospital referral region had been reduced to the level of the Birmingham benchmark, the calculated surplus number of generalists in the United States would be 28,816.

This approach to benchmarking was used in developing the maps and tables in this chapter. The benchmark question can, of course, be framed differently. One strategy poses the obverse question: if all regions with lower rates were brought up to the benchmark (and those with higher rates were left the same), how many additional visits or physicians or admissions would be required? And the benchmark question can also be framed in a another way: If all regions with higher rates were brought down to the benchmark, and those with lower rates were brought up to the benchmark, how many physicians, admissions, or visits would there be in excess (or deficit) of the current supply or rate?

The Dartmouth Atlas Data Viewer makes it possible to calculate, using any of the above strategies, the surpluses or deficits in the resources and utilization of any hospital referral region, including such measures as hospital beds, employees, physicians, surgical procedures, admissions to hospitals and to intensive care units, and the use of preventive and ambulatory care.

CHAPTER SEVEN TABLE

The Quality of Medical Care in the United States

Hospital Referral Region	Hospitalizations for All Medical Conditions per 1,000 Medicare Enrollees (1995-96)	Rank of Region	Excess Hospitalizations in U.S. According to HRR Benchmark	Percent of Medicare Enrollees Admitted to Intensive Care in the Last Six Months of Life (1995-96)	Rank of Region	Excess Admissions in U.S. According to HRR Benchmark	Medical Specialist Visits per Enrollee in the Last Six Months of Life (1995-96)	Rank of Region	Excess Visits in U.S. According to HRR Benchmark	Generalists per 100,000 Residents (1996)	Rank of Region	Excess Generalists in U.S. According to HRR Benchmark	Selected Specialists per 100,000 Residents (1996)	Rank of Region	Excess Selected Specialists in U.S. According to HRR Benchmark
Alabama															
Birmingham	259.4	46	91,218	34.4	68	24,767	8.5	146	300,500	54.9	217	28,816	90.3	189	49,447
Dothan	291.6	9	9,085	30.4	145	60,662	7.2	203	402,548	53.0	244	32,839	84.1	250	63,045
Huntsville	236.2	106	370,100	37.6	36	10,892	8.4	153	307,030	54.3	226	30,023	80.4	273	71,975
Mobile	268.2	27	45,093	38.7	24	8,020	11.5	73	156,364	51.3	259	36,829	99.7	128	32,638
Montgomery	250.9	58	161,516	33.4	84	31,689	7.9	167	341,650	49.6	272	41,063	82.2	259	67,575
Tuscaloosa	264.5	35	62,106	36.3	44	15,532	6.2	232	488,804	56.6	194	25,341	87.2	230	56,008
Alaska															
Anchorage	230.4	125	512,366	25.9	235	133,818	5.1	260	600,346	73.0	42	6,576	101.9	112	29,507
Arizona															
Mesa	176.6	286	2,868,348	33.3	88	32,512	12.6	53	122,318	53.0	246	32,984	87.3	228	55,611
Phoenix	196.0	247	1,834,841	30.9	135	54,758	8.7	138	290,235	59.5	158	20,328	103.9	98	26,864
Sun City	163.7	300	3,599,418	14.2	306	391,049	10.6	93	194,400	64.3	105	13,426	121.4	40	11,720
Tucson	194.5	251	1,910,846	28.5	186	87,231	8.6	141	293,140	63.3	118	14,810	102.7	107	28,407
Arkansas															
Fort Smith	252.9	54	142,740	32.4	103	39,616	12.5	55	126,763	57.7	185	23,293	78.8	280	76,083
Jonesboro	271.3	24	36,414	29.2	168	76,691	7.2	199	399,688	53.9	235	30,821	72.5	296	92,284
Little Rock	254.0	50	132,399	32.0	111	43,474	8.7	135	287,634	57.7	188	23,310	93.6	169	42,997
Springdale	221.3	153	782,490	30.9	133	54,486	5.5	250	559,283	58.4	174	22,100	78.9	279	75,767
Texarkana	271.5	23	35,721	41.5	9	3,862	10.9	85	181,721	53.4	239	31,874	75.9	290	83,434
California															
Orange Co.	214.9	175	1,003,880	39.3	22	6,869	20.1	11	15,520	73.1	40	6,489	121.7	39	11,572
Bakersfield	218.2	161	885,994	34.8	59	22,752	12.9	47	114,630	49.5	273	41,173	86.1	236	58,342
Chico	198.7	235	1,702,575	28.8	182	82,807	7.1	205	406,033	55.3	207	27,972	104.6	96	26,086
Contra Costa Co.	176.5	287	2,871,468	23.8	263	175,194	8.5	148	302,580	69.2	61	8,949	128.5	31	8,465
Fresno	189.2	265	2,186,645	29.4	166	75,014	8.7	137	289,207	54.6	220	29,457	87.5	224	55,281
Los Angeles	245.7	70	219,436	45.8	3	679	22.9	3	2,437	64.9	98	12,816	115.1	53	15,690
Modesto	212.6	184	1,090,369	36.9	41	13,225	9.2	123	259,013	54.3	225	29,948	84.9	241	61,130
Napa	199.1	233	1,684,861	23.6	265	181,083	5.8	244	528,332	89.0	9	997	143.6	18	3,269
Alameda Co.	193.9	254	1,943,814	26.7	224	118,049	9.9	108	223,277	82.2	24	2,446	122.7	37	11,083
Palm Spr/Rancho Mir	204.2	216	1,448,300	38.6	25	8,199	14.9	26	72,004	55.5	206	27,628	125.4	35	9,811
Redding	193.2	255	1,979,724	29.5	163	73,038	5.3	255	578,896	68.4	70	9,551	106.3	85	24,042
Sacramento	198.7	237	1,705,581	27.1	209	110,991	8.0	162	338,248	64.9	97	12,731	105.3	92	25,180
Salinas	177.8	283	2,804,834	36.7	42	14,245	8.9	130	278,376	60.4	144	18,841	117.8	48	13,896
San Bernardino	237.6	95	341,396	38.4	26	8,627	11.1	82	173,114	49.8	271	40,645	81.9	263	68,355
San Diego	190.2	260	2,130,707	31.0	131	53,558	13.2	44	105,949	61.1	140	17,822	115.8	52	15,253
San Francisco	183.9	277	2,469,960	28.3	190	90,601	9.4	117	249,167	102.1	3	37	157.7	7	670
San Jose	181.8	279	2,584,935	29.4	164	74,583	8.6	140	291,798	69.2	62	9,001	111.9	64	18,491
San Luis Obispo	169.6	296	3,261,167	33.2	90	33,363	6.9	212	426,725	77.6	30	4,387	137.9	23	5,115
San Mateo Co.	161.2	301	3,739,649	32.5	101	38,981	7.2	201	401,094	72.3	45	6,958	140.5	21	4,228
Santa Barbara	174.9	289	2,962,490	25.8	237	136,324	7.8	179	351,913	73.3	39	6,373	125.6	34	9,752

Hospital Referral Region	Hospitalizations for All Medical Conditions per 1,000 Medicare Enrollees (1995-96)	Rank of Region	Excess Hospitalizations in U.S. According to HRR Benchmark	Percent of Medicare Enrollees Admitted to Intensive Care in the Last Six Months of Life (1995-96)	Rank of Region	Excess Admissions in U.S. According to HRR Benchmark	Medical Specialist Visits per Enrollee in the Last Six Months of Life (1995-96)	Rank of Region	Excess Visits in U.S. According to HRR Benchmark	Generalists per 100,000 Residents (1996)	Rank of Region	Excess Generalists in U.S. According to HRR Benchmark	Selected Specialists per 100,000 Residents (1996))	Rank of Region	Excess Selected Specialists in U.S. According to HRR Benchmark
Santa Cruz	184.1	275	2,458,066	33.3	85	32,014	10.7	90	188,000	73.9	37	6,079	133.7	24	6,557
Santa Rosa	192.4	257	2,018,708	17.7	299	311,441	11.4	75	162,985	84.1	18	1,807	130.9	25	7,518
Stockton	204.5	215	1,435,501	28.8	181	82,604	10.0	107	222,491	50.3	266	39,446	89.7	194	50,637
Ventura	192.8	256	1,998,713	31.1	127	52,684	20.1	10	15,345	68.4	69	9,548	119.0	46	13,120
Colorado															
Boulder	196.4	245	1,815,897	30.6	142	58,832	11.7	69	151,016	85.0	11	1,594	129.7	29	7,988
Colorado Springs	202.9	221	1,506,668	23.2	273	189,215	5.1	257	596,035	59.0	165	21,142	101.9	111	29,433
Denver	199.6	231	1,659,901	26.7	222	117,643	8.3	156	311,246	69.1	64	9,055	114.7	57	16,043
Fort Collins	198.4	239	1,721,790	23.6	264	180,839	7.8	172	346,986	61.8	135	16,898	97.8	140	35,616
Grand Junction	189.9	262	2,150,714	17.4	301	318,057	2.6	305	869,330	71.3	50	7,593	100.9	121	30,836
Greeley	211.1	193	1,149,650	22.4	282	204,971	7.4	193	382,406	62.6	128	15,757	97.8	141	35,631
Pueblo	201.2	230	1,585,419	33.0	95	35,020	12.6	54	122,652	70.9	53	7,860	106.9	82	23,430
Connecticut															
Bridgeport	188.7	266	2,209,327	29.6	162	72,103	13.6	39	96,467	83.2	20	2,091	153.5	11	1,054
Hartford	188.4	267	2,227,003	27.3	205	107,798	8.4	154	307,095	68.3	72	9,655	130.6	26	7,625
New Haven	198.7	236	1,705,372	28.7	184	84,174	7.9	163	338,649	74.6	34	5,742	140.7	20	4,177
Delaware															
Wilmington	217.0	166	926,698	33.5	81	30,691	12.8	52	117,733	65.5	89	12,169	105.5	89	24,933
District of Columbia															
Washington	232.2	119	464,645	31.0	129	53,396	12.4	59	130,006	84.5	15	1,681	157.8	6	662
Florida															
Bradenton	181.7	280	2,588,722	38.1	28	9,426	10.6	95	195,083	48.3	280	44,174	102.7	106	28,407
Clearwater	210.0	199	1,193,084	34.5	66	24,561	13.9	37	91,764	63.9	110	13,968	111.4	65	18,925
Fort Lauderdale	210.5	197	1,172,183	40.2	18	5,339	21.8	6	6,320	68.4	71	9,603	130.1	28	7,795
Fort Myers	194.4	252	1,915,783	33.1	92	33,692	12.0	64	140,286	54.5	222	29,682	106.3	84	24,015
Gainesville	226.8	138	612,502	32.4	104	39,805	8.8	132	281,226	61.8	134	16,854	93.6	170	43,089
Hudson	243.6	72	246,967	41.2	10	4,143	10.8	88	185,903	55.0	213	28,497	97.3	144	36,565
Jacksonville	246.9	67	205,060	39.9	19	5,854	14.8	29	73,888	59.9	152	19,662	105.8	88	24,667
Lakeland	213.7	178	1,048,579	32.3	105	41,115	10.8	89	186,666	48.8	278	43,043	88.3	209	53,459
Miami	252.8	56	143,462	49.3	1	0	25.1	1	0	83.0	21	2,141	129.2	30	8,189
Ocala	197.3	244	1,774,368	28.2	191	92,385	9.9	109	226,432	45.6	291	51,264	91.8	182	46,587
Orlando	212.0	186	1,110,407	38.9	23	7,543	13.1	45	109,184	54.0	231	30,669	97.0	147	37,034
Ormond Beach	184.1	276	2,459,087	37.8	33	10,285	11.9	68	145,441	54.9	216	28,729	95.0	157	40,533
Panama City	261.2	41	80,151	31.2	126	51,790	9.6	114	239,345	45.2	292	52,311	89.7	195	50,727
Pensacola	245.2	71	225,924	33.9	73	27,951	10.6	92	194,033	58.5	171	21,883	102.7	105	28,384
Sarasota	181.3	281	2,611,958	34.5	67	24,603	12.9	50	115,650	61.4	137	17,469	128.0	32	8,692
St Petersburg	213.1	181	1,069,682	44.2	4	1,653	12.2	60	135,857	69.0	67	9,165	113.0	62	17,524
Tallahassee	231.3	120	488,190	26.2	230	128,171	7.8	180	352,872	57.7	187	23,309	88.2	211	53,720
Tampa	209.4	202	1,217,099	40.8	12	4,534	15.2	22	68,245	60.0	151	19,530	105.4	90	25,069
Georgia															
Albany	234.9	113	401,705	29.4	165	75,009	9.4	119	249,844	40.6	301	64,179	74.4	294	87,216
Atlanta	237.5	96	343,832	32.0	113	43,936	11.0	83	175,045	56.6	196	25,471	101.3	115	30,261
Augusta	236.7	101	359,533	26.9	218	114,915	7.9	166	340,039	56.6	195	25,469	107.7	77	22,547
Columbus	215.9	172	965,584	31.5	121	48,216	7.4	191	377,950	52.0	253	35,214	81.0	269	70,465
Macon	241.7	80	272,821	29.7	158	70,062	7.6	188	367,912	58.3	178	22,292	98.1	137	35,265
Rome	239.3	90	312,509	34.0	71	27,268	6.6	220	455,615	63.2	119	14,942	88.5	206	53,123

Hospital Referral Region	Hospitalizations for All Medical Conditions per 1,000 Medicare Enrollees (1995-96)	Rank of Region	Excess Hospitalizations in U.S. According to HRR Benchmark	Percent of Medicare Enrollees Admitted to Intensive Care in the Last Six Months of Life (1995-96)	Rank of Region	Excess Admissions in U.S. According to HRR Benchmark	Medical Specialist Visits per Enrollee in the Last Six Months of Life (1995-96)	Rank of Region	Excess Visits in U.S. According to HRR Benchmark	Generalists per 100,000 Residents (1996)	Rank of Region	Excess Generalists in U.S. According to HRR Benchmark	Selected Specialists per 100,000 Residents (1996)	Rank of Region	Excess Selected Specialists in U.S. According to HRR Benchmark
Savannah	249.4	61	177,441	31.4	124	49,170	10.5	96	195,791	54.2	229	30,274	102.1	109	29,152
Hawaii															
Honolulu	170.5	294	3,210,535	23.5	267	182,249	7.7	183	358,973	75.8	32	5,211	114.8	56	15,998
Idaho															
Boise	185.7	271	2,369,265	23.4	268	183,532	4.9	266	622,131	51.0	262	37,517	94.7	160	40,992
Idaho Falls	172.0	292	3,128,362	24.9	250	153,496	4.7	273	643,270	37.9	302	71,248	84.4	248	62,410
Illinois															
Aurora	210.4	198	1,176,766	29.2	169	77,124	9.5	115	243,919	45.1	293	52,613	82.4	258	67,116
Bloomington	203.5	219	1,482,951	15.2	305	368,143	5.6	248	549,396	50.2	269	39,599	83.7	251	63,921
Blue Island	250.5	59	165,796	36.0	50	16,923	15.2	23	68,297	67.0	79	10,784	103.0	102	28,080
Chicago	278.2	18	20,544	40.5	16	4,863	13.9	35	90,295	84.5	16	1,693	120.1	42	12,452
Elgin	230.3	126	512,703	40.9	11	4,384	10.5	97	198,995	51.8	257	35,684	90.1	191	49,784
Evanston	237.0	98	353,367	34.7	63	23,470	11.6	70	154,223	98.1	5	178	156.0	9	800
Hinsdale	206.5	209	1,343,663	33.6	80	30,461	11.2	79	167,352	89.0	10	1,006	143.8	17	3,213
Joliet	264.6	34	61,740	34.6	65	23,621	15.3	20	66,033	54.7	219	29,086	100.7	124	31,196
Melrose Park	229.3	131	540,841	34.8	61	22,924	11.6	71	154,613	81.2	25	2,815	121.8	38	11,514
Peoria	211.6	190	1,128,421	24.9	251	153,554	7.9	170	344,878	53.3	241	32,110	83.7	252	64,122
Rockford	217.8	163	900,235	29.2	171	77,839	6.6	221	456,503	52.8	248	33,364	89.6	196	50,829
Springfield	238.2	92	330,278	26.9	214	113,990	5.3	254	577,606	52.0	254	35,274	79.7	278	73,709
Urbana	221.1	155	789,179	27.1	211	111,758	6.6	219	448,172	56.5	198	25,626	89.5	197	50,960
Indiana															
Evansville	253.7	51	135,304	31.9	114	44,881	5.7	247	538,862	53.8	236	30,994	78.3	284	77,352
Fort Wayne	190.5	259	2,116,937	32.0	110	43,325	7.8	176	349,847	48.2	282	44,500	74.3	295	87,625
Gary	266.7	30	51,353	34.2	69	26,006	16.7	17	46,289	50.6	265	38,676	84.6	242	61,777
Indianapolis	228.8	135	554,166	30.3	146	61,865	9.2	124	260,036	58.9	166	21,205	97.5	143	36,232
Lafayette	188.2	268	2,235,769	25.3	245	144,975	7.0	207	414,066	46.4	288	49,227	82.8	257	66,189
Muncie	241.0	84	282,715	35.1	58	21,129	10.1	105	216,941	59.0	164	21,053	88.2	212	53,799
Munster	276.0	19	25,010	48.7	2	95	12.4	57	128,150	58.4	177	22,218	88.4	208	53,326
South Bend	198.4	238	1,717,424	27.1	210	111,352	6.3	226	480,317	55.9	200	26,857	80.5	272	71,874
Terre Haute	224.7	141	676,616	39.4	21	6,688	12.1	62	138,111	55.2	209	28,165	87.5	221	55,134
Iowa															
Cedar Rapids	188.2	269	2,238,461	22.5	280	202,876	10.1	104	216,908	51.3	260	37,018	83.1	254	65,448
Davenport	210.5	196	1,171,804	29.1	172	78,220	8.6	142	293,901	52.9	247	33,195	92.5	178	45,244
Des Moines	229.3	130	540,384	27.5	203	103,873	7.6	187	364,596	63.3	117	14,739	80.1	275	72,864
Dubuque	205.6	214	1,384,526	21.7	288	221,044	4.1	284	697,977	48.9	277	42,881	90.3	190	49,461
Iowa City	229.6	128	533,339	23.2	270	187,682	4.1	285	702,389	58.5	173	22,038	99.2	130	33,467
Mason City	177.4	284	2,824,435	16.9	302	327,853	2.0	306	931,671	64.1	108	13,784	74.8	293	86,261
Sioux City	213.2	180	1,066,929	30.3	148	62,406	3.7	292	740,300	52.4	250	34,190	66.5	304	107,711
Waterloo	201.7	227	1,565,932	24.8	254	155,929	3.8	291	735,337	60.2	147	19,267	76.4	288	82,157
Kansas															
Topeka	190.2	261	2,134,977	17.6	300	312,774	7.8	178	351,051	52.1	252	35,108	91.7	183	46,732
Wichita	236.5	105	365,064	25.7	239	138,296	6.9	210	420,585	61.2	138	17,704	76.0	289	83,066
Kentucky															
Covington	251.2	57	158,259	33.7	76	29,462	10.2	100	210,157	58.7	169	21,705	89.7	193	50,596
Lexington	280.2	15	17,492	29.1	175	79,106	7.7	185	359,708	57.4	190	23,831	84.4	247	62,409
Louisville	255.3	48	122,048	31.5	120	48,214	10.6	94	194,746	59.6	156	20,075	103.0	101	27,982

Hospital Referral Region	Hospitalizations for All Medical Conditions per 1,000 Medicare Enrollees (1995-96)	Rank of Region	Excess Hospitalizations in U.S. According to HRR Benchmark	Percent of Medicare Enrollees Admitted to Intensive Care in the Last Six Months of Life (1995-96)	Rank of Region	Excess Admissions in U.S. According to HRR Benchmark	Medical Specialist Visits per Enrollee in the Last Six Months of Life (1995-96)	Rank of Region	Excess Visits in U.S. According to HRR Benchmark	Generalists per 100,000 Residents (1996)	Rank of Region	Excess Generalists in U.S. According to HRR Benchmark	Selected Specialists per 100,000 Residents (1996)	Rank of Region	Excess Selected Specialists in U.S. According to HRR Benchmark
Owensboro	266.7	31	51,627	33.2	89	33,343	10.3	99	205,615	40.9	300	63,343	87.5	223	55,232
Paducah	282.2	13	15,217	33.4	82	31,497	7.2	200	400,871	50.2	267	39,460	80.6	271	71,490
Louisiana															
Alexandria	307.0	6	3,506	27.5	202	103,791	9.8	111	231,862	59.5	159	20,370	94.1	163	42,227
Baton Rouge	254.1	49	132,159	36.1	47	16,460	9.0	127	268,850	52.7	249	33,666	86.9	231	56,477
Houma	278.8	17	19,524	29.1	173	78,862	9.8	112	232,010	37.0	303	73,608	88.9	200	52,305
Lafayette	262.1	38	74,852	32.1	108	42,713	7.2	202	402,454	48.2	283	44,645	81.9	262	68,309
Lake Charles	296.8	8	6,935	27.0	212	113,584	10.9	87	182,160	43.9	295	55,483	83.0	255	65,630
Metairie	275.4	20	26,263	31.6	118	47,121	14.5	31	80,347	68.5	68	9,542	158.6	5	632
Monroe	327.9	2	133	37.8	34	10,311	10.1	103	214,278	49.9	270	40,330	80.0	276	73,096
New Orleans	253.6	52	135,820	32.8	99	36,640	15.1	24	68,673	59.4	161	20,404	138.6	22	4,889
Shreveport	265.9	32	55,480	31.3	125	50,778	8.5	149	302,778	47.9	284	45,197	97.0	148	37,042
Slidell	320.8	3	992	33.6	77	29,867	12.4	58	128,354	46.7	287	48,334	105.4	91	25,085
Maine															
Bangor	248.0	65	192,476	26.7	221	117,495	5.8	243	525,875	65.4	90	12,312	94.3	161	41,800
Portland	215.9	174	967,725	23.1	274	190,744	6.2	233	490,472	73.0	41	6,554	111.4	66	18,946
Maryland															
Baltimore	260.2	42	85,814	30.1	150	64,273	8.7	134	286,294	82.6	23	2,263	145.6	16	2,697
Salisbury	223.9	144	700,104	25.4	244	144,269	12.9	48	115,202	62.6	126	15,651	114.6	58	16,154
Takoma Park	213.7	177	1,046,500	33.2	91	33,409	21.5	7	8,094	92.2	7	656	156.4	8	764
Massachusetts															
Boston	237.7	94	339,924	28.1	192	94,684	9.0	126	267,806	84.7	12	1,644	151.4	12	1,346
Springfield	202.3	224	1,535,969	22.5	279	202,650	5.7	245	535,768	71.9	47	7,221	114.9	55	15,862
Worcester	235.2	111	393,703	26.9	217	114,651	6.3	229	483,960	81.2	26	2,826	117.6	49	14,025
Michigan															
Ann Arbor	230.5	124	508,666	37.1	40	12,633	8.4	151	305,057	66.3	81	11,435	105.9	86	24,502
Dearborn	240.4	87	292,848	42.6	7	2,850	12.0	63	140,098	60.9	142	18,199	97.7	142	35,890
Detroit	240.7	86	288,876	34.1	70	26,704	11.3	77	165,828	61.2	139	17,713	99.0	132	33,788
Flint	240.9	85	284,766	36.0	51	16,933	12.0	65	142,470	71.6	48	7,361	78.8	281	76,099
Grand Rapids	185.6	272	2,376,003	28.4	187	89,054	4.4	280	671,148	57.4	192	23,877	84.5	245	62,179
Kalamazoo	196.4	246	1,816,626	27.7	199	100,345	6.3	227	481,179	60.2	146	19,173	93.2	173	43,767
Lansing	216.3	171	953,021	27.7	197	100,172	6.8	215	436,213	68.0	75	9,927	93.3	172	43,569
Marquette	219.2	158	852,027	24.8	255	156,334	3.4	299	783,301	59.5	157	20,276	82.9	256	65,938
Muskegon	171.0	293	3,181,685	24.0	261	172,337	3.1	300	813,048	63.7	113	14,239	82.1	260	67,876
Petoskey	196.0	248	1,835,973	28.3	189	90,415	5.4	253	567,470	65.3	92	12,425	91.5	185	47,048
Pontiac	249.0	63	181,125	30.3	147	62,125	10.9	86	182,081	84.2	17	1,772	146.5	15	2,435
Royal Oak	223.9	143	698,564	30.1	152	64,414	13.9	34	90,123	102.9	2	23	160.9	3	563
Saginaw	242.8	74	257,852	33.0	93	34,554	7.2	197	395,854	59.9	153	19,731	85.1	240	60,810
St Joseph	201.8	226	1,557,220	27.7	198	100,184	3.0	302	818,916	58.1	180	22,691	93.9	167	42,479
Traverse City	221.9	151	762,683	26.9	219	115,248	5.8	242	523,258	70.1	56	8,338	98.9	133	33,880
Minnesota															
Duluth	202.4	223	1,531,151	26.3	229	124,843	4.0	287	710,080	69.4	60	8,869	86.3	235	58,006
Minneapolis	205.9	213	1,372,215	22.8	276	196,491	3.8	290	730,748	68.0	76	9,951	87.4	226	55,395
Rochester	202.2	225	1,542,457	25.8	236	134,422	3.7	294	749,826	70.4	54	8,139	110.5	70	19,718
St Cloud	215.9	173	966,582	25.3	246	145,352	7.3	195	390,958	64.6	101	13,154	77.2	287	80,097
St Paul	217.2	164	921,296	28.7	185	85,347	5.5	249	553,911	80.4	28	3,143	91.9	181	46,239

Hospital Referral Region	Hospitalizations for All Medical Conditions per 1,000 Medicare Enrollees (1995-96)	Rank of Region	Excess Hospitalizations in U.S. According to HRR Benchmark	Percent of Medicare Enrollees Admitted to Intensive Care in the Last Six Months of Life (1995-96)	Rank of Region	Excess Admissions in U.S. According to HRR Benchmark	Medical Specialist Visits per Enrollee in the Last Six Months of Life (1995-96)	Rank of Region	Excess Visits in U.S. According to HRR Benchmark	Generalists per 100,000 Residents (1996)	Rank of Region	Excess Generalists in U.S. According to HRR Benchmark	Selected Specialists per 100,000 Residents (1996)	Rank of Region	Excess Selected Specialists in U.S. According to HRR Benchmark
Mississippi															
Gulfport	301.4	7	5,274	37.9	32	9,990	14.9	27	72,789	46.1	289	50,040	112.9	63	17,601
Hattiesburg	311.3	4	2,455	27.2	207	109,961	12.8	51	117,146	42.6	297	58,984	87.2	229	55,998
Jackson	285.0	11	12,554	27.1	208	110,887	7.5	189	372,772	52.3	251	34,535	85.4	239	60,057
Meridian	330.3	1	0	26.9	215	114,527	12.9	49	115,331	54.3	224	29,941	78.1	285	77,880
Oxford	310.3	5	2,662	26.7	223	118,022	8.3	158	315,753	50.2	268	39,572	81.6	265	68,990
Tupelo	273.7	22	30,151	31.5	122	48,440	7.3	194	389,942	46.1	290	50,042	69.6	302	99,651
Missouri															
Cape Girardeau	218.1	162	890,492	33.6	79	30,335	4.7	270	636,278	48.4	279	43,977	79.9	277	73,223
Columbia	233.7	115	430,803	31.7	116	46,605	9.3	122	254,088	59.4	160	20,390	86.0	237	58,592
Joplin	259.6	44	89,739	28.4	188	89,351	4.6	276	651,916	58.4	176	22,151	83.1	253	65,376
Kansas City	235.8	108	379,217	34.0	72	27,448	9.3	121	252,957	65.1	94	12,585	99.5	129	32,970
Springfield	210.6	195	1,169,280	27.6	200	102,195	6.2	231	484,962	55.7	205	27,134	78.6	282	76,502
St Louis	231.3	121	488,456	33.4	83	31,522	6.7	218	442,549	63.5	116	14,501	104.7	95	25,922
Montana															
Billings	226.8	139	614,420	21.0	293	237,123	4.8	269	630,802	65.0	96	12,716	100.8	122	30,930
Great Falls	261.2	40	80,105	26.8	220	116,599	7.8	173	347,179	61.8	133	16,833	104.4	97	26,287
Missoula	232.5	117	458,640	22.5	281	203,962	6.0	239	511,382	64.3	107	13,535	116.6	50	14,711
Nebraska															
Lincoln	179.4	282	2,712,169	20.6	295	245,725	4.9	264	614,980	56.3	199	25,939	70.7	300	96,796
Omaha	212.9	182	1,077,999	29.1	174	78,931	8.8	131	280,492	58.6	170	21,706	88.7	202	52,631
Nevada															
Las Vegas	206.1	210	1,363,077	34.7	62	23,131	15.3	21	66,257	47.4	286	46,532	88.2	210	53,676
Reno	189.5	263	2,171,316	24.4	257	163,592	7.7	182	358,942	59.6	155	20,074	107.0	81	23,301
New Hampshire															
Lebanon	201.5	229	1,573,602	21.9	287	216,835	2.6	303	867,490	74.2	35	5,940	114.3	59	16,364
Manchester	186.7	270	2,319,474	22.7	277	198,690	5.2	256	587,632	64.4	103	13,319	110.7	68	19,569
New Jersey															
Camden	240.1	88	297,346	35.9	52	17,406	16.7	18	46,955	73.5	38	6,293	126.0	33	9,537
Hackensack	228.8	136	554,854	32.6	100	37,829	17.3	15	39,288	99.9	4	104	173.1	2	294
Morristown	218.3	160	881,308	31.6	119	47,495	15.6	19	62,265	83.7	19	1,908	142.5	19	3,631
New Brunswick	237.5	97	344,621	40.3	17	5,087	22.5	4	3,885	82.8	22	2,216	130.3	27	7,734
Newark	262.7	37	71,718	43.9	6	1,833	23.8	2	1,016	74.7	33	5,694	119.4	45	12,861
Paterson	237.8	93	337,953	32.9	97	35,280	21.9	5	5,996	69.0	66	9,092	104.8	94	25,765
Ridgewood	234.9	112	400,572	29.6	161	71,100	21.0	8	10,213	84.6	14	1,651	159.3	4	610
New Mexico															
Albuquerque	212.5	185	1,093,014	26.6	225	119,567	5.0	262	605,717	71.0	52	7,755	108.5	74	21,697
New York															
Albany	223.1	147	723,103	26.4	228	124,737	11.5	72	156,202	66.2	82	11,480	118.5	47	13,421
Binghamton	224.2	142	690,106	25.1	248	148,868	7.5	190	375,326	58.5	172	21,894	102.9	103	28,108
Bronx	246.1	68	214,002	26.9	216	114,588	14.0	32	89,003	66.7	80	11,045	113.3	61	17,230
Buffalo	216.9	167	929,139	28.8	183	83,778	7.8	177	350,918	67.1	78	10,717	108.1	76	22,106
Elmira	238.3	91	329,699	28.9	179	81,945	7.7	184	359,541	59.1	163	21,005	113.4	60	17,162
East Long Island	222.7	149	735,222	30.6	141	58,573	18.3	13	27,898	96.4	6	269	154.3	10	949
New York	237.0	99	353,598	30.5	143	58,981	18.0	14	30,904	84.6	13	1,651	150.0	13	1,603
Rochester	211.8	188	1,120,098	25.7	238	137,279	4.6	274	643,712	72.6	43	6,807	108.3	75	21,906

Hospital Referral Region	Hospitalizations for All Medical Conditions per 1,000 Medicare Enrollees (1995-96)	Rank of Region	Excess Hospitalizations in U.S. According to HRR Benchmark	Percent of Medicare Enrollees Admitted to Intensive Care in the Last Six Months of Life (1995-96)	Rank of Region	Excess Admissions in U.S. According to HRR Benchmark	Medical Specialist Visits per Enrollee in the Last Six Months of Life (1995-96)	Rank of Region	Excess Visits in U.S. According to HRR Benchmark	Generalists per 100,000 Residents (1996)	Rank of Region	Excess Generalists in U.S. According to HRR Benchmark	Selected Specialists per 100,000 Residents (1996)	Rank of Region	Excess Selected Specialists in U.S. According to HRR Benchmark
Syracuse	218.7	159	868,431	26.2	231	128,473	8.3	157	311,733	57.7	186	23,301	102.0	110	29,292
White Plains	241.3	82	278,478	30.0	155	65,946	13.8	38	93,523	105.1	1	0	200.8	1	0
North Carolina															
Asheville	211.4	192	1,135,972	28.0	194	96,401	4.9	265	620,285	67.6	77	10,280	101.1	118	30,494
Charlotte	205.9	212	1,370,282	33.9	74	28,125	6.1	236	502,803	53.2	243	32,422	94.0	165	42,262
Durham	199.1	234	1,685,373	29.7	160	70,904	7.2	198	398,671	53.6	238	31,612	100.8	123	31,038
Greensboro	202.5	222	1,525,586	31.5	123	48,474	6.0	240	511,983	55.2	210	28,185	92.9	175	44,307
Greenville	222.5	150	742,119	33.0	94	34,610	5.9	241	522,621	52.0	255	35,348	93.1	174	44,057
Hickory	201.6	228	1,568,720	33.8	75	28,902	6.0	237	505,552	47.7	285	45,826	80.9	270	70,753
Raleigh	214.4	176	1,020,262	32.1	109	42,939	7.2	196	395,693	53.9	234	30,773	92.8	176	44,528
Wilmington	217.1	165	925,304	30.1	149	64,078	7.0	209	418,935	54.0	230	30,666	98.8	135	34,017
Winston-Salem	223.8	145	702,647	32.2	106	41,685	7.9	168	342,090	49.1	275	42,290	87.9	217	54,394
North Dakota															
Bismarck	236.6	102	362,567	21.7	289	221,950	6.1	234	494,971	54.4	223	29,784	88.7	204	52,729
Fargo Moorhead -Mn	194.5	250	1,910,273	22.1	284	212,602	4.8	268	630,536	60.4	145	18,895	68.8	303	101,767
Grand Forks	212.8	183	1,082,637	21.0	292	235,493	4.0	286	708,990	65.8	86	11,870	71.8	299	93,975
Minot	231.0	123	496,755	23.5	266	181,884	4.4	279	666,225	69.1	63	9,053	88.4	207	53,239
Ohio															
Akron	256.1	47	115,766	35.3	56	20,081	11.9	67	142,978	65.3	91	12,404	101.0	119	30,657
Canton	209.9	200	1,196,836	36.0	49	16,904	8.5	147	301,463	54.2	227	30,124	84.6	244	61,969
Cincinnati	216.4	170	947,922	26.4	227	124,499	8.4	152	305,476	64.8	100	12,944	110.2	71	20,045
Cleveland	236.7	100	359,242	37.2	38	12,255	11.2	80	168,378	71.0	51	7,742	120.6	41	12,156
Columbus	229.2	132	541,940	32.9	98	35,812	7.0	208	415,114	57.9	184	22,996	87.5	222	55,206
Dayton	211.6	189	1,126,675	30.1	153	65,152	8.7	136	288,081	55.3	208	28,006	80.3	274	72,308
Elyria	236.5	104	363,791	40.6	15	4,701	12.5	56	126,905	56.6	197	25,496	95.1	155	40,298
Kettering	197.5	243	1,761,760	31.0	130	53,444	11.3	78	166,038	76.7	31	4,781	116.2	51	14,954
Toledo	231.1	122	493,531	36.2	45	15,990	11.4	74	161,104	63.6	115	14,416	100.1	127	31,987
Youngstown	241.2	83	280,748	38.3	27	9,000	10.9	84	181,612	66.1	83	11,563	95.7	152	39,227
Oklahoma															
Lawton	225.9	140	640,071	26.9	213	113,967	6.4	223	466,616	62.6	125	15,641	81.5	267	69,282
Oklahoma City	229.0	134	549,709	27.7	196	99,944	8.1	159	325,324	58.0	181	22,881	90.8	188	48,508
Tulsa	208.1	208	1,277,154	25.9	234	133,499	8.9	129	275,405	62.8	124	15,377	87.7	220	54,873
Oregon															
Bend	155.5	304	4,068,473	16.6	304	336,088	4.6	275	649,914	60.2	148	19,271	101.6	113	29,886
Eugene	173.9	290	3,019,201	18.4	298	294,055	3.4	298	777,216	70.1	57	8,359	96.8	149	37,450
Medford	160.3	302	3,796,427	20.8	294	241,532	3.9	289	717,918	62.5	130	15,817	92.2	180	45,795
Portland	172.2	291	3,115,819	21.9	286	216,319	3.7	293	743,457	68.0	74	9,902	107.6	78	22,637
Salem	134.3	306	5,294,317	29.0	178	80,849	5.1	261	601,231	57.4	191	23,832	98.0	139	35,414
Pennsylvania															
Allentown	242.4	77	262,761	32.1	107	42,521	13.9	33	89,905	64.0	109	13,856	101.4	114	30,166
Altoona	242.3	78	264,674	33.3	86	32,181	7.1	204	405,454	53.2	242	32,328	84.5	246	62,243
Danville	230.3	127	513,627	25.6	241	140,230	7.6	186	361,908	60.9	141	18,092	94.8	159	40,942
Erie	241.4	81	277,651	28.9	180	82,168	8.1	160	329,739	54.2	228	30,272	93.9	166	42,442
Harrisburg	208.3	207	1,267,621	29.3	167	75,436	7.8	174	348,097	65.6	87	12,098	93.7	168	42,871
Johnstown	286.7	10	11,571	32.5	102	39,001	6.9	211	421,152	66.1	84	11,647	101.0	120	30,677
Lancaster	206.0	211	1,366,285	29.9	157	67,715	12.2	61	136,303	59.3	162	20,669	87.7	219	54,866

Hospital Referral Region	Hospitalizations for All Medical Conditions per 1,000 Medicare Enrollees (1995-96)	Rank of Region	Excess Hospitalizations in U.S. According to HRR Benchmark	Percent of Medicare Enrollees Admitted to Intensive Care in the Last Six Months of Life (1995-96)	Rank of Region	Excess Admissions in U.S. According to HRR Benchmark	Medical Specialist Visits per Enrollee in the Last Six Months of Life (1995-96)	Rank of Region	Excess Visits in U.S. According to HRR Benchmark	Generalists per 100,000 Residents (1996)	Rank of Region	Excess Generalists in U.S. According to HRR Benchmark	Selected Specialists per 100,000 Residents (1996))	Rank of Region	Excess Selected Specialists in U.S. According to HRR Benchmark
Philadelphia	250.3	60	167,774	38.1	30	9,527	19.3	12	20,233	89.4	8	948	147.4	14	2,193
Pittsburgh	268.5	26	43,930	35.3	55	19,824	13.3	43	105,113	64.5	102	13,251	110.6	69	19,638
Reading	221.3	152	780,993	28.0	193	95,477	7.7	181	356,590	62.4	131	16,032	91.4	186	47,205
Sayre	252.8	55	143,093	25.4	242	142,304	5.7	246	535,990	58.1	179	22,639	89.5	198	50,991
Scranton	236.6	103	362,740	25.6	240	139,520	13.9	36	90,345	69.6	59	8,674	104.9	93	25,623
Wilkes-Barre	229.2	133	542,000	29.7	159	70,359	10.7	91	191,358	78.6	29	3,929	107.4	80	22,843
York	197.8	242	1,750,269	31.8	115	45,287	6.1	235	502,547	64.3	106	13,445	86.6	233	57,261
Rhode Island															
Providence	216.9	168	930,383	24.7	256	157,504	9.3	120	252,188	72.4	44	6,902	122.7	36	11,068
South Carolina															
Charleston	221.2	154	787,072	31.7	117	46,633	9.4	116	248,244	57.9	183	22,994	108.7	73	21,545
Columbia	196.0	249	1,838,067	29.1	176	79,408	8.4	150	304,298	55.1	211	28,378	95.9	151	38,926
Florence	259.5	45	90,941	32.0	112	43,652	7.9	164	339,159	50.9	263	37,807	72.0	298	93,535
Greenville	194.4	253	1,919,753	30.5	144	59,449	8.0	161	338,061	58.8	167	21,389	94.2	162	41,984
Spartanburg	211.0	194	1,152,531	37.2	39	12,274	8.6	144	296,025	51.4	258	36,737	84.6	243	61,779
South Dakota															
Rapid City	220.4	157	812,580	23.2	272	188,640	6.2	230	484,645	71.6	49	7,387	88.6	205	52,957
Sioux Falls	223.1	148	724,204	24.2	259	167,629	4.2	282	690,714	63.6	114	14,326	74.8	292	86,136
Tennessee															
Chattanooga	248.4	64	188,442	35.2	57	20,464	8.7	133	285,769	55.8	203	27,016	92.5	177	45,182
Jackson	247.8	66	194,330	36.0	48	16,904	8.5	145	298,126	55.0	214	28,592	72.1	297	93,183
Johnson City	239.9	89	301,480	31.0	128	53,353	6.7	217	438,309	72.0	46	7,114	103.5	99	27,442
Kingsport	280.9	14	16,591	36.1	46	16,412	4.8	267	624,765	62.5	129	15,800	88.7	203	52,650
Knoxville	259.9	43	88,240	33.3	87	32,367	9.8	110	230,318	60.1	149	19,283	91.0	187	48,063
Memphis	242.5	76	261,811	30.9	134	54,632	13.4	42	102,397	49.5	274	41,288	87.9	215	54,369
Nashville	267.5	29	47,898	33.6	78	29,963	7.8	175	349,114	57.7	189	23,453	98.1	136	35,232
Texas															
Abilene	253.3	53	138,863	30.0	156	66,628	7.9	165	339,312	55.8	202	27,011	88.1	213	53,991
Amarillo	232.3	118	462,499	30.8	138	56,410	8.4	155	309,247	54.0	232	30,695	86.4	234	57,649
Austin	203.7	217	1,472,228	25.3	247	145,386	10.2	101	211,039	62.6	127	15,737	103.4	100	27,550
Beaumont	284.8	12	12,747	43.9	5	1,796	14.9	25	71,936	55.7	204	27,090	93.5	171	43,238
Bryan	208.8	206	1,244,076	26.0	232	132,266	4.7	272	639,314	58.7	168	21,574	77.9	286	78,376
Corpus Christi	264.2	36	63,828	35.5	53	18,900	9.7	113	236,644	55.1	212	28,406	87.7	218	54,691
Dallas	213.3	179	1,060,831	30.7	139	56,869	11.9	66	142,670	54.0	233	30,712	100.3	125	31,703
El Paso	211.8	187	1,119,654	38.1	29	9,454	11.3	76	163,255	41.6	299	61,527	87.9	216	54,380
Fort Worth	197.8	241	1,750,181	32.9	96	35,199	9.4	118	249,538	53.0	245	32,976	87.5	225	55,298
Harlingen	235.8	109	381,320	42.6	8	2,910	13.6	40	96,652	34.0	305	81,334	58.1	305	129,698
Houston	241.8	79	271,774	37.8	35	10,342	14.8	30	73,956	53.4	240	32,046	101.2	116	30,384
Longview	220.8	156	799,220	40.8	13	4,580	13.6	41	98,023	48.9	276	42,766	81.7	264	68,862
Lubbock	265.2	33	58,486	37.9	31	9,845	12.9	46	113,516	54.5	221	29,534	87.4	227	55,469
McAllen	245.8	69	217,908	40.7	14	4,597	20.4	9	13,796	33.8	306	81,956	46.7	306	159,637
Odessa	249.3	62	177,743	39.8	20	5,887	6.8	216	436,949	36.4	304	75,153	78.4	283	77,058
San Angelo	243.4	73	248,955	30.6	140	57,763	6.4	225	473,684	50.7	264	38,317	95.4	153	39,823
San Antonio	223.3	146	717,369	34.7	64	23,494	11.1	81	170,626	55.9	201	26,866	107.5	79	22,761
Temple	209.2	203	1,225,776	25.1	249	149,699	5.4	252	563,294	44.9	294	53,043	70.4	301	97,511
Tyler	235.6	110	385,494	30.8	136	56,247	6.8	213	429,355	57.9	182	22,987	95.1	154	40,278

Hospital Referral Region	Hospitalizations for All Medical Conditions per 1,000 Medicare Enrollees (1995-96)	Rank of Region	Excess Hospitalizations in U.S. According to HRR Benchmark	Percent of Medicare Enrollees Admitted to Intensive Care in the Last Six Months of Life (1995-96)	Rank of Region	Excess Admissions in U.S. According to HRR Benchmark	Medical Specialist Visits per Enrollee in the Last Six Months of Life (1995-96)	Rank of Region	Excess Visits in U.S. According to HRR Benchmark	Generalists per 100,000 Residents (1996)	Rank of Region	Excess Generalists in U.S. According to HRR Benchmark	Selected Specialists per 100,000 Residents (1996)	Rank of Region	Excess Selected Specialists in U.S. According to HRR Benchmark
Victoria	279.5	16	18,499	30.1	154	65,286	9.2	125	260,880	54.9	215	28,712	90.1	192	49,917
Waco	189.3	264	2,179,725	23.4	269	185,313	4.0	288	717,450	54.9	218	28,852	86.0	238	58,656
Wichita Falls	234.7	114	406,913	27.5	204	104,394	10.1	106	217,934	60.1	150	19,423	102.4	108	28,777
Utah															
Ogden	151.7	305	4,290,892	22.6	278	200,693	2.6	304	869,130	41.7	298	61,359	84.1	249	63,014
Provo	168.0	298	3,355,438	23.2	271	188,046	6.0	238	508,691	43.5	296	56,600	81.6	266	69,200
Salt Lake City	165.0	299	3,525,545	20.6	296	246,328	3.6	297	760,829	48.3	281	44,271	99.1	131	33,537
Vermont															
Burlington	227.2	137	600,059	26.5	226	121,473	4.5	277	656,035	74.0	36	6,024	106.6	83	23,735
Virginia															
Arlington	202.9	220	1,506,342	27.9	195	96,721	14.9	28	72,811	70.2	55	8,307	119.6	44	12,739
Charlottesville	233.7	116	430,837	29.1	177	79,463	7.0	206	411,881	63.1	120	15,022	110.7	67	19,528
Lynchburg	199.4	232	1,672,441	34.8	60	22,910	6.3	228	482,293	53.6	237	31,476	82.0	261	68,101
Newport News	203.6	218	1,474,344	36.6	43	14,592	17.2	16	40,166	62.3	132	16,088	105.9	87	24,561
Norfolk	216.8	169	933,133	35.5	54	19,213	8.9	128	273,521	63.1	121	15,027	115.1	54	15,754
Richmond	229.4	129	536,469	30.1	151	64,312	10.2	102	212,987	63.7	112	14,212	98.0	138	35,372
Roanoke	236.0	107	376,131	30.8	137	56,249	8.6	143	295,890	63.0	122	15,166	101.2	117	30,435
Winchester	269.5	25	41,183	24.3	258	164,719	7.8	171	346,202	51.2	261	37,075	98.9	134	33,926
Washington															
Everett	169.8	295	3,251,734	21.3	290	229,004	5.1	258	597,799	65.1	93	12,532	97.1	145	36,861
Olympia	169.3	297	3,280,593	27.3	206	107,895	5.4	251	562,501	63.0	123	15,188	95.1	156	40,420
Seattle	176.1	288	2,895,287	25.9	233	133,251	7.4	192	382,245	80.9	27	2,942	119.7	43	12,680
Spokane	184.8	274	2,417,748	22.9	275	195,025	5.1	259	600,116	65.8	85	11,865	94.9	158	40,671
Tacoma	157.4	303	3,962,530	29.2	170	77,292	6.4	224	467,036	59.8	154	19,843	102.8	104	28,312
Yakima	183.1	278	2,509,846	25.4	243	143,125	4.7	271	636,944	63.7	111	14,190	88.1	214	54,013
West Virginia															
Charleston	274.2	21	29,067	31.0	132	53,663	7.9	169	343,362	65.5	88	12,154	89.5	199	51,101
Huntington	268.1	28	45,688	24.8	253	155,828	10.5	98	199,444	61.5	136	17,257	94.1	164	42,239
Morgantown	262.0	39	75,506	37.5	37	11,221	6.8	214	433,627	64.9	99	12,834	97.0	146	36,986
Wisconsin															
Appleton	176.8	285	2,858,701	21.3	291	230,642	4.5	278	657,408	58.4	175	22,132	75.2	291	85,239
Green Bay	192.4	258	2,021,101	24.1	260	169,013	4.9	263	614,055	51.9	256	35,419	81.3	268	69,763
La Crosse	208.9	204	1,240,753	22.3	283	208,401	3.0	301	816,987	60.8	143	18,278	86.8	232	56,720
Madison	208.8	205	1,243,247	23.9	262	172,913	4.2	283	692,502	69.1	65	9,066	88.8	201	52,562
Marshfield	211.4	191	1,134,262	22.0	285	213,600	6.5	222	461,261	68.2	73	9,735	91.5	184	47,033
Milwaukee	209.6	201	1,210,704	27.6	201	103,246	8.6	139	291,303	64.4	104	13,352	109.5	72	20,717
Neenah	198.2	240	1,727,092	18.5	297	293,222	4.3	281	675,170	57.0	193	24,724	96.4	150	38,109
Wausau	185.1	273	2,403,888	16.9	303	329,864	3.6	296	751,325	65.0	95	12,641	92.3	179	45,550
Wyoming															
Casper	242.6	75	259,849	24.9	252	153,762	3.7	295	749,990	69.6	58	8,672	100.2	126	31,926
HMO															
										46.2		49,600	80.1		72,898
United States															
	227.1		604,007	31.4		49,829	10.3		205,094	65.0		12,646	108.4		21,841

Appendices

Appendix on Methods

1. The Geography of Health Care in The United States

1.1 Files Used in the Atlas

The Atlas depends on the integrated use of databases provided by the American Hospital Association (AHA), the American Medical Association, the American Osteopathic Association, and several federal agencies, including the Agency for Health Care Policy and Research, the Bureau of the Census, the Health Care Financing Administration, the National Center for Health Statistics, and the Department of Veterans Affairs. Table 1 lists these files and provides a short description of the uses made of them in the Atlas.

TABLE 1.

Data Files Used in Analysis

File	Year Used (Sample)	Source / Provider	Description and Use in Analyses
Medicare Files			
Denominator File	1995 & 1996 (100%)	HCFA	Contains one record for each Medicare beneficiary, and includes demographic information (age, sex, race), residence (ZIP Code), program eligibility and mortality. Used to determine denominators for utilization rates and to determine mortality.
MEDPAR File	1995 & 1996 (100%)	HCFA	One record for each hospital stay by Medicare beneficiaries. Includes data on dates of admission / discharge, diagnoses, procedures and Medicare reimbursements to the hospital. Used for (1) allocation of acute care resources and physicians and (2) numerators for utilization rates.
Continuous Medicare History Sample File	1995 (5%)	HCFA	Includes a record for each beneficiary in a 5% sample for each year. Includes summary expenditure data. Used to estimate Medicare spending by program component.
Medicare Provider of Services File	1997	HCFA	Includes a record for each hospital eligible to provide inpatient care through Medicare. Includes location and resource data. Used in measuring acute care resource investments.
Medicare Cost Reports	1994	HCFA	Includes a record for each hospital and provides detailed accounting data for the specified year. Used in measuring acute care resource investments.
Part B Standard Analytical Variable Length File	1995 & 1996 (5%)	HCFA	Includes physician/supplier claims for services paid by the Part B program in 1995b and 96. A majority of services are provided in office, inpatient, outpatient, home, and nursing home settings. Used to measure physician visit rates, and rates of certain diagnostic procedures and preventive services.

TABLE 1. (CONTINUED)

File	Year Used	Source/Provider	Description and Use in Analyses
Resource Files			
American Hospital Association Annual Survey of Hospitals	1996	American Hospital Association	Includes a record for each hospital registered with the AHA. Used in measuring acute care resources (beds, personnel).
Physician File	1995	American Medical Association	Includes one record for each allopathic physician with practice ZIP Code, self-designated specialty, major professional activities, and federal / non-federal status. Used to determine specialty-specific counts of physicians in each health care market.
Osteopath File	1995	American Osteopathic Association	Includes one record for each osteopathic physician with practice ZIP Code, self-designated specialty, major professional activities, and federal / non-federal status. Used to determine specialty-specific counts of physicians in each health care market.
Federal hospital utilization and resources	1993-1994	U.S. Medicine Directory 1993-94 ISSN 0890-6637	Provides location, counts and occupancy rates of federal hospital beds.
VA patient travel pattern file	1989	VA Outcomes Group, White River Jct VA	ZIP Code level patient origin file for veterans using VA hospitals in 1989. Used to allocate VA physicians to appropriate HSAs.
UPIN File	1996	HCFA	Provides unique physician identifier, their primary and secondary specialties and zip code locations of practice, credentials, age, and licensing state. Used in the analysis of physician visit rates.
Other Files			
Geographic Practice Cost Index	1993	HCFA	Records for each MSA and non-MSA area of each state. Records include area-level values for each of the components of the GPCI (physician work, practice cost, malpractice) and summary index value. Used for price adjustment.
National Hospital Discharge Survey	1989	NTIS	Provides age-sex specific hospital discharge rates for the U.S. as a whole, which were used as the basis for the age-sex adjustment of acute care resources.
National Ambulatory Medical Care Survey (NAMCS)	1989-1994	NTIS	Ambulatory services from samples of patient records selected from a national sample of office-based physicians. Allows estimation of age-sex specific use rates by specialty. Used for age-sex adjustment of physician workforce.
Population files	1998	Claritas, Inc., Arlington, VA	1990 STF3 data from the U.S. Bureau of the Census was adapted by Claritas, Inc. to 1997 ZIP Code geography; includes 1998 age-sex specific estimated counts of residents in the ZIP Code. Used (1) for age-sex adjustment, (2) as denominator for rates of allocated and adjusted resources.
ZIP Code boundary files	1997	Geographic Data Technology, Lebanon, NH	Includes records for each ZIP Code with the coordinates of the boundary precisely specified. Used as basis for mapping HSAs and HRRs and for assigning ZIP Codes appropriately.

1.2 Defining Hospital Service Areas

Hospital Service Areas (HSAs) represent local health care markets for community-based inpatient care. The definitions of HSAs used in the 1996 edition of the Atlas were retained in the 1999 edition. HSAs were originally defined in three steps using 1993 provider files and 1992-93 utilization data. First, all acute care hospitals in the 50 states and the District of Columbia were identified from the American Hospital Association Annual Survey of Hospitals and the Medicare Provider of Services files and assigned to a location within a town or city. The list of towns or cities with at least one acute care hospital (N=3,953) defined the maximum number of possible HSAs. Second, all 1992 and 1993 acute care hospitalizations of the Medicare population were analyzed according to ZIP Code to determine the proportion of residents' hospital stays that occurred in each of the 3,953 candidate HSAs. ZIP Codes were initially assigned to the HSA where the greatest proportion (plurality) of residents were hospitalized. Approximately 500 of the candidate HSAs did not qualify as independent HSAs because the plurality of patients resident in those HSAs were hospitalized in other HSAs.

The third step required visual examination of the ZIP Codes used to define each HSA. Maps of ZIP Code boundaries were made using files obtained from Geographic Data Technologies (GDT) and each HSA's component ZIP Codes were examined. In order to achieve contiguity of the component ZIP Codes for each HSA, "island" ZIP Codes were reassigned to the enclosing HSA, and/or HSAs were grouped into larger HSAs (See the Appendix on the Geography of Health Care in the United States for an illustration). Certain ZIP Codes used in the Medicare files were restricted in their use to specific institutions (e.g., a nursing home) or a post office. These "point ZIPs" were assigned to their enclosing ZIP Code based on the ZIP Code boundary map.

This process resulted in the identification of 3,436 HSAs, ranging in total 1996 population from 604 (Turtle Lake, North Dakota) to 3,067,356 (Houston) in the 1999 edition of the Atlas. Thus, the HSA boundaries remained the same but the HSA populations might have changed between the two editions of the Atlas. In most HSAs, the majority of Medicare hospitalizations occurred in a hospital or hospitals located within the HSA. See the Appendix on the Geography of Health Care in the United States for further details.

1.3 Defining Hospital Referral Regions

Hospital referral regions (HRRs) represent health care markets for tertiary medical care. As defined previously in the 1996 Atlas, each HRR contained at least one HSA that had a hospital or hospitals that performed major cardiovascular procedures and neurosurgery in 1992-93. Three steps were taken to define HRRs.

First, the candidate hospitals and HRRs were identified. A total of 862 hospitals performed at least 10 major cardiovascular procedures (DRGs 103-107) on Medicare enrollees in both years. These hospitals were located within 458 HSAs, thereby defining the maximum number of possible HRRs. Further checks verified that all 458 HSAs included at least one hospital performing the specified major neurosurgical procedures (DRGs 1-3 and 484).

Second, we calculated in each of the 3,436 HSAs in the United States the proportion of major cardiovascular procedures performed in each of the 458 candidate HRRs in 1992-93. Each HSA was then assigned provisionally to the candidate HRR where most patients went for these services.

Third, HSAs were reassigned or further grouped to achieve (a) geographic contiguity, unless major travel routes (e.g., interstate highways) justified separation (this occurred in only two cases, the New Haven, Connecticut, and Elmira, New York, HRRs); (b) a minimum population size of 120,000; and (c) a high localization index. Because of the large number of hospitals providing cardiovascular services in California, several candidate California HRRs met the above criteria but were found to perform small numbers of cardiovascular procedures. These HRRs were further aggregated according to county boundaries to achieve stability of cardiovascular surgery rates within the areas.

The process resulted in the definition of 306 hospital referral regions which ranged in total 1996 population from 126,329 (Minot, North Dakota) to 9,288,694 (Los Angeles) in the 1999 edition of the Atlas. See the Appendix on the Geography of Health Care in the United States for further details.

1.4 Populations of HSAs and HRRs

Total population counts were estimated for residents of all ages in each HSA using either 1995 or 1998 ZIP Code level files obtained from GDT and Claritas, Inc. The Claritas file is based on the latest U.S. Census STF3B ZIP Code file, updated to account for changes in ZIP Code definitions. Population counts for HRRs are the sum of the counts of the constituent HSAs. These serve as denominators for estimating rates for hospital resource (1998) and physician workforce (1995) allocations.

For rates that apply to the Medicare population for the years 1995-96, enrollee counts were obtained from the Medicare Denominator file. The 1995 and 1996 Medicare enrollee population included those alive and age 65 to age 99 on June 30, 1995 and 1996, respectively. For preventive services and physician visit rates, the population above was further restricted to a 5% sample of Medicare enrollees having Medicare part B physician claims for 1995-96, who were selected on the basis of the terminal digits in the Social Security number; for each year, we included only those enrolled in Medicare part B on June 30, 1995 and 1996, respectively. For Medicare reimbursement rates, the Medicare population above was restricted to a 5% sample of 1996 enrollees, selected on the basis of Social Security numbers, belonging to both Medicare A and B programs. For all rates, the numerator and the denominator counts exclude those who were enrolled in risk bearing HMOs on June 30.

2. Medicare Program Reimbursement Rates

The numerators for Medicare reimbursement rates are from the 1996 Continuous Medicare History Sample (CMHS), which documents reimbursements by calendar year for each component of the Medicare program. The data are for a 5% sample of Medicare enrollees selected on the basis of the terminal digits in the Social Security

TABLE 2.

Definitions for Categories of Reimbursement

Category of Reimbursement	For each service, the specified components were selected from the file and summed as indicated. All fields refer to packed-decimal, variable length, EBCDIC, mainframe record layout locations.
All Services	Sum of Individual Services
Professional and Laboratory Services	File: Payment trailer 1. Total Reimb., cols. 11-13 2. Medical line items, cols. 14-15 (TOS=1, 3, Y, Z) 3. Medical Reimb., cols. 19-21 4. Surgical line items, cols. 22-23 (TOS=2, 8) 5. Surgical Reimb., cols. 27-29 6. Lab/X-ray line items, cols. 30-31 (TOS=4, 5) 7. Lab/X-ray Reimb., cols. 35-37 Professional and Lab. reimb. = 3+5+7
Acute Care Hospital Services	File: Short Stay trailer Stays, cols. 6-7 LOS, cols. 10-11 Reimbursement, cols. 20-23 Passthrough amount, cols. 64-67
Outpatient Hospital Services	Outpatient trailer Total bills, cols. 6-7 Total Reimb., cols. 11-13 Outpatient POS bills, cols. 14-15 Outpatient POS Reimb., cols. 19-21 Inpatient POS bills, cols. 22-23 Inpatient POS Reimb., cols. 27-29 Total Reimb. = Outpatient POS Reimb. + Inpatient POS Reimb.
Home Health Care Services	HHA trailer Part A Reimb., cols. 11-13 Part B Reimb., cols. 19-21 Total Reimb. = Part A + Part B

number. The denominator for rates is the corresponding 5% sample of the enrollment file for persons enrolled in both Medicare parts A and B (see Section 1.4).

2.1 Categories of Medicare Reimbursement

Categories of Medicare reimbursement in the Atlas are listed in Table 2 with their definitions from the CHMS file.

2.2 Calculation of Adjusted Medicare Reimbursement Rates

Medicare reimbursement rates were indirectly adjusted for sex, race and age, with the corresponding 1996 Medicare population as the standard, as described in Section 9.1, and were further adjusted for illness, as described in Section 9.2, and regional differences in price, as described in Section 9.3. Total noncapitated Medicare reimbursement rates were computed as the sum of the component rates.

2.3 Precision of the Aggregate Medicare Reimbursement Rates

The precision of the HRR-specific aggregate Medicare reimbursement rates varies according to the population of the HRR but in general, these rates are precisely determined. For all HRRs with at least 12,000 Medicare enrollees, the width of the approximate 95% confidence interval for the reimbursement rate is 20% of the corresponding national rate. For HRRs with a minimum Medicare population of 48,000 enrollees, it is 10% of the national average.

3. Hospital Resources.

Acute care hospital resources consist of hospital beds and personnel. Three tasks were required to estimate the hospital resource rates. First, the resources for each hospital were determined; second, resources were allocated to populations, proportionate to their rates of use; third, rates were computed and adjusted to take into account differences in age, sex and illness among regions.

3.1 Measuring Hospital Resources

Hospitals were eligible for inclusion if they were located within the 50 states or the District of Columbia and were classified either by Medicare or the AHA as short term general medical and surgical hospitals (AHA service code = 10), specialty hospitals listed as obstetrics and gynecology (code 44), eye, ear, nose and throat (code 45), orthopedic (code 47), or other specialty (code 49); and children's hospitals (codes 50,59). For inclusion in this study, hospitals must have been open on June 30, 1996. Certain specialty hospitals were excluded if additional information gathered from external sources (e.g., telephone calls) indicated they did not meet the inclusion criteria, or if they fell into the following categories: Shriners' hospitals, crippled children's hospitals, hospital units of institutions (prisons, colleges, etc.), institutions for mental retardation, psychiatric facilities, rehabilitation or chronic disease facilities, addiction treatment facilities, communication disorders facilities, podiatry facilities, small surgery centers, obstetrics and gynecology clinics, and hospices. Department of Veterans' Affairs hospitals were excluded from this edition of the Atlas because of the non-comparability of expenditure and personnel data.

The 1996 American Hospital Association Annual Survey file and the Medicare Provider file were searched to identify all non-federal hospitals (AHA control code = 12-33) and federal PHS Indian Service hospitals (control code = 47) that met the criteria for inclusion. Short term general hospitals (N= 4912), children's hospitals (N=48), and specialty hospitals (N=52) located in the 50 states or the District of Columbia as of June 30, 1996 were identified.

The resources for each hospital were determined as follows:

Hospital beds were ascertained primarily from the AHA file. The field selected was "hospital beds (including cribs, pediatric and neonatal bassinets) that were set up and staffed at the end of the reporting period". Our measure of intensive care beds included both "medical/surgical intensive care" and "cardiac intensive care" beds. For the 699 hospitals that were non-reporting in 1996, we used data from the Medicare Cost Reports for "total beds available in the hospital" and "intensive care" plus "coronary care beds" as the measure of intensive care beds. For 37 remaining non-reporting hospitals (including 16 PHS Indian Service hospitals) that also lacked

Cost Report data, AHA data were used to measure all resources, even though the data came from a prior year's Annual Survey. For 27 hospitals lacking both AHA and Cost Report data, Medicare Provider file data were used, supplemented by previous years' AHA and Cost Report data, when available.

Full time equivalent hospital personnel were defined as the sum of full time employees and 1/2 of the part time employees. Hospital employees do not include medical or dental interns or residents or trainees. For the 699 hospitals that were non-reporting in 1996, the Medicare Cost Report value for "average number of employees, hospital total" was used to estimate hospital personnel at these hospitals.

Full time equivalent registered nurses were defined as the sum of full time nurses and 1/2 of the part time nurses. For the 699 hospitals that were non-reporting for 1996, the Medicare Provider of Services file count of "licensed registered nurses" was used to estimate the number of registered nurses at these hospitals.

3.2 Allocation of Hospital Resources

In order to account for the use of care by patients who live in one HSA but obtain care in another, hospital resources for acute care short-term hospitals have been allocated to the HSAs in proportion to the actual patterns of use. This was accomplished using the proportion of all Medicare patient days (1996) provided by each specific hospital to each HSA. For example, if 60% of total Medicare inpatient days at a hospital were used by residents of the HSA where the hospital was located, then 60% of that hospital's resources would be assigned to its HSA. If 20% of the Medicare patient days provided by that hospital were used by a neighboring HSA, 20% of the hospital's resources would be assigned to that neighboring HSA.

Children's hospitals and specialty hospitals were found to have too little actual utilization data in the Medicare files to allow their allocation based on hospital-specific proportionate utilization. These hospitals were allocated according to the utilization patterns of all Medicare enrollees residing in the HSA. In other words, if 80% of the patient days in an HSA were provided by hospitals within the HSA, then 80% of the resources of any specialty or children's hospital located within that HSA would be assigned to it.

The use of Medicare data to estimate resources allocated to populations of all ages is justified by studies which show that the geographic patterns of use of hospital care by patients under and over sixty-five years of age are similar. Our own analyses of data from both New York and New England revealed that travel patterns for those under age 65 are nearly identical to those over age 65. Radany and Luft (1993) found similar results in California.

Once each of the hospital resources had been allocated to HSAs, the allocated resources were summed. For example, the allocated beds of each HSA were equal to the sum of allocated acute short-term beds and allocated specialty/children's beds. For the HSAs located in a given HRR, resources were further summed to obtain the total for the HRR. Crude rates were then calculated for HRRs using the 1998 population for all ages described in Section 1.4.

3.3 Calculation of Adjusted Per Capita Hospital Resource Rates

The resource allocation rates were adjusted for differences in age and sex, and age, sex and illness using the indirect method as described in Sections 9.1 and 9.2, using the 1998 U.S. population as the standard.

4. Physician Workforce Rates

The methods for allocating and estimating the per capita rates of physicians serving HSAs and HRRs are analogous to the methods used for estimating and allocating hospital resources described in Section 3.2. The sources of information on physicians are the American Medical Association (AMA; January 1, 1996) and the American Osteopathic Association (AOA; June 1, 1996) Physician Masterfiles. These files have been used extensively to study physician supply and are the only comprehensive data available on physician location, specialty and level of effort devoted to clinical practice. Both the AMA and the AOA physician files classify physicians according to self-reported level of effort devoted to clinical practice. In this study, we excluded physicians who reported that they worked the majority of the time in medical teaching, administration or research, and part time physicians working fewer than 20 hours a week in clinical practice. Both files also list ZIP Code fields indicating the physician's primary place of practice, which was complete in more than 90% of records. When this information was not available, we used the physician's preferred professional address to indicate location. Based on these criteria, 495,510 physicians resident in the 50 states and District of Columbia constituted the clinically active physician workforce for 1996. There were also 99,972 physicians in residency or fellowship programs.

4.1 Physician Specialties

The AMA and AOA physician files include the physician's primary self-designated specialty from a list of 243 specialties. We grouped these into the categories in Table 3.

TABLE 3.

Categories of Clinically Active Physicians

Classification of physician specialties and type of utilization used for allocation and age adjustment

Dartmouth Specialty	AMA or AOA Specialty	AMA/AOA Code	Allocation	Age Adjustment
All Physicians	All except Unspecified (Codes US, T)			
Primary Physicians	Adolescent Medicine-GP	AGP	Medical	Family Practice
	Family Practice	FP		
	Geriatrics Medicine (Family Practice)	FPG		
		FSM		
	General Practice	GP		
	Sports Medicine-GP	SGP		
	Internal Medicine-Emergency Medicine	IEM	Medical	Internal Medicine
	Internal Medicine	IM		
	Internal Medicine-Pediatrics	IPD		
	Pediatrics	PD	Medical	Pediatrics
Specialty Physicians	All except Primary Physicians and Unspecified (Codes US, T)			
Anesthesiology	Anesthesiology	AN	Surgical	Surgery
	Cardiothoracic Anesthesiology	CAN		
	Obstetrics Anesthesiology	OBA		
	Pediatric Anesthesiology	PAN		
Cardiology	Cardiology	C	Medical	Cardiology
	Cardiovascular Diseases	CD		
		CVD		
	Cardiac Electrophysiology	ICE		
General Surgery	Abdominal Surgery	AS	Surgical	General Surgery
	Colon and Rectal Surgery	CRS		
	General Surgery	GS		
	Surgery-General	S		
Obstetrics/ Gynecology	Gynecological Oncology	GO	Surgical	Ob/Gyn
	Gynecological Surgery	GS		
	Gynecology	GYN		
	Maternal & Fetal Medicine	MFM		
	Obstetrics & Gynecology	OBG		
	Obstetrics	OBS		
	Obstetrics/Gynecology Surgery	OGS		
	Reproductive Endocrinology	RE		
	Reproductive Endocrinology	REN		
Ophthalmology	Ophthalmology	OPH	Surgical	Ophthalmology

TABLE 3. (CONTINUED)

Dartmouth Specialty	AMA or AOA Specialty	AMA/AOA Code	Allocation
Orthopedic Surgery	Hand Surgery (Ortho Surgery)	HSO	Surgical
	Adult Reconstructive Orthopedics	OAR	
	Pediatric Orthopedics	OP	
	Orthopedics	OR	
	Orthopedic Surgery	ORS	
	Sports Medicine (Orthopedic Surgery)	OSM	
	Orthopedic Surgery - Spine	OSS	
	Orthopedic Trauma	OTR	
Psychiatry	Child Psychiatry	CHP	Medical
	Psychiatry	P	
	Pediatric Psychiatry	PDP	
	Psychoanalysis	PYA	
	Geriatric Psychiatry	PYG	
	Psychosomatic Medicine	PYM	
Radiology	Angiography/Interventional Radiology	ANG	All
	Diagnostic Radiology	DR	
	Diagnostic Ultrasound	DUS	
	Nuclear Medicine	NM	
	Nuclear Radiology	NR	
	Neuroradiology	NRA	
	Pediatric Radiology	PDR	
	Radiology	R	
	Diagnostic Roentgenology	RTD	
Urology	Urological Surgery	U	Surgical
	Urology	URS	

4.2 Allocation of Clinically Active Physicians

Clinically active Physicians were assigned to the HSA of their primary place of practice or preferred professional address. Since physicians, like hospitals, provide services to patients residing outside of the HSA in which their practices are located, the physician workforce was allocated to adjust for patient migration. Unfortunately, allocations could not be based on information about the travel patterns of the patients of individual physicians or information about the use of care outside acute hospitals. For clinically active non-federal physicians (N = 480,761), the adjustments are closely analogous to the method used for hospital resources, with an important exception. Since the hospital affiliations of the physicians were not determined, the physicians were allocated on the basis of the patterns of inpatient care of all the hospitals located in their HSAs. The 1995-96 MEDPAR records selected for allocation, which depended on the physician's specialty, are given in Table 3. For example, primary physicians were allocated on the basis of medical DRGs. If an HSA had 4 primary care physicians and if 25% of the medical DRG patient days at the local hospital(s) in 1995-96 were for residents of a neighboring HSA, then the four primary physicians would be estimated to contribute 1.0 FTE primary care physician to the neighboring HSA.

We included clinically active federal physicians (N = 14,749) in the study, since these physicians serve populations counted by the U.S. census, such as veterans, residents of Indian reservations, residents of medically underserved areas, and military personnel and their dependents. Federal physicians were assigned to either the Department of Defense/Public Health Service (DoD/PHS) or the Department of Veterans Affairs (VA) in proportion to the mix of staffed federal beds within each HSA (U.S. Medicine; DoD technical document). All federal pediatricians and obstetrician/gynecologists were assigned to the DoD/PHS. DoD/PHS physicians were allocated to HSAs in the same proportion as the non-federal physicians. Since VA utilization data were available that were analogous to the Medicare Part A data, VA physicians were allocated to areas in proportion to VA inpatient utilization (e.g., if 25% of the patient days of VA hospitals in Manhattan were provided to veterans residing in the Bronx, then 25% of the VA physicians in New York were assigned to the Bronx). If no federal inpatient facility (DoD, VAH, PHS, Indian Health Service) was present within the HSA, then the physicians were assumed to represent primary care and were allocated in the same proportion as non-federal primary care physicians (using inpatient medical days).

When all physician specialty groups had been allocated to HSAs, their allocated FTEs were summed. The physicians allocated to an HSA represent the total of all federal and non-federal FTE physicians allocated from local as well as remote HSAs. For the HSAs in a given HRR, physician resources were further summed to obtain the total for the HRR. Crude rates were then calculated for HRRs using the 1995 population for all ages described in Section 1.4. Measures of physicians in residency training programs used in the Atlas were prepared separately using similar methods. The allocated physician rates were adjusted for age and sex using the indirect method, as described in Section 9.1 using the 1995 U.S. population as the standard.

5. Medicare Hospitalization and Surgical Procedure Rates

Hospitalization rates represent counts of the number of discharges that occurred in a defined time period (the numerator) for a specific population (the denominator). The counts of discharges for specific conditions are based on the MEDPAR files for 1995-96. The denominator is the 1995-96 Medicare enrollee population defined in Section 1.4 that was enrolled in Medicare part A on June 30, 1995 or 1996. In order to ensure that the events counted in the numerator correspond to the denominator population, certain records were excluded, including MEDPAR records with a length of stay over 365 days; hospitalizations in psychiatric, rehabilitation or long term care units (provider codes = S, T, U or V; facility type not equal to S; third digit of Medicare provider number not equal to 0); records where an HMO paid the provider (MEDPAR GHO paid code 1).

5.1 Procedures and Conditions Examined in the Atlas

The specific procedures and conditions, or "numerator events", and the codes used to identify the event in the file are given in Table 4. The "modified diagnosis-related group" (M-DRG) Classification System used in Chapter Three to examine the pattern of variation in hospitalizations among the Medicare population is given in Table 5. "Ambulatory Care Sensitive Conditions" refer to hospitalizations, such as asthma, pneumonia, chronic pulmonary obstructive disease and congestive heart failure, that are preventable when access to primary care is adequate, and are defined in Table 6.

TABLE 4.

Conditions and Procedures	Codes Used to Define Conditions and Procedures[1]
All Discharges	
Inhospital Deaths	(Discharge status = 'B')
Medical Discharges	
Low/moderate variation medical	DRGs 174, 175, 14, 121-123
High variation medical	DRGs 9-13, 15-35, 43-48, 64-74, 78-102, 124-145, 172-173, 176-190, 202-208, 235-256, 271-284, 294-301, 316-333, 346-352, 366-369, 372, 373, 376, 378-391, 395-399, 403-405, 409-414, 416-423, 425-437, 444-457, 460, 462-467, 473, 475, 487, 489, 490, 492
Surgical Discharges	DRGs 1-8, 36-42, 49-63, 75-77, 103-108, 110-120, 146-171, 191-201, 209-234, 257-270, 285-293, 302-315, 334-345, 353-365, 370, 371, 377, 392-394, 400-402, 406-408, 415, 424, 439-443, 458, 459, 461, 468, 471-472, 476-486, 488, 491, 493, 494, 495
General Surgery	
cholecystectomy	Procedure code 51.2-51.23
resection for colorectal cancer	Procedure code 45.7-45.79, 45.8, 48.5, 48.6-48.69 and Diagnosis code 153-153.9, 154-154.1
mastectomy for cancer[f]	Procedure code 85.41, 85.43, 85.45, 85.47 and Diagnosis code 174-174.9 (but not 233.0)
partial mastectomy[f]	Procedure code 85.20 - 85.23 and Diagnosis code 174-174.9, not (233.0)
Vascular Surgery	
carotid endarterectomy	Procedure code 38.12
abdominal aortic aneurysm repair	Procedure code 38.44, 39.25 and Diagnosis code 441.3-441.9
lower extremity revascularization	Procedure code 39.25, 39.29 and Diagnosis codes not = 441.3-441.9
major leg amputation	Procedure code 84.15-84.17
Cardiothoracic Surgery	
Coronary artery bypass surgery	Procedure code 36.10-36.19
aortic / mitral valve replacement	Procedure code 35.20-35.24
lung resection	Procedure code 32.29-32.5 and Diagnosis code 162-162.9
PTCA	Procedure code 36.01, 36.02, 36.05
coronary angiography	Procedure code 37.22, 37.23, 88.55-88.57
Urology	
radical prostatectomy[m]	Procedure code 60.5
TURP for BPH[m]	Procedure code 60.2 and Diagnosis code (1-5) = 600-601.4, 601.8, 601.9, 602-602.1, 602.3, 602.8, 602.9, 788.2-788.29
radical nephrectomy	Procedure code 55.5-55.51 and Diagnosis code 189-189.1

TABLE 4. (CONTINUED)

Conditions and Procedures	Codes Used to Define Conditions and Procedures[1]
Orthopedic Surgery	
back surgery	Procedure code 03.0, 03.1, 03.2, 03.32, 03.39, 03.4, 03.5, 03.6, 03.93, 03.94, 03.96, 80.5-80.59, 81.0-81.09
hip replacement	Procedure code 81.51 and Diagnosis codes not = (820-821.39, 996.0-996.99)
knee replacement	Procedure code 81.54
hip fracture repair (by type) for*	
a) femoral neck fracture	Diagnosis code 820-820.19, 820.8-820.9 and
- total hip replacement	-Procedure code 81.51
- partial hip replacement	-Procedure code 81.52
- internal fixation	-Procedure code 78.55, 79.10, 79.15, 79.30, 79.35
- other treatment-	-None of the above procedure codes
b) other hip fracture	Diagnosis code 820.2-820.32 and
- total hip replacement	-Procedure code 81.51
- partial hip replacement	-Procedure code 81.52
- internal fixation	-Procedure code 78.55, 79.10, 79.15, 79.30, 79.35
- other treatment	-None of the above procedure codes

*Records were excluded if codes were present which indicated malunion or nonunion of fracture, aseptic necrosis of the hip, evidence of old fractures, or cancer in bone.

Fractures	
Hip	Primary diagnosis code 820-820.9
Shaft of femur	Primary diagnosis code 821-821.39
Patella	Primary diagnosis code 822.0-822.1
Tibia	Primary diagnosis code 823-823.92
Ankle	Primary diagnosis code 824-824.9
Foot	Primary diagnosis code 825-825.29
Proximal humerus	Primary diagnosis code 812-812.19
Elbow	Primary diagnosis code 812.4-812.59
Radius/ulna	Primary diagnosis code 813-813.93
Distal radius/ulna	Primary diagnosis code 813.4-813.55
Radius/ulna/wrist	Primary diagnosis code 813-813.93, 814-814.19
Diagnostic Procedures	
Carotid duplex	CPT code 93875-93888
Cardiac cathererization	CPT code 93510-93529, 93539, 93540, 93545

NOTES:
1. Unless otherwise specified, all codes are ICD-9-CM; up to 10 diagnoses and 6 procedures were coded on 1994-95 MEDPAR records, and all fields were searched for the presence of the conditions specified. CPT refers to Current Procedure Terminology codes used for the reporting of physician procedures and services on Medicare Part B data.
2. (f) refers to procedures for which counts of women served as the denominator; (m) refers to procedures for which counts of men served as the denominator.

TABLE 5.

MDRG	DRG Description	DRGs
Nervous System		
1	Craniotomy, Other Cranial and Nervous System Procedures	1-4, 7-8, 484
2	Extracranial Vascular Procedures (Carotid Endarterectomy)	5
3	Specific Cerebrovascular Disorders Except TIA	14
4	Transient Ischemic Attack (TIA)	15
5	Seizure and Headache	24-26
6	Coma and Concussion	27-33
7	Residual Nervous System Diagnoses	9-13, 16-23, 34-35
Eye		
8	Eye Procedures	36-42
112	Eye Diagnoses	43-48
Ear, Nose and Throat		
9	Tonsillectomy and/or Adenoidectomy	57-60
10	Sinus Procedures	53-55
11	Residual Ear-Nose-Throat Procedures	49-52, 56, 61-63, 168-169, 185-187
12	Ear-Nose-Throat Diagnoses	64-74
Respiratory System		
13	Major Chest and Other Respiratory Procedures	75-77
14	Respiratory Neoplasms	82
15	Pleural Effusion and Respiratory Failure	85-87
16	Adult Respiratory Infections	79-80
109	Adult Simple Pneumonia	89-90
17	Pediatric Respiratory Infections and Pneumonia	81, 91
18	Chronic Obstructive Pulmonary Disease	88
19	Adult Bronchitis and Asthma	96-97
20	Pediatric Bronchitis and Asthma	98
21	Residual Respiratory Diagnoses	78, 83-84, 92-95, 99-102
Circulatory System		
22	Valve Procedures Other Than CABG	104-105
23	Coronary Artery Bypass Graft	106-107
110	Other Heart Procedures	108
24	Major Vascular Procedures	110-111, 478-479
25	Vascular Procedures Other Than Major (PTCA)	112
26	Cardiac Pacemaker Procedures	115-118
27	Residual Circulatory System Procedures	109, 113-114, 119-120
28	Acute Myocardial Infarction	121-123
29	Cardiac Catheterization Except for AMI	124-125
30	Heart Failure and Shock (Congestive Heart Failure)	127
31	Peripheral Vascular Disorders	130-131

Table 5. (continued)

MDRG	DRG Description	DRGs
Circulatory System, Continued		
32	Cardiac Arrhythmia	138-139
33	Angina Pectoris	140
34	Syncope and Collapse	141-142
35	Chest Pain	143
36	Residual Circulatory System Diagnoses	126, 129, 132-137, 144-145
111	Deep Vein Thrombosis	128
Digestive System		
37	Major Small and Large Bowel Procedures	146-149
38	Stomach, Esophageal and Duodenal Procedures	154-156
39	Anal Procedures	157-158, 267
40	Inguinal and Femoral Hernia Procedures	159-163
41	Appendectomy	164-167
42	Residual Digestive System Procedures	150-153, 170-171
43	Gastro-Intestinal Hemorrhage	174-175
44	Gastro-Intestinal Obstruction	180-181
45	Adult Gastroenteritis	182-183
46	Pediatric Gastroenteritis	184
47	Residual Digestive System Diagnoses	172-173, 176-179, 188-190
Hepatobiliary System		
48	Cholecystectomy	195-198, 493, 494
49	Other Hepatobiliary Procedures	191-194, 199-201
50	Biliary Tract Disorders	207-208
51	Other Hepatobiliary System Diagnoses	202-206
Musculoskeletal and Connective Tissue		
52	Major Joint Procedures	209, 471
53	Hip and Femur Procedures Other Than Major Joint	210-211
54	Back and Neck Procedures	214-215
55	Lower Extremity Procedures	218-219
56	Knee Procedures	221-222
57	Upper Extremity Procedures	223-224, 491
58	Residual Musculoskeletal Procedures	6, 212-213, 216-217, 220, 225-234
59	Hip, Femur, Pelvis Fracture	235-236
60	Medical Back Problems	243
61	Misc. Fracture/Sprain/Strain/Dislocation	250-255
62	Residual Musculoskeletal Diagnoses	237-242, 244-249, 256
Skin, Subcutaneous Tissue and Breast		
63	Total and Subtotal Mastectomy	257-260
64	Other Skin/Tissue/Breast Procedures	261-266, 268-270
65	Cellulitis	277-279
66	Other Skin/Tissue/Breast Diagnoses	271-276, 280-284

TABLE 5. (CONTINUED)

MDRG	DRG Description	DRGs
Endocrine, Nutritional and Metabolic		
67	Endocrine/Nutritional/Metabolic Procedures	285-293
68	Diabetes Age >=35	294
69	Adult Nutritional and Metabolic Disorders	296-297
70	Pediatric Nutritional and Metabolic Disorders	298
71	Residual Endocrine/Nutrional/Metabolic Diagnoses	295, 299-301
Kidney and Urinary System / Male Reproductive System		
72	Major Genito-Urinary Procedures	302-307, 334-335
73	Transurethral Prostatectomy	336-337
74	Transurethral Procedures Except TURP	310-311
75	Major Genito-Urinary Procedures	308-309, 312-315, 338-345
76	Kidney-Urinary Tract Infections	320-321
77	Urinary Tract Stones	323-324
78	Residual Kidney/Urinary System Diagnoses	316-319, 322, 325-333
79	Male Reproductive System Diagnoses	346-352
Female Reproductive System		
80	Uterus and Adnexa Procedures for Non-Malignant Conditions	358-359
81	Female Reproductive System Reconstructive Procedures	356
82	Residual Female Reproductive System Procedures	353-355, 357, 360-365
83	Female Reproductive System Diagnoses	366-369
Pregnancy-Related		
84	Cesarean Delivery	370-371
85	Vaginal Delivery	372-375
86	Pregnancy Not Delivered	376-384
Newborns and Neonates		
87	Newborns and Neonates	385-391
Blood and Blood Forming Organs		
88	Diagnoses of Blood and Blood Forming Organs	395-399
Myeloproliferative Diseases		
89	Chemotherapy	410, 492
90	Myeloproliferative/Lymphoma/Leukemia Diagnoses Other Than Chemotherapy	403-405, 409, 411-414
Infectious and Parasitic Diseases		
91	Septicemia	416
92	Adult Viral Disease and Fever of Unknown Origin	419-421
93	Pediatric Viral Disease and Fever of Unknown Origin	422
94	Residual Infectious and Parasitic Diseases	417-418, 423, 489-490
Mental Diseases and Disorders		
95	Psychoses	430
96	Other Mental Diseases and Disorders	425-429, 431-432

Table 5. (continued)

MDRG	DRG Description	DRGs
Substance Use		
97	Substance Use Treatment, Left Against Medical Advice	433
98	Substance Use Detoxification (w/o Rehab)	434-435
99	Substance Use Rehabilitation (with or w/o Detox)	436-437
Injuries and Adverse Effects		
100	Operating Room Procedures for Injuries	439-443
101	Toxic Effects of Drugs	449-450
102	Other Injury Diagnoses w/o Procedure	444-448, 451-457, 487
Health Status Factors		
103	Rehabilitation (Other Than for Substance Abuse)	462
104	Other Health Status Diagnoses	463-467
Residual MDRGs		
105	Unrelated Operating Room Procedures	468
106	Respiratory Disease with Ventilator	475
107	Residual O.R. Procedures with Case Mix Index >=3.0	103, 392, 415, 458, 472-474, 480-483, 485-486, 488
108	Residual O.R. Procedures with Case Mix Index <3.0	393-394, 400-402, 406-408, 424, 459-461

Table 6 – Ambulatory Care-Sensitive Conditions

CONDITION	ICD – 9 – CM CODES
Convulsions	780.3
Chronic obstructive pulmonary disease	491, 492, 494, 496, 466.0 Acute bronchitis (466.0) only with secondary diagnosis of 491, 492, 494, 496
Bacterial pneumonia	481, 482.2, 482.3, 482.9, 483, 485, 486 Excluding cases with secondary diagnosis of sickle cell (282.6)
Asthma	493
Congestive heart failure	428, 402.01, 402.11, 402.91, 518.4 Excluding cases with the following surgical procedures: 36.01, 36.02, 36.05, 36.1, 37.5, or 37.7
Hypertension	401.0, 401.9, 402.00, 402.10, 402.90 Excluding cases with the following surgical procedures: 36.01, 36.02, 36.05, 36.1, 37.5, or 37.7
Angina	411.1, 411.8, 413 Excluding cases with a surgical procedure (01-86.99)
Cellulitis	681, 682, 683, 686 Excluding cases with a surgical procedure (01-86.99), except incision of skin and subcutaneous tissue (86.0) where it is the only listed surgical procedure
Diabetes	250.0 250.1, 250.2, 250.3, 250.8, 250.9
Gastroenteritis	558.9
Kidney/urinary infection	590, 599.0, 599.9
Dehydration – volume depletion	276.5

5.2 Surgical Procedure Rates

The rates of inpatient surgery in Chapter Five are based on the MEDPAR files for 1995 and 1996. The denominators are the 1995-96 Medicare enrollee population described in Section 1.4, with the same restrictions as for utilization rates above. The procedure codes used in the MEDPAR file are based on the International Classification of Disease, ICD-9-CM. Selection of procedure codes was based on review of the literature and/or consultation with clinical experts. The rates of carotid duplex diagnostic procedures and cardiac catheterization are derived from Medicare part B data and are described in Section 6. Some rates were suppressed for reasons of data confidentiality. Suppression rules meet current HCFA standards. rates with fewer than 26 expected events were suppressed for reasons of statistical precision.

5.3 Adjusted Procedure and Utilization Rates

Utilization rates were adjusted using the indirect method for age, sex and race, and further adjusted for illness using the corresponding 1995-96 national Medicare population as the standard, as described in Section 9.1 and 9.2. Surgical procedure rates were similarly adjusted, except that sex-specific population estimates were used for prostate and breast procedures. Although the majority of events occurred at most once per person during the study period, we included multiple events to the same person to allow the rates to reflect total health care utilization.

Although standard errors of the rates were not reported, these estimates are, for the most part, precisely determined. The minimum Medicare population in an HRR is 14,497 residents in Boulder, CO. The following precisions were obtained in the smallest HRR (the "worst case scenario") for an event rate of 5 per 1,000:

- For procedures related exclusively to males or females in this smallest HRR, the precision would be ±16% of the true rate.
- For procedures related to the entire HRR, the precision would be ±12%.
- For procedures in a median-sized HRR (N=64,000) the precision would be ±6%.

In general, if we denote the event rate as p and the population size as N, the standard error is $(p/N)^{0.5}$ and the precision, expressed as a percent of the true rate, is $(s.e.(p)/p)*100\%$.

6. Preventive Services and Continuity of Care

Preventive service rates are counts of Medicare enrollees receiving at least one medical service of a particular type divided by the target Medicare population. The data were derived from Medicare part B physician claims files for 1995-96 for a 5% sample of Medicare enrollees (see Section 1.4). Mammography rates were computed for women age 65 to 69; eye examinations, HgbA1c and LDL blood lipid monitoring were computed for diabetics. Diabetics were defined as enrollees with two outpatient evaluation and management visits or one inpatient visit, with a diagnosis of diabetes (see the Endnote). We counted the number of people obtaining these services at least once in any year and then computed the average annual rate after combining years, as described in Section 9.1 and 9.2. The preventive services examined in the Atlas for Medicare enrollees are defined in Table 7 and are based on HEDIS recommendations (see the Endnote).

Table 7 – Preventive Services

Preventive Services CPT Codes	
Pneumococcal Immunization	90732
Mammogram	76090-76092
Occult Blood Test	82270
Sigmoidoscopy	45300-45320,45330-45336,45338-45339
Eye Exam	92002,92004,92012,92014,92018,92019,9222,92226,92235,92250
HgbAlc	83036
Blood Lipids	83715-83721,80061

NOTE:
CPT refers to Current Procedure Terminology codes used for the reporting of physician procedures and services on Medicare Part B data.

Access to care is defined as the percent of Medicare enrollees who had one or more visits to a physician in 1996. Continuity of care was defined as the percent of Medicare patients who received at least 50% of their ambulatory care visits from one provider in 1996. Ambulatory visits are those whose place of service was a physician office, patient home, hospital outpatient setting, hospital emergency room, or rural health clinic. Physician visits were defined as those that were for the purpose of evaluation and management only, not including pathology, and were based on BETOS codes (see the Endnote). The data and Medicare enrollee populations are as defined above.

The rates of carotid duplex diagnostic procedures and cardiac catheterizations are derived from the Medicare part B physician claims files for 1995-96 using the population described above. The codes for these procedures are listed in Table 4.

7. Quality of Care in the Last Six Months of Life

For all rates pertaining to the last six months of life, the denominator was the 18 month 1995-96 deceased Medicare population, defined as the Medicare enrollee population who died between July 1, 1995 and December 31, 1996 (see Section 1.4). Percent of Medicare deaths occurring in a hospital was computed using as numerator event, death in a hospital (discharge status='B' in MEDPAR file). For the percent of Medicare deaths who were admitted to the ICU in the last 6 months of life, the numerator event was death in a hospital with admission to an ICU within 6 months of the death date using MEDPAR files. Rates were age, sex, and race adjusted as described in Section 9.1 and were expressed as a percentage of deaths.

Average days in the hospital, average days in the ICU and average reimbursements for inpatient care per capita were computed using only the portion of the event (hospital stay or ICU stay) falling within the 6 month period prior to death. Rates were age, sex and race adjusted as described in Section 9.1. Inpatient reimbursement rates were also price adjusted as described in Section 9.3.

Number of physician visits during the last six months of life were computed for physician visits with any place of service, that were for the purpose of evaluation and management only, not including pathology, and were based on BETOS codes. The number of physicians seen in the last six months of life was computed based on linkage with the Medicare Physician Identification Master File (UPIN) For both these measures, data were derived from Medicare part B files, as described in Section 6, and the population was the 18 month 1995-96 deceased Medicare population, as defined above, that was enrolled in Medicare part B in the month of death and belonged to the 5% sample of Medicare part B physician claims files for 1995-96.

8. The Medicare Current Beneficiary Survey (MCBS)

Chapter Three considers the correspondence among hospital bed capacity, utilization and self-reported health. This issue was also addressed by Ashby et al (1986) who found that states with higher Medicare expenditures also had lower levels of self-reported health. We turned to the Medicare Current Beneficiary Survey (MCBS) to reexamine this issue.

The MCBS is a continuous multi-purpose survey of a representative sample of the entire Medicare population, with oversampling of the old-old, the disabled, those living in institutional settings (HCFA, 1992). Survey participants complete three rounds of surveys each year throughout their participation in the study. The sample was drawn from 107 primary sampling units (PSU) consisting of counties or groups of counties intended to be representative of the U.S. Within those PSUs, sampling was further restricted to certain geographic areas (sub-PSUs, N = 1163), based on the ZIP Code of residence of the beneficiary, again with the goal of maintaining representativeness while economizing on interviewer travel. Beneficiaries within each area were then sampled randomly within age strata, with oversampling of the disabled under age 65 and the oldest beneficiaries (age 85 and over).

Participants are interviewed three times each year, wherever they reside and with the interview tailored to reflect the setting and using proxy respondents where necessary.

Survey items include a core of data that are repeated at each subsequent interview on utilization, charges and payments for health care and a supplement that focuses on other domains. Critical to this analysis is the Supplement on Access and Satisfaction, which was carried out on Round 1 (Fall 1991) and is repeated annually thereafter (Rounds 4, 7, 10 etc.). In addition to data on access and satisfaction, this supplement includes detailed questions on self-assessed health status, current health conditions and physical function.

The study population for this analysis (N=8860) was created by taking Round 4 of the 1992 wave of the MCBS and excluding persons under age 65, those who were institutionalized and answered questions by proxy, and those enrolled in risk-bearing HMOs. We matched each individual with his or her 1993 Medicare claims data on health care utilization and appended regional-level information about health resources from the Atlas database. This made it possible for us to measure health characteristics of people who live in regions with relatively high, and relatively low, levels of hospital beds or Medicare spending.

Individuals' total 1993 hospital days were summed and hospital days per capita were computed by self-reported health status (poor, fair, good, very good, and excellent). To assess the dependence on hospital resources, they were also computed separately by hospital bed supply in the region (above vs. below the median). These were indirectly standardized by age and sex using the 1993 Medicare population as the standard, as described in Section 9.1.

To compute the expected number of hospital days as predicted by self-reported health status, according to quintile of hospital beds, we used regression analysis to predict hospital days based on self-reported health, age and sex in each quintile of hospital beds. Quintiles (20th percentiles) were computed by taking (weighted) intervals of the sorted data for MCBS respondents and ranged from the lowest quintile with the fewest hospital beds to the highest quintile with the most hospital beds.

9. Calculation of Adjusted Rates

9.1 Calculation of Age, Sex and Race Adjusted Rates

Medicare procedure, condition, preventive services and reimbursement rates were adjusted using the indirect method for the following strata: sex, race (black, non-black) and age (65-69, 70-74, 75-79, 80-84, 85-99). The standard population for reimbursement rates was the 1996 Medicare population, and for procedure, condition, and preventive services rates, the 1995-96 Medicare population corresponding to the numerator (see Section 1.4). The expected counts within HSAs were computed as weighted averages of the stratum-specific crude rates in the standard population and were obtained using weighted least squares regression, weighting by the stratum-specific population. Observed and expected counts at the HSA level were summed to the HRR level. Procedures, counts and preventive services were obtained separately for each year and summed across years before summing to the HRR level. Indirectly standardized rates for HRRs were then computed from observed and expected counts (Breslow and Day, 1987).

This procedure was slightly modified for hospital resource and physician workforce rates. The hospital resource rates were adjusted for differences in age and sex using the indirect method using the 1998 U.S. population as the standard. Since the national age-sex specific bed supply rates are not obtainable, these were estimated using the national age-sex specific patient day rates obtained from the 1989 National Hospital Discharge Survey. These estimates were used to calculate the expected bed supply in each HSA and HRR. Under the assumption that employee allocations across age and sex groups are also proportionate to patient days, a similar strategy was used to adjust employees.

The allocated physician rates were adjusted for age and sex using the indirect method using the 1995 U.S. population as a standard. As with hospital bed supply rates, the national age-sex specific physician workforce rates are not known. These were estimated using outpatient age, sex and specialty specific physician visit rates from the combined 1989-1994 National Ambulatory Care Survey (NAMCS). These estimates were used to calculate the expected physician supply in each HSA, by specialty. Specialties that had too few visits to reliably estimate age-sex specific visit rates (< 800 total NAMCS) used the visit rates of allied specialties, as indicated in Table 3. Four NAMCS specialty categories could not be age and sex adjusted because of the low frequency of ambulatory visits and the lack of allied specialties: pathology, radiology, critical care and "unspecified". Expected counts of resident physicians were prepared separately using similar methods. The expected counts were summed to the HRR level and were used to calculate indirectly standardized rates. Rates for combined generalists, combined specialists and combined total physicians were obtained by first summing expected counts of the component specialties to the HRR level.

9.2 Calculation of Illness Adjusted Rates

Rates published in the Atlas were further adjusted for the Medicare population illness characteristics. The measures of illness used were the 1995 and 1996 HSA age-sex-race stratum specific mortality and incidence rates for five conditions. The conditions selected consisted of specific events for which hospitalization is a proxy for the incidence of disease: hospitalizations for hip fracture, cancer of the colon or lung treated surgically, gastro-intestinal hemorrhage, acute myocardial infarction or stroke (Wennberg, NEJM 1984; Wennberg, Lancet 1987; see the Endnote).

For procedures, conditions and reimbursements, we obtained age-sex-race-illness adjusted rates using regression methods as follows. For each outcome, we regressed the crude HSA stratum-specific rate against age, sex, race and all higher order interactions as well as the crude HSA age-sex-race specific illness rates, for each year separately, weighting by the HSA stratum Medicare population. The resulting expected counts and dollars were summed across years and across strata to the HSA level. The observed and expected counts were then summed to the HRR level and used to calculate age-sex-race-illness standardized rates using the usual formula for indirectly standardized rates (Breslow and Day, 1987; see the Endnote).

This procedure was modified for hospital resource and physician workforce rates. Here, we first obtained HSA-level age-sex adjusted rates, as described in Section 9.1.

These rates were then regressed against the age-sex-race adjusted HSA mortality and incidence rates of the five conditions above, weighting by the HSA Medicare population, to produce predicted physician and resource rates for each HSA. The expected counts were obtained from the predicted rates, corrected for bias so that the sum of the observed and expected counts were equal, and then used in the usual formula for indirect standardization. This technique was used because of the lack of information on stratum-specific national resource and physician counts. The estimated rates correlated very highly with the usual regression-based rates for variables where this information was obtainable.

9.3 Calculation of Price Adjusted Rates
Medicare program expenditure rates were further adjusted to account for regional differences in price. Two different price adjustors were used, depending on the category of Medicare spending, the Dartmouth Price Index and the HCFA Part B Index, both of which are based on the Geographic Practice Cost Index (GPCI) developed by Zuckerman, Welch, and Pope (1990) (see the Endnote). These price indexes are described below.

Dartmouth (Modified GPCI) Price Index. Seeking to avoid a price adjustment that depended on physician or hospital market conditions, we focused on cost of living indices using non-medical regional price measures. We relied on the Geographic Practice Cost Index (GPCI) applicable to fiscal year 1995 Medicare physician claims. The index is the weighted sum of three components: the relative cost of non-physician professional labor across areas, the relative cost of physician practice inputs (principally rents and wages to office employees) and the relative cost of malpractice. The weights are based on the national proportions of these costs in physician services. We re-weighted the index, excluding the malpractice costs. We also used the full professional labor component in our revised index (HCFA used only one-quarter of the professional labor component). While not perfectly exogenous to health care (as it includes physician office expenses), this modified GPCI index is both available at the level of geographic analysis needed in this study, and is preferable to the major alternative, Medicare's hospital wage index. (The hospital wage index is based on actual wages paid to hospital employees in each area and is thus distorted by differences in occupational mix and market conditions. Hospitals that hire more highly paid staff have those costs reflected in the wage index.) The Dartmouth index was available for each metropolitan statistical area (MSA) and for non-MSA areas of each state. The values for the area-specific modified GPCI were assigned to each HSA according to the location of the principal city or town of each HSA.

HCFA Part B Index. Because Medicare Part B payments compensate for only one-quarter of the difference in professional wage adjustments across areas and include an adjustment for malpractice insurance costs, these adjustments were made in reverse to recover the original value of the Part B billings.

For both indexes, HRR-level modified GPCIs were calculated as weighted sums of the HSA-specific indexes, using the number of Medicare enrollees in the HSA as the weight. The Dartmouth Price Index was used to adjust all components of Medicare expenditures except professional and laboratory services. This latter component was adjusted using the HCFA Part B regional price measure.

To implement the adjustment, each component of the Medicare program was first either age-sex-race adjusted or age-sex-race-illness adjusted at the HSA level. Observed and expected dollars were then summed to the HRR level and indirectly standardized rates were computed. HRR-specific Medicare expenditure rates were then divided by the index for that HRR to adjust for regional differences in price.

9.4 Predicted Rates
Predicted rates were computed as the expected counts or dollars in an area divided by the corresponding HSA or HRR population count (see Section 1.4). These were used to measure the rate that would have been observed if age, sex and race or age, sex, race and illness alone determined the variations in that outcome.

10. Measures of Variation and Association

10.1 The Distribution Graph

The distribution graphs used in the Atlas provide a simple way to show the dispersion in particular rates of health care resources and utilization across the 306 hospital referral regions. For example, Figure 2.2 shows the distribution of hospital employees per thousand residents for each of the 306 hospital referral regions. The vertical axis shows the rate of hospital employees per thousand residents. The Bronx, which had 25.7 employees per thousand residents, is represented by the highest point on the graph. Hattiesburg, Mississippi, which had 19.34 employees per 1,000 residents, and Bismarck, North Dakota, which had 19.26 employees per 1,000 residents, are represented by two points that are side by side on the graph. Areas which did not have exactly the same number of hospital employees per thousand residents are arrayed on a single line because their rates fall into a "bin" between two values.

This chart summarizes two features of the data. The first is a measure of dispersion; if the number of employees per thousand (or whatever measure is on the vertical axis) for the highest hospital referral region is two or three times higher than the number of employees per thousand for the lowest hospital referral region, it suggests substantial variation in health care resources. Second, the distribution graph shows whether the variation is caused by just a few outliers — hospital referral regions that for various reasons are very different from the rest of the country — or whether the variation is pervasive and widespread across the country. In the example above, there is widespread dispersion across the country, but one area, the Bronx, does stand apart from all other areas.

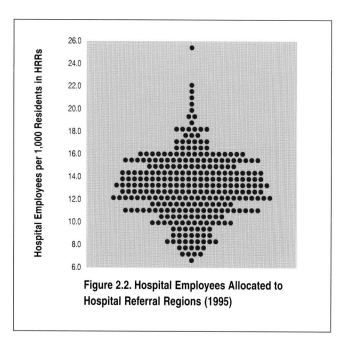

Figure 2.2. Hospital Employees Allocated to Hospital Referral Regions (1995)

10.2 Measures of Association (R^2 and Regression Lines)

In this Atlas, we often suggest that some factors may be related in a systematic way to other factors. For example, in Chapter Three we hypothesize that regions with high rates of beds per thousand residents also have high rates of hospitalization for medical conditions. To capture the degree and extent of the association between hospital beds and medical hospitalizations in Figure 3.5, we put hospital beds per thousand residents on the hori-

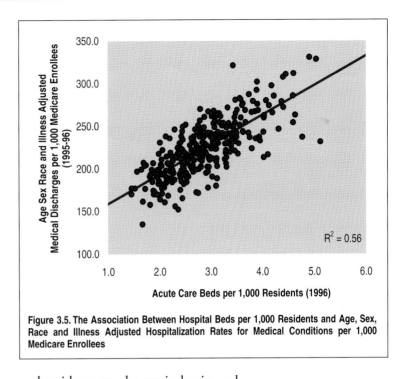

Figure 3.5. The Association Between Hospital Beds per 1,000 Residents and Age, Sex, Race and Illness Adjusted Hospitalization Rates for Medical Conditions per 1,000 Medicare Enrollees

zontal axis and hospitalization rates per thousand residents on the vertical axis, and placed a point on the graph for each of the 306 hospital referral regions. If hospital beds and hospitalization rates were negatively correlated, so that regions with higher beds per thousand residents had lower per capita expenditures, then we might expect to see the cloud of points tilted downward, running from northwest to southeast. Conversely, if they were positively correlated — as they in fact are — the cloud of points would run from southwest to northeast on the graph, as seen in Figure 3.5.

It is sometimes difficult to discern from this cloud of points the relationship between two variables. A linear regression line provides the best fit of the data and summarizes the relationships between them. A measure of the "goodness of fit" or the extent to which hospital beds per 1,000 predicts hospitalizations per 1000 residents is R^2, which is defined as the proportion of total variation in the vertical axis (hospitalizations) that is explained by variation in the horizontal axis (beds). It ranges from 0 to 1, where 1 is perfect correlation and 0 means that the two variables are completely unrelated. In Figure 3.5, the R^2 for the relationship between medical hospitalizations and hospital beds is 0.56, which means that the two are closely related — that 56% of the variation in medical hospitalizations per 1000 residents is related to the bed supply.

The regression lines and R^2 statistics given in the text are not weighted for the size of the population. Weighted and unweighted R^2 statistics were similar.

10.3 Index of Variation: the SCV

The Systematic Component of Variation (SCV) was developed as a measure of the variation among the rates of admission across different areas that is not affected by the mean rate or the size of the population studied, as are other measures of variation. It can, therefore, be used to compare relative variations of different procedures or conditions, even when the mean rates differ substantially. It is typically used to classify procedures into categories of low, moderate, high and very high variation. Differences in the SCV among causes of admission can be tested by computing ratios of two SCVs and comparing them to the F distribution. The SCV is computed by subtracting the random component of variation from the total variance. Further details on the computation of the SCV and its use are given in McPherson et al. (1982) and Wennberg et al (1984) (see the Endnote).

Appendix on the Geography of Health Care in the United States*

The use of health care resources in the United States is highly localized. Most Americans use the services of physicians whose practices are nearby. Physicians, in turn, are usually affiliated with hospitals that are near their practices. As a result, when patients are admitted to hospitals, the admission generally takes place within a relatively short distance of where the patient lives. This is true across the United States. Although the distances from homes to hospitals vary with geography – people who live in rural areas travel farther than those who live in cities – in general most patients are admitted to a hospital close to where they live which provides an appropriate level of care.

The Medicare program maintains exhaustive records of hospitalizations, which makes it possible to define the patterns of use of hospital care. When Medicare enrollees are admitted to hospitals, the program's records identify both the patients' places of residence (by ZIP Code) and the hospitals where the admissions took place (by unique numerical identifiers). These files provide a reliable basis for determining the geographic pattern of health care use, because research shows that the migration patterns of patients in the Medicare program are similar to those for younger patients.

Medicare records of hospitalizations were used to define 3,436 geographically distinct hospital service areas in the United States. In each hospital service area, most of the care received by Medicare patients is provided in hospitals within the area. Based on the patterns of care for major cardiovascular surgery and neurosurgery, hospital service areas were aggregated into 306 hospital referral regions; this Atlas reports on patterns of care in these hospital referral regions.

How Hospital Service Areas Were Defined

Hospital service areas were defined through a three-step process. First, all acute care hospitals in the 50 states and the District of Columbia were identified from the American Hospital Association and Medicare provider files and assigned to the town or city in which they were located. The name of the town or city was used

---

*Abstracted from the 1996 edition of the Dartmouth Atlas of Health Care

as the name of the hospital service area, even though the area might have extended well beyond the political boundary of the town. For example, the Mt. Ascutney Hospital is in Windsor, Vermont. The area is called the Windsor hospital service area, even though the area serves several other communities.

In the second step, all 1992 and 1993 Medicare hospitalization records for each hospital were analyzed to ascertain the ZIP Code of each of its patients. When a town or city had more than one hospital, the counts were added together. Using a plurality rule, each ZIP Code was assigned on a provisional basis to the town containing the hospitals most often used by local residents.

The analysis of the patterns of use of care by Medicare patients led to the provisional assignment of five post office ZIP Codes to the Windsor hospital service area.

ZIP Code	Community Name	1990 Population	% of Medicare Discharges to Mt. Ascutney Hospital
05037	Brownsville	415	52.8
05048	Hartland	1,730	46.8
05053	Pomfret	245	52.6
05062	Reading	614	36.8
05089	Windsor	5,406	63.2

The third step involved the visual examination of the ZIP Codes using a computer-generated map to make sure that the ZIP Codes included in the hospital service areas were contiguous. In the case of the Windsor area, inspection of the map led to the reassignment of Pomfret to the Lebanon hospital service area. In the final determination, the Windsor hospital service area contained four communities and a total population of 8,165. (See Map A)

Details about the method of constructing hospital service areas are given in The Appendix on Methods.

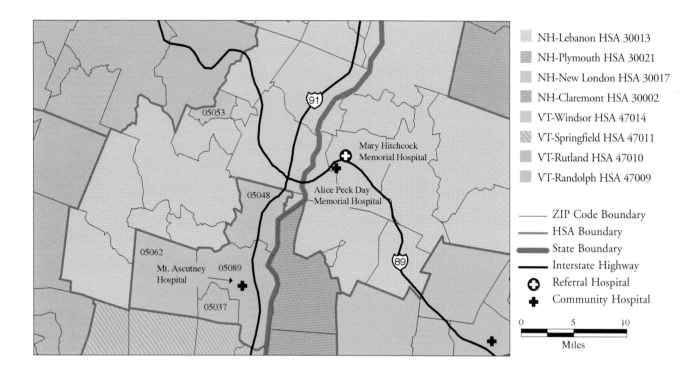

Map A. ZIP Codes Assigned to the Windsor, Vermont, Hospital Service Area

The analysis of the pattern of use of hospitals revealed that Medicare enrollees living in the five ZIP Code areas in light blue most often used the Mt. Ascutney Hospital in Windsor, Vermont. To maintain geographic continuity of hospital service areas, the Pomfret ZIP Code 05053 was reassigned to the Lebanon hospital service area. The Windsor hospital service area contained four communities, with a 1990 census of 8,165. During 1992-93, there were 679 hospitalizations among the Medicare population; 394 (58%) were to Mt. Ascutney Hospital, 131 to the Mary Hitchcock Memorial Hospital, and 154 to other hospitals.

Hospital Service Areas in the United States

The documentation of the patterns of use of hospitals according to Medicare enrollee ZIP Codes during 1992-93 led to the aggregation of approximately 42,000 ZIP Codes into 3,436 hospital service areas. In each area, more Medicare patients were hospitalized locally than in any other single hospital service area. The propensity of patients to use local hospitals is measured by the localization index, which is the percentage of all residents' hospitalizations that occur in local hospitals (the number of local hospitalizations of residents divided by all hospitalizations of residents). This index varied from a low of 17.9% to over 94%. More than 85% of Americans lived in hospital service areas where the majority of Medicare hospitalizations occurred locally. More than 51% lived in areas where the localization index exceeded 70%.

In 1993, most Americans lived in hospital service areas with three or fewer local hospitals. Eighty-two percent, or 2,830, of all hospital service areas, which comprised 39% of the population in 1990, had only one hospital. Four hundred twenty-eight hospital service areas, which comprised 23% of the United States population, had either two or three hospitals. One hundred seventy-eight, or less than 6% of hospital service areas, had four or more local hospitals and comprised about 37% of the population of the United States.

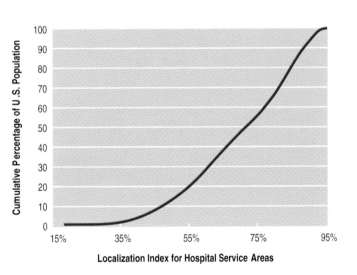

Figure A. Cumulative Percentage of Population of the United States According to the Hospital Service Area Localization Index (1992-93)

The localization index is the proportion of all hospitalizations for area residents that occur in a hospital or hospitals within the area. The figure shows the localization index for Medicare patients in 3,436 hospital service areas, according to the cumulative proportion of the population living in the region. Most of the population lived in regions where more than 50% of hospitalizations occurred locally.

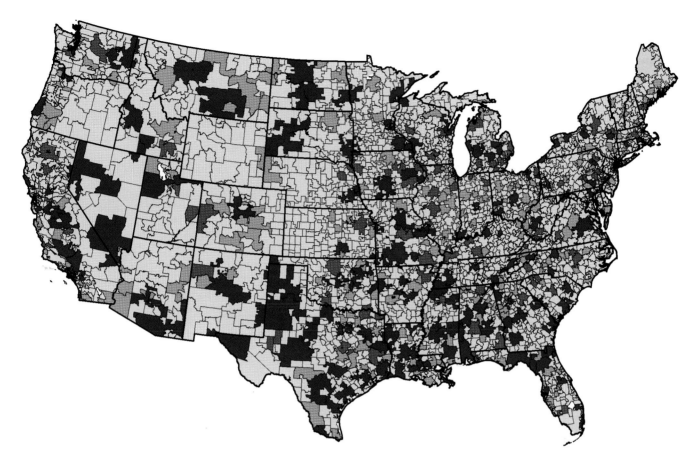

Map B. Hospital Service Areas According to the Number of Acute Care Hospitals

Thirty-nine percent of the population of the United States lived in areas with one hospital (buff); 15% lived in areas with two hospitals (light orange); 8.4% lived in areas with three hospitals (bright orange); and 37% of the population lived in areas with four or more hospitals within the hospital service area (red).

Count of Acute Care Hospitals
by Hospital Service Area (1993)

- 4 or more (178 HSAs)
- 3 (106)
- 2 (322)
- 1 (2,830)
- Not Populated

How Hospital Referral Regions Were Defined

Hospital service areas make clear the patterns of use of local hospitals. A significant proportion of care, however, is provided by referral hospitals that serve a larger region. Hospital referral regions were defined in this Atlas by documenting where patients were referred for major cardiovascular surgical procedures and for neurosurgery. Each hospital service area was examined to determine where most of its residents went for these services. The result was the aggregation of the 3,436 hospital service areas into 306 hospital referral regions. Each hospital referral region had at least one city where both major cardiovascular surgical procedures and neurosurgery were performed. Maps were used to make sure that the small number of "orphan" hospital service areas – those surrounded by hospital service areas allocated to a different hospital referral region – were reassigned, in almost all cases, to ensure geographic contiguity. Hospital referral regions were pooled with neighbors if their populations were less than 120,000 or if less than 65% of their residents' hospitalizations occurred within the region.

Hospital referral regions were named for the hospital service area containing the referral hospital or hospitals most often used by residents of the region. The regions sometimes cross state boundaries. The Evansville, Indiana, hospital referral region (Map C) provides an example of a region that is located in three states: Illinois, Indiana, and Kentucky. In this region, three hospitals provided cardiovascular surgery services. Two were in Evansville; a third hospital, in Vincennes, Indiana, also provided cardiovascular surgery, but in the years of this study residents of the Vincennes area used cardiovascular and neurosurgery procedures provided in Evansville more frequently than those in Vincennes, resulting in the assignment of the Vincennes hospital service area to the Evansville hospital referral region.

Map C also provides an example of a region with a population too small to meet the minimum criterion for designation as a hospital referral region. The Madisonville, Kentucky, hospital service area met the criterion as a hospital referral region on the basis of the plurality rule, but its population was less than 57,000. The area was assigned to the Paducah, Kentucky, hospital referral region because hospitals in Paducah were the second most commonly used place of care for cardiovascular and neurosurgical procedures.

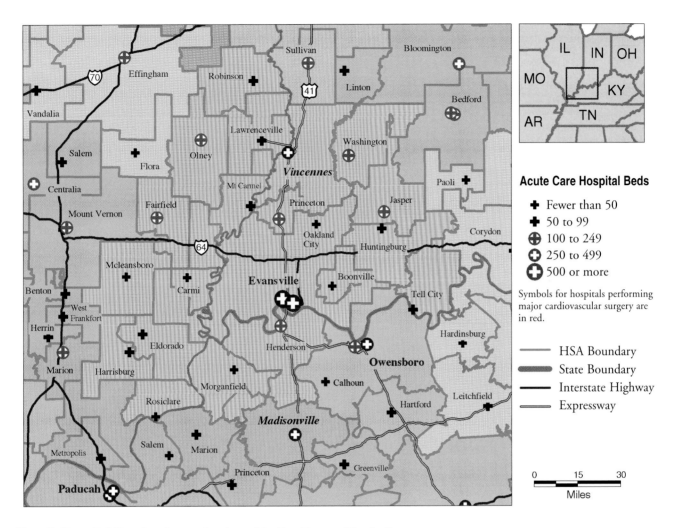

Map C. Hospital Service Areas Assigned to the Evansville, Indiana, Hospital Referral Region

Hospital referral regions are named for the hospital service area containing the referral hospital or hospitals most often used by residents of the region. Hospital referral regions overlap state boundaries in every state except Alaska and Hawaii. The Evansvillle, Indiana, hospital referral region is in parts of three states: Illinois, Indiana, and Kentucky.

Maps of Hospital Referral Regions in the United States

The maps on the following pages outline the boundaries of the hospital referral regions. Although in some regions more than one city provided referral care, each hospital referral region was named for the city where most patients receiving major cardiovascular surgical procedures and neurosurgery were referred for care.

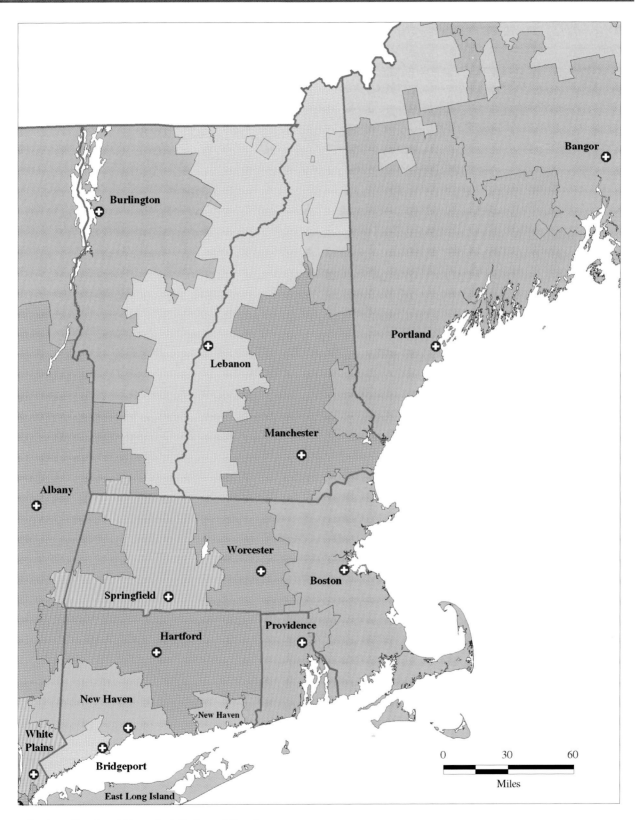

Map D. New England Hospital Referral Regions

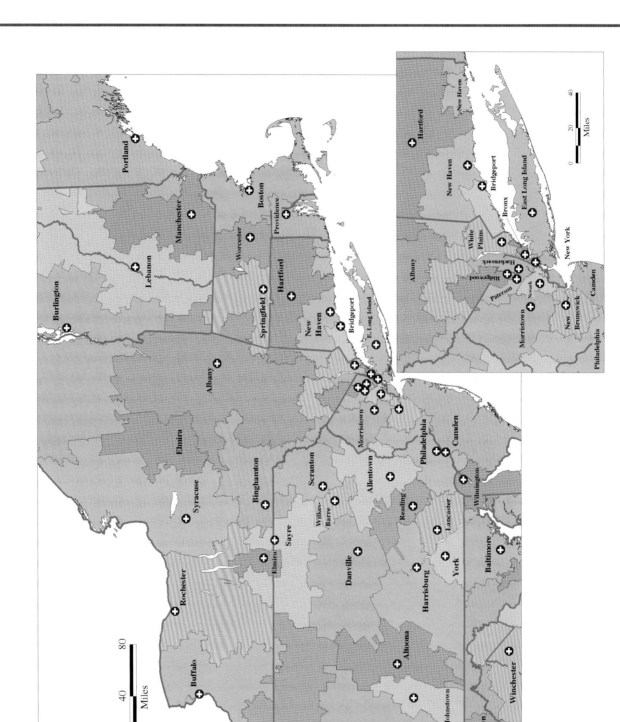

Map E. Northeast Hospital Referral Regions

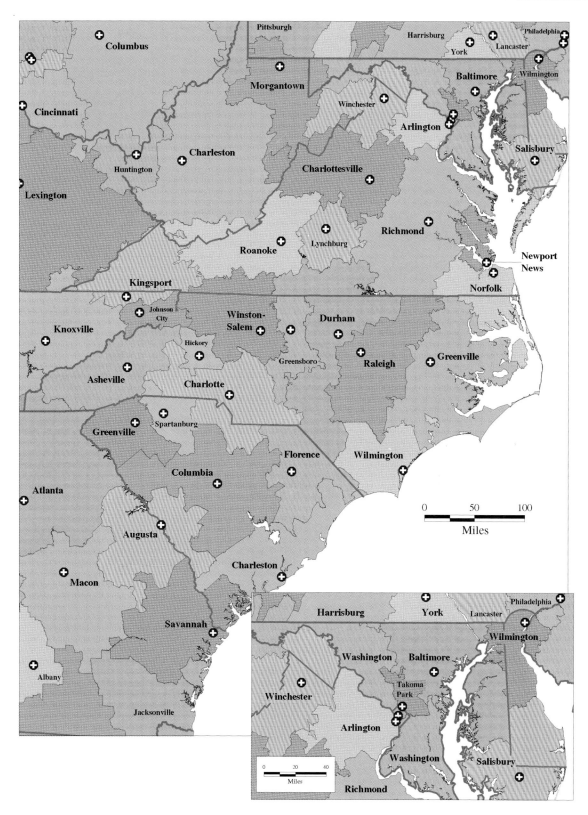

Map F. South Atlantic Hospital Referral Regions

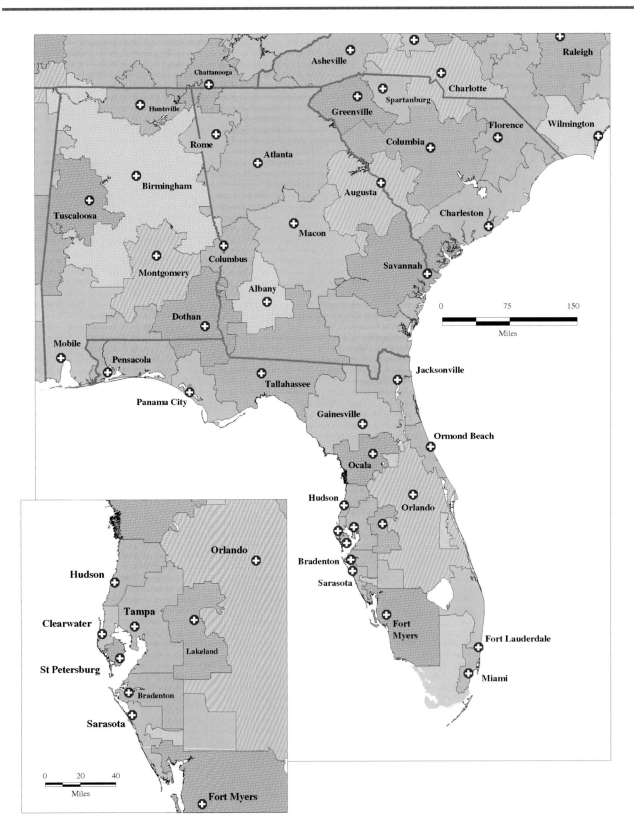

Map G. Southeast Hospital Referral Regions

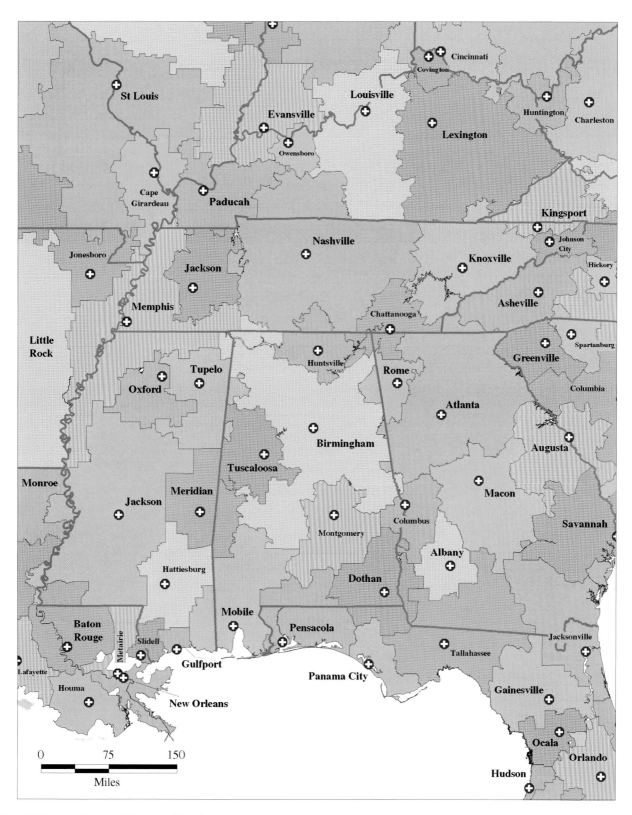

Map H. South Central Hospital Referral Regions

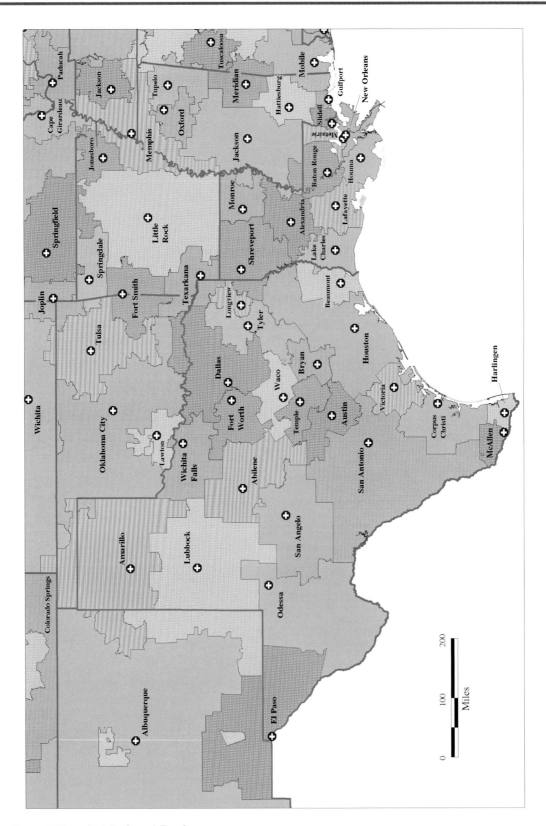

Map I. Southwest Hospital Referral Regions

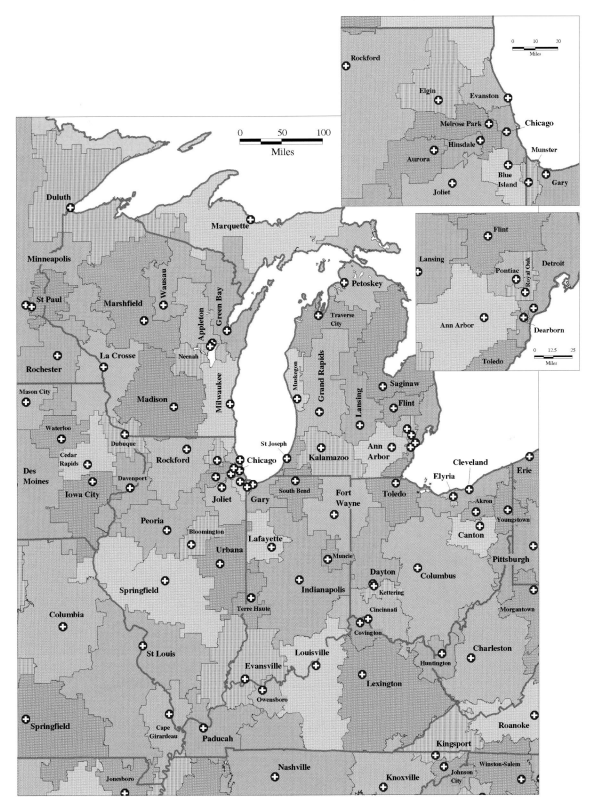

Map J. Great Lakes Hospital Referral Regions

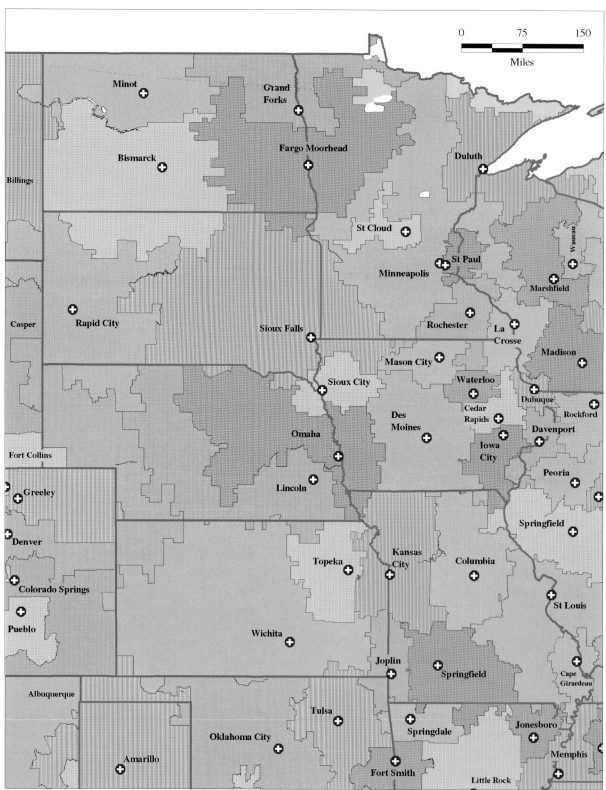

Map K. Upper Midwest Hospital Referral Regions

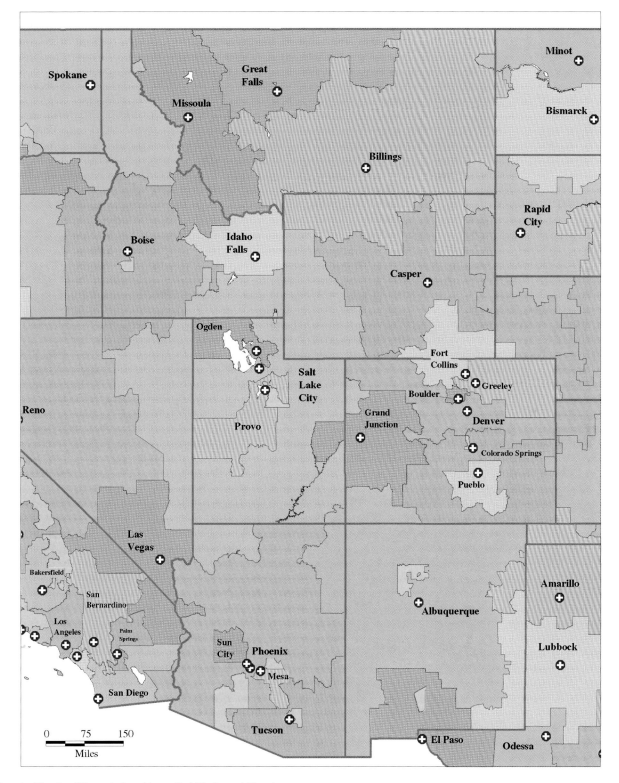

Map L. Rocky Mountains Hospital Referral Regions

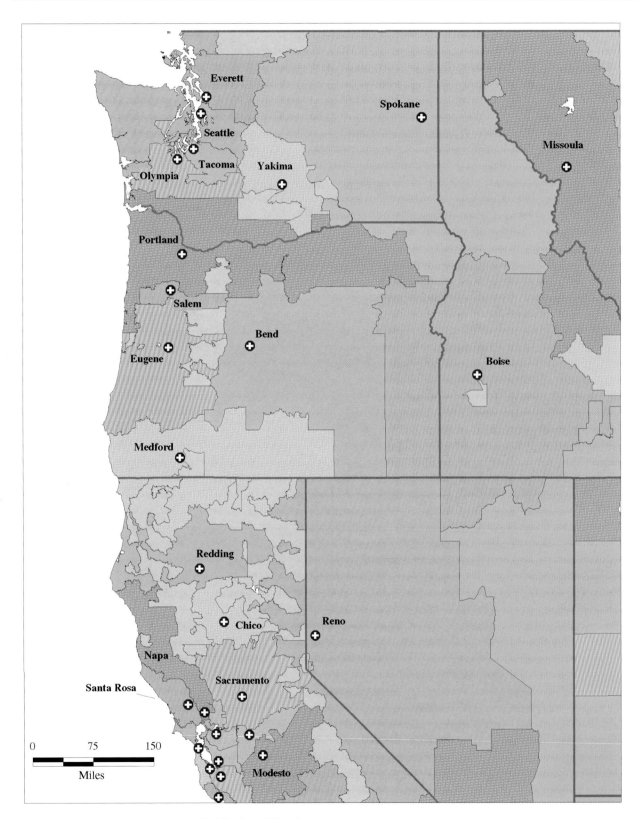

Map M. Pacific Northwest Hospital Referral Regions

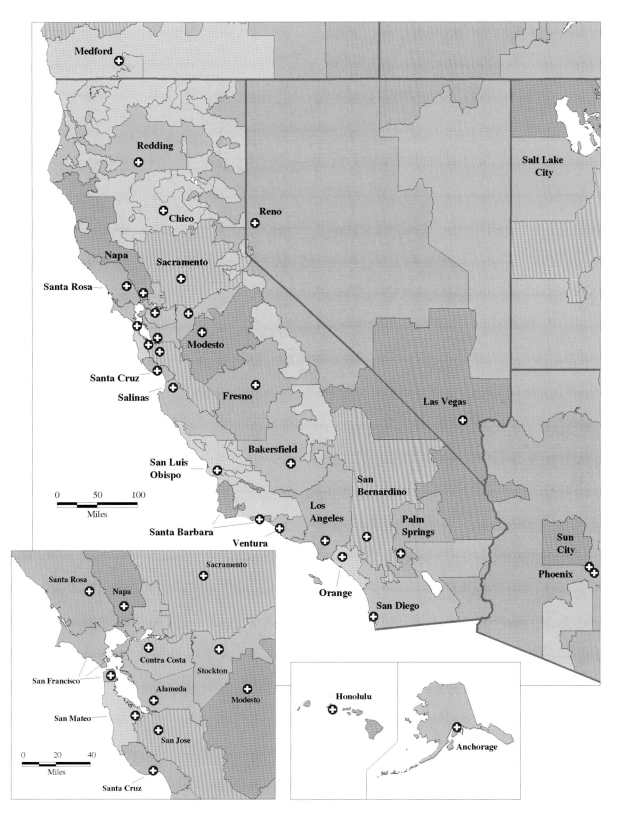

Map N. Pacific Coast Hospital Referral Regions

Endnote

Page 2

Chassin MR, Galvin RW, the National Roundtable on Health Care Quality. The urgent need to improve health care quality. Institute of Medicine National Roundtable on Health Care Quality. *JAMA.* 1998;280(11):1000-1005.

Page 3

For a further description of the systematic coefficient of variation see: McPherson K, Wennberg JE, Hovine OB, Clifford P. Small-area variations in the use of common surgical procedures: an international comparison of New England, England and Norway. *N Eng J Med.* 1982;307:1310-1314.

The American Hospital Association's "Reality Check" report was issued in 1997. Contact the American Hospital Association Resource Center, One North Franklin, Chicago, IL 60606.

Page 6

Wennberg, JE, Cooper MM, editors, *The Dartmouth Atlas of Health Care.* American Hospital Publishing, Inc. Chicago, IL 1998.

Page 72

Milton I. Roemer first posited Roemer's law around 1960. In 1993, he reiterated this observation in *National Health Systems of the World, Volume Two* (Oxford University Press): "The optimal supply of hospital beds needed by each country, for planning purposes, has been a subject of study and debate everywhere. If there is an assured payment system, it seems that almost any additional hospital beds provided will tend to be used, up to a ceiling not yet determined."

Pages 82-85

Fisher ES, Wennberg JE, Stukel TA, Skinner JS, Sharp SM, Freeman JL, Gittelsohn AM. Associations between hospital capacity, utilization and medicare mortality in the United States: might more be worse? Center for the Evaluative Clinical Sciences Working Paper, 1993.

Page 93

For a general discussion of whether more medical care results in better outcomes, see:
Fisher ES, Welch HG. Avoiding the unintended consequences of growth in medical care: how might more be worse? *JAMA.* 1999;281(5):446-453.

A note on the influence of the acute care hospital bed supply on utilization:
The influence of supply is largely subliminal — it is not recognized as an influence on their practices by the physicians themselves. Before they were informed about comparative levels of supply and utilization in their hospital service areas, clinicians in New Haven were asked if they were aware of any differences in their practice styles and those of their colleagues at Boston's teaching hospitals. Clinicians in Boston were asked the same question — how did their practice style differ from that of their colleagues in New Haven? Physicians in New Haven did not report that they were constrained by a lack of resources, or practiced any differently from their colleagues in Boston; physicians in Boston did not feel that they had an oversupply of resources, or that they practiced any differently from their colleagues in New Haven. Then the physicians in each community were asked to look at the information in Table 3.9, with the names of hospitals and cities obscured, and asked to identify which hospital they thought was their own. It became clear from these discussions that

all of the clinicians — in both Boston and New Haven — were unaware of their own areas' supplies of beds or of any differences in practice style.

The comparison of the propensity to hospitalize patients at Boston University Hospital and patients at Boston City Hospital provides additional insight into the subliminal effect of supply on utilization. These two hospitals have the same house officers and attendings and are located physically within the same structure. The principal difference is that Boston City Hospital serves the indigent of Boston. Boston University Hospital serves non-indigent, higher-income, mostly insured patients. No one, when the medical staff was asked to guess, guessed that propensity to hospitalize was actually lower at the institution serving the poorest and presumably most sick segment of the population of Boston. As a corollary to this point, they were not aware of danger, harm, or even scarcity. When asked, clinicians in New Haven did not believe that they were withholding valued and necessary hospital care because of a lack of resources. Indeed, they did not profess to have more conservative treatment theories or to exercise conscious choice that it was better to treat seriously ill patients outside of the hospital. *(J.E.W.)*

Page 94
For a specific study of mortality outcomes of variations in intensive care during the last six months of life, see:
Skinner JS, Wennberg JE. How much is enough? Efficiency and Medicare spending in the last six months of life. National Bureau of Economic Research Working Paper # 6513, April 1998. Available from the NBER at 1050 Massachusetts Avenue, Cambridge, Massachusetts 02138. (http://www.nber.org/papers/w6513)

Brennan TA, Leape LL, Laird NM, Hebert L, Localio AR, Lawthers AG, Newhouse JP, Weiler PC, Hiatt HH. Incidence of adverse events and negligence in hospitalized patients: results of the Harvard medical practice study I. *N Eng J Med.* 1991;324(6):370-376.

Wennberg JE, Feeman JL, Shelton RM, Bubolz TA. Hospital use and mortality among Medicare beneficiaries in Boston and New Haven. *N Eng J Med.* 1989;321:1168-1173.

Page 107
U.S. Preventive Services Task Force: Guide to Clinical Preventive Services: Report of the U.S. Preventive Services Task Force, Second Edition. Williams & Wilkins, Baltimore, 1996.

Page 126
For a study of ambulatory care sensitive conditions or preventable hospitalizations among the Medicare population, see:
Blustein J, Hanson K, Shea S. Preventable hospitalizations and socioeconomic status. *Health Affairs.* 1998;17(2):177-189.
Note that this study controlled for socioeconomic status but not for hospital capacity.

Page 146
For reports on the NASCET and ACAS trials, see:
North American Symptomatic Carotid Surgery Trial Steering Committee. Beneficial effect of carotid endarterectomy in symptomatic patients with high-grade carotid stenosis. *N Engl J Med.* 1991;325:445-453.
and
Executive Committee for the Asymptomatic Carotid Atherosclerosis Study. Endarterectomy for asymptomatic carotid artery stenosis. *JAMA.* 1995;273:1421-1428.
and
Wennberg DE, Lucas FL, Birkmeyer JD, Bredenberg CE, Fisher ES. Variation in carotid endarterectomy mortality in the Medicare population: Trial hospitals, volume, and patient characteristics. *JAMA.* 1998;279(16):1278-1281.

Page 153

Figure 5.6. Adapted from the JAMA.
Wennberg DE, Lucas FL, Birkmeyer JD, Bredenberg CE, Fisher ES. Variation in carotid endarterectomy mortality in the Medicare population: Trial hospitals, volume, and patient characteristics. *JAMA.* 1998;279(16):1278-1281.

Page 165

O'Connor GT, Quinton HB, Traven N, Ramunno LD, Dodds TA, Marciniak TA, Wennberg JE. Geographic variation in the treatment of acute myocardial infarction: The cooperative cardiovascular project. *JAMA.* 1999;281(7):627-633.

Page 196

Skinner JS, Wennberg JE. How much is enough? Efficiency and Medicare spending in the last six months of life. National Bureau of Economic Research Working Paper # 6513, April 1998. Available from the NBER at 1050 Massachusetts Avenue, Cambridge, Massachusetts 02138 (http://www.nber.org/papers/w6513).

Page 198

For a report on the principal findings of the SUPPORT study, see:
The SUPPORT Principal Investigators for the SUPPORT Project. A controlled trial to improve care for seriously ill hospitalized patients: The Study to Understand Prognoses and Preferences for Outcomes and Risks of Treatments (SUPPORT). *JAMA.* 1995;274:1591-1598.

Page 199

For a study of the relationship between hospital capacity and the place of death, see:
Pritchard RS, Fisher ES, Teno JM, Sharp SM, Reding DJ, Knaus WA, Wennberg JE, Lynn J. Influence of patient preferences and local health system characteristics on the place of death. *JAGS.* 1998;46:1242-1250.

For further information on the role of capacity in influencing care in the last six months of life, see:
Mor V, Hiris J. Determinants of the site of death among hospice cancer patients. *J Health Soc Behav.* 1983;24:375-385.
and
Moinpour C, Polissar L. Factors affecting place of death of hospice and non-hospice cancer patients. *Am J Public Health.* 1989;79(11):1549-1551.

Page 213

Best practices benchmarks are from an audited study of compliance with HEDIS guidelines conducted by the Pacific Business Group on Health.

Page 217

O'Connor GT, Quinton HB, Traven N, Ramunno LD, Dodds TA, Marciniak TA, Wennberg JE. Geographic variation in the treatment of acute myocardial infarction: The cooperative cardiovascular project. *JAMA.* 1999;281(7):627-633.

Page 223

Chassin MR, Galvin RW, and the National Roundtable on Health Care Quality. The urgent need to improve health care quality. Institute of Medicine National Roundtable on Health Care Quality. *JAMA.* 1998;280(11):1000-1005.

Page 224-227

For more on shared decision making, see:
Barry MJ, Fowler FJ, Mulley AG, Henderson JV, Wennberg JE. Patient reactions to a program designed to facilitate patient participation in treatment decisions for benign prostatic hyperplasia. *Med Care.* 1995;33:771-782.

Wagner EH, Barrett P, Barry MJ, Barlow W, Fowler FJ. The effect of a shared decisionmaking program on rates of surgery for benign prostatic hyperplasia: pilot results. *Med Care.* 1995;33:765-770.

Barry MJ, Cherkin DC, Chang YC, Fowler FJ, Skates S. A randomized trial of a multimedia shared decision-making program for men facing a treatment decision for benign prostatic hyperplasia. *Disease Management and Clinical Outcomes.* 1997;1:5-14.

For a broader discussion of the role of outcomes research and shared decision making in resolving surgical practice variations for benign prostatic hyperplasia and prostate cancer, see:
Prostate Disease Patient Outcomes Research Team (PORT) Final Report. Agency for Health Care Policy and Research Pub. No. 95-N010; July 1995:1-59.

Appendix on Methods

The National Committee for Quality Assurance (NCQA) internet site can be accessed at: www.ncqa.org

The Health Plan Employer Data and Information Set (HEDIS) can be accessed at the NCQA internet site: www.ncqa.org

The Berenson-Eggers Type of Service File (BETOS) can be accessed at the internet site of the Health Care Financing Administration: www.hcfa.gov

See also:
Wennberg JE, Freeman JL, Culp WJ. Are hospital services rationed in New Haven or over-utilized in Boston? *Lancet.* 1987;1(8543):1185-1188.

Breslow NE, Day NE. Statistical Methods in Cancer Research. Volume II - The Design and Analysis of Cohort Studies. Lyon: IARC, 1987.

On the Geographic Practice Cost Index (GPCI) developed by Zuckerman, Welch, and Pope. See:
Pope GC, Welch WP, Zuckerman S, Henderson MG, Cost of practice and geographic variation in Medicare fees. *Health Affairs.* 1989;8(3):117-28.

The Dartmouth Atlas of Health Care is based, in part, on data supplied by
The American Hospital Association
The American Medical Association
The American Osteopathic Association
The Health Care Financing Administration
The National Center for Health Statistics
The United States Census
The United States Department of Defense
Claritas, Incorporated

Data analyses were performed using
Software developed by the Center for the Evaluative Clinical Sciences
using SAS® on HP® equipment running the UNIX® system software

Maps and map databases were generated using
MapInfo® software
Highway map coordinates from MapInfo®
ZIP Code map coordinates from GDT®
Claritas 3H. Custom Dataset for US ZIP Codes from Claritas®

Interested in applying what you've learned in this book to your specific region?

Order The Dartmouth Atlas of Health Care Data Viewer, version 1.2

With the *Dartmouth Atlas of Health Care Data Viewer* on CD-Rom, you can create your own scenarios and analyze how different areas of the country compare. For example:

- Study trends and differences in care delivery from market to market

- Understand how geography affects care delivery

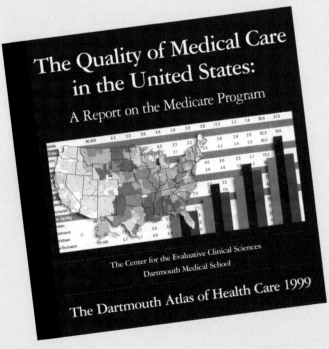

- Use underlying utilization patterns in negotiating agreements under capitated rates

- Study variations in practice patterns to improve outcomes and reduce costs

- Compare geographic variations in treatment of a disease to better understand the impact of treatment options.

The Dartmouth Atlas Health Care database, provided in Access format, contains the five years of national data used in the *Dartmouth Atlas* research. The included *Data Viewer* is a software interface that allows you to seamlessly view the *Dartmouth Atlas Health Care* database, and to easily map and chart the data, and perform benchmark, statistical and market share analyses.

Price $1,295/$1,095 for AHA members
+ applicable tax, shipping and handling
(Includes 90 days of free technical support)

Interested in purchasing the Book and Data Viewer, and in saving money?
Ask for The Combo - Item #044453.

*It's Customizable -enabling you to "drill down"
to your specific area of focus, whether that is a
specific local market or 1 of more than 140
clinical diagnoses variables!*

For more information or to
order this product or additional copies of this book (Item # 044452)

Call (800) AHA-2626 or visit our website at www.healthforum.com